Girls and Aggression

Contributing Factors and Intervention Principles

Perspectives in
Law & Psychology

Girls and Aggression

Contributing Factors and Intervention Principles

Edited by

Marlene M. Moretti
Simon Fraser University, Burnaby, British Columbia, Canada

Candice L. Odgers
University of Virginia, Charlottesville, Virginia, U.S.A.

Margaret A. Jackson
Simon Fraser University, Burnaby, British Columbia, Canada

KLUWER ACADEMIC / PLENUM PUBLISHERS
NEW YORK / BOSTON / DORDRECHT / LONDON / MOSCOW

Library of Congress Cataloging-in-Publication Data

ISBN   0-306-48224-X

© 2004 by Kluwer Academic/Plenum Publishers, New York
233 Spring Street, New York, New York 10013

http://www.kluweronline.com

10 9 8 7 6 5 4 3 2 1

A C.I.P. record for this book is available from the Library of Congress.

To Sean and Sarah, with much love always.—**MMM**

To Nicole and Natasah, for their courage and great
success in the face of adversity.—**CLO**

For my parents.—**MAJ**

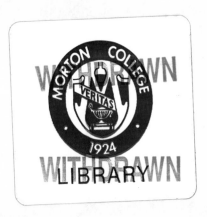

Contributors

JILL ANTONISHAK • Department of Psychology, University of Virginia, Charlottesville, Virginia, United States, 22901.

SIBYLLE ARTZ • School of Child and Youth Care, University of Victoria, Victoria, British Columbia, Canada, V8W 2Y2.

LEENA K. AUGIMERI • Earlscourt Child & Family Centre, Toronto, Ontario, Canada, M6E 3V4.

OZLEM AYDUK • Psychology Department, University of California, Berkeley, California, United States, 94720.

ERIN M. BOONE • Department of Psychology, University of Victoria, Victoria, British Columbia, Canada,V8P 5C2.

DEBORAH A. CONNOLLY • Department of Psychology, Simon Fraser University, Burnaby, British Columbia, Canada, V5A 1S6.

NICKI R. CRICK • Institute of Child Development, University of Minnesota, Minneapolis, Minnesota, United States, 55455.

KIMBERLEY DaSILVA • Department of Psychology, Simon Fraser University, Burnaby, British Columbia, Canada, V5A 1S6.

MANDEEP K. DHAMI • Department of Psychology, University of Victoria, Victoria, British Columbia, Canada,V8P 5C2.

GERALDINE DOWNEY • Department of Psychology, Columbia University, New York, New York, United States, 10027.

CATHERINE ÉMOND • School of Criminology, University of Montréal, Montréal, Québec, Canada, H3C 3J7.

TASHA C. GEIGER • Institute of Child Development, University of Minnesota, Minneapolis, Minnesota, United States, 55455.

WENDY L. HOGLUND • Department of Psychology, University of Victoria, Victoria, British Columbia, Canada,V8P 5C2.

ROY HOLLAND • Maples Adolescent Treatment Centre, Burnaby, British Columbia, Canada, V5G 3H4.

SHELLEY HYMEL • Faculty of Education, University of British Columbia, Vancouver, British Columbia, Canada, V6T 1Z4.

LAUREN IRWIN • Department of Psychology, Columbia University, New York City, New York, United States, 10027

MARGARET A. JACKSON • School of Criminology, Simon Fraser University, Burnaby, British Columbia, Canada, V5A 1S6.

NADINE LANCTÔT • School of Criminology, University of Montréal, Montréal, Québec, Canada, H3C 3J7.

BONNIE J. LEADBEATER • Department of Psychology, University of Victoria, Victoria, British Columbia, Canada,V8P 5C2.

MARC LE BLANC • School of Criminology, University of Montréal, Montréal, Québec, Canada, H3C 3J7.

ZINA LEE • Department of Psychology, Simon Fraser University, Burnaby, British Columbia, Canada, V5A 1S6.

KATHRYN S. LEVENE • Earlscourt Child & Family Centre, Toronto, Ontario, Canada, M6E 3V4.

MARLENE M. MORETTI • Department of Psychology, Simon Fraser University, Burnaby, British Columbia, Canada, V5A 1S6.

CARRIE FRIED MULFORD • Department of Psychology, University of Virginia, Charlottesville, Virginia, United States, 22901.

CANDICE L. ODGERS • Department of Psychology, University of Virginia, Charlottesville, Virginia, United States, 22901.

DEBRA J. PEPLER • Department of Psychology, York University, Toronto, Ontario, Canada M3J 1P3.

MELISSA RAMSAY • Department of Psychology, Columbia University, New York City, New York, United States, 10027.

MARGE REITSMA-STREET • Studies in Policy and Practice in Health and Social Services, Faculty of Human and Social Development, University of Victoria, Victoria, British Columbia, Canada, V8W 2Y2.

N. Dickon Reppucci • Department of Psychology, University of Virginia, Charlottesville, Virginia, United States, 22901.

Melinda G. Schmidt • Department of Psychology, University of Virginia, Charlottesville, Virginia, United States, 22901.

Tracy Vaillancourt • Department of Psychology, McMaster University, Hamilton, Ontario, Canada, L8S 4L8.

Margaret M. Walsh • Earlscourt Child & Family Centre, Toronto, Ontario, Canada, M6E 3V4.

Tristin M.Wayte • Department of Psychology, Simon Fraser University, Burnaby, British Columbia, Canada, V5A 1S6.

Jennifer L. Woolard • Department of Psychology, Georgetown University, Washington, DC, United States, 20057.

Marion K. Underwood • School of Behavioral and Brain Sciences, University of Texas at Dallas, Richardson, Texas, United States, 75083.

Melanie J. Zimmer-Gembeck • School of Applied Psychology, Griffith University, Gold Coast, Queensland, Australia, 9726.

Preface

Despite decades of research on the involvement of boys and men in aggressive and violent behavior, little attention has been directed toward these issues in girls and women. The increasing involvement of young women in violence, both as perpetrators and victims, has led to urgent calls for more information on what causes aggression and violence in girls and what we can do about it. Indeed, both the Canadian Department of Justice and the Office of Juvenile Delinquency and Prevention in the United States have openly expressed concern regarding the lack of information and programming for young females. In addition, recent media portrayals of high profile cases involving young women participating in brutal acts of violence have heighten public concern over the emergence of a new wave of "violent and aggressive girls".

This book presents a collection of cutting edge interdisciplinary perspectives that address risk and protective factors, developmental pathways and intervention principles specific to the problem of aggression and violence in the lives of young women. The collection seeks to represent the full social-psychological context in which girls lives unfold with the goal of leading the field to a developmental-ecological understanding of the issue. With this goal in mind, perspectives were sought from the disciplines of psychology, criminology, education and sociology. In the first section of the book, the question of gender specificity in the form and function of aggression is addressed from a psychological perspective. Downey, Irwin, Ramsay and Ayduk discuss the significance of rejection sensitivity in determining how girls interpret and respond to experiences in close relationships, and how this in turn can lead to engagement in aggressive behavior. Next, Geiger, Zimmer-Gembeck and Crick examine the definition, measurement and prevalence of relational aggression, its causes and consequences, and the importance of identifying relational aggression as a target of therapeutic intervention. The function of aggression from an attachment perspective is then considered by Moretti, DaSilva and Holland, who suggest that aggression may develop in girls under conditions of adversity as a desperate attempt to coerce others into meeting attachment needs.

Turning to the importance of social-interpersonal context, Vaillancourt and Hymel review research on the complex processes through which peer relationships contribute to aggressive behavior. They suggest that future research must go beyond the examination of family influences to more fully consider how aggressive behavior is promoted and maintained within peer groups. Finally, Lanctôt, Émond and LeBlanc present research that illustrates the diversity of developmental trajectories among aggressive girls. Their findings challenge researchers to further investigate the complex relationship between risk factors, both psychological and social, over development.

In the next section of the book, the importance of social-cultural context is discussed with attention to the factors that contribute to discrimination and victimization of girls. In her chapter, Jackson references three studies which consider the voices of young immigrant and refugee girls and their service providers in the identification of racial and gender factors that impact both on girls being targeted for violence and/or on girls becoming violent themselves. Artz offers insights into the importance of the social conditions of young girls which shape their sexual and gender identity, their moral identity and their action. From her analysis of girls lived experiences, she argues we must move away from the traditional deficit model to a model of inclusion, relationship building and community partnership. Reitsma-Street examines restrictive welfare and punitive justice policies that increase the vulnerabilities of girls to violence, especially if they live in low income communities.

Section three of the book presents perspectives on intervention, linking risk factors and early identification with specific treatment programs. Applications to both juvenile justice system and school based programming are presented. Pepler, Walsh and Levene review the process of developing and evaluating a promising new gender specific program, the Earlscourt Girls Connection, which addresses young troubled girls' developmental issues within multiple relationship contexts. Levene, Walsh and Augimeri describe a risk assessment instrument specifically for girls that guides the delivery of clinical intervention. They also provide more in-depth information on the intervention programs provided at the Earlscourt center. The ability of the Earlscourt group to translate developmental theory and research into practice serves as an excellent model for the development of future interventions and programming for girls. Leadbeater and her colleagues also provide an example of an intervention that, while not specifically designed for girls, demonstrates differential outcomes and highlights the importance of poverty in understanding the development of antisocial behavior during childhood. The chapter by Antonishak, Fried and Reppucci provides a rationale for the development of gender specific programming based on the profiles of girls within the justice system. Despite the unique profiles of female offenders evident in this review, the authors detail the paucity of treatment options in general, and gender based programs specifically, that exist for girls within juvenile justice settings.

Finally, we turn our attention to the issues of risk assessment and juvenile justice policy as these relate to the issue of aggression and violence in girls. Odgers, Reppucci and Schmidt argue that we cannot empirically or ethically justify the current use of male based forensic assessment tools with adolescent female populations due to the limitations in our research and the serious decisions that may be made based on these assessments. Connelly, Wayte and Lee emphasize the problems that are created by the lack of empirically and developmentally sound research in anticipating the effects that major policy changes, such as the Youth Criminal Justice Act in Canada, will have on female offenders. Woolard describes how policy makers and researchers might approach the phenomenon of girls' delinquency from different vantage points and identifies areas that might benefit from policy-relevant empirical research. In the closing chapter, the themes that draw together the diverse disciplinary perspectives and research presented in this volume are succinctly summarized by Underwood, highlighting the accomplishments we achieved to date and pointing to the challenges of the future.

It is our hope that this volume offers a starting point for the emergence of a truly transdisciplinary understanding of aggression and violence in the lives of girls—a perspective that goes beyond the mere recognition of the independent contribution of researchers from distinct disciplines. Although this may seem challenging and beyond what is reasonable to set as a goal for the field, it is our view that to settle for anything less will ultimately lead us to fail. If we have achieved our goal of putting forth a point of departure for the field, this book will stimulate dialogue and debate. For this we thank our contributors who have shown great dedication and cooperation throughout this endeavor. We also thank Dr. Ron Roesch, our series editor, for his recognition of the importance of this work and his support in seeing it to publication in a timely manner. Finally, we thank the girls who we have all come to know through our work. Their insights and willingness to discuss their experiences of victimization and violence have had a profound effect upon us as individuals and scientists, and it is our deepest hope that this work produces understanding and change which ultimately benefits them.

Contents

Girls and Aggression
A Point of Departure

MARLENE M. MORETTI, CANDICE L. ODGERS, AND MARGARET A. JACKSON

On the evening of November 14, 1997, a group of teenage girls in Victoria, British Columbia participated in the brutal beating death of Reena Virk, an adolescent girl whom they all knew well, and alternately befriended and ostracized. The murder was not an accident, nor was it the result of impulsive lashing out that caused death without intention. On the contrary, the murder of Reena Virk was well planned, and it required vicious beatings that took place over several hours before she was left to drown. News of her death was a wake up call to Canadians. Although similar events involving teenage girls as the perpetrators of violent crime had occurred in the United States, Canada had remained relatively insulated in this regard. Reena's murder provoked the public and academic researchers to ask whether rates of violence and aggression in girls were increasing, what factors contributed to such acts being carried out, and how we could intervene to prevent further tragedies. In response to these questions, we organized a conference in Vancouver during May 2001. The Vancouver Conference on Aggressive and Violent Girls brought together leading experts from across Canada and the U.S., representing knowledge from a diverse range of disciplines, to speak to the question of girls' involvement in aggression and

MARLENE M. MORETTI • Department of Psychology, Simon Fraser University, Burnaby, British Columbia, Canada, V5A 1S6. CANDICE L. ODGERS • Department of Psychology, University of Virginia, Charlottesville, Virginia, United States, 22901. MARGARET A. JACKSON • School of Criminology, Simon Fraser University, Burnaby, British Columbia, Canada, V5A 1S6.

violence (*www.sfu.ca/gap/*). This book grew out of that conference, and it reflects the current knowledge in the field, and importantly, the fundamental
questions that remain unanswered.

What is clear is that rates of girls' involvement in aggressive acts are
increasing. During the last decade in the United States the growth in person offense cases was greater for females (157%) than for males (71%)
(Puzzanchera, Stahl, Finnegan, Tierney, & Snyder, 2003). Similarly, between
1990 and 2001, charges for violent crimes against Canadian youths increased 68% among females versus 22% among males (Statistics Canada,
2001). Self report data also support the decreasing gender gap among adolescents' participation in violent acts (U.S. Department of Health and Human Services, 2001). Despite the fact that adolescent girls are the only
sub-group of individuals that have displayed a consistent increase in rates
of violent crime, boys still far outnumber girls as the perpetrators of the
most severe violent acts. Nonetheless, the number of girls involved in serious aggressive acts represents a significant social and mental health issue.
Furthermore, as research has progressed, it has become clear that a sizeable minority of girls are involved in other forms of persistent aggressive
behavior, namely social and relational forms of aggression, which has for
years persisted as a relatively invisible but destructive behavior. Unfortunately, because the vast majority of studies on aggression and violence
have focused on boys and men, relatively little is known about the factors
that precipitate and sustain such behavior in girls.

There are several important themes that emerge from the chapters of
this book. The first is that there is no single perspective or linear combination of risk factors that explains aggression in girls, or for that matter, aggression in boys. The contributors to this book represent perspectives from a diverse range of disciplines. The chapters that follow address
the interaction between gender and a variety of individual (see Geiger,
Zimmerman-Gembeck, & Crick; Downey, Irwin, Ramsay, & Ayduk), family (see Moretti, Da Silva, & Holland), peer (see Vaillancourt & Hymel),
school (see Leadbeater, Dhami, & Hogland), socio-cultural (see Artz; Jackson; Reitsma-Street) and legal (see Connolly, Wayte, & Lee; Woolard) factors that contribute to aggressive and violent behavior. In this way, the
current volume encompasses a multi-level ecological approach in understanding girls' involvement in aggressive and violent behavior. Some may
argue that such an approach is too complex to offer useful guidance about
violence and aggression. In response, we would say that human behavior
is complex. As such, our responsibility as researchers and clinicians is to
enter into dialogue across disciplines, with the goal of understanding the
complexity of factors in which human behavior is embedded, so that we
can offer meaningful rather than overly simplistic contributions to science
and public welfare.

The second theme that emerges from this work is the value of integrating knowledge across different populations of youths. While a tremendous amount of research has been conducted with adolescent males, there are very few studies that have focused on aggressive and violent behavior among girls. The central question that arises, therefore, is how, and perhaps whether, existing knowledge can be applied to the study of aggression among girls. In particular, questions are raised regarding the utility of existing measurement instruments, risk assessment tools (see Odgers, Schmidt, & Reppucci) and intervention programs (see Antonishak, Fried, & Reppucci) within samples of high risk female adolescents.

Third, research increasingly points out that there is no single pathway across development. What we have learned in the larger field of aggressive and antisocial behavior is that there are multiple developmental trajectories; while some children who appear aggressive early on in life desist as they grow older, others continue on. As well, aggressive behavior may be associated with a diversity of mental health problems in adulthood, including serious depression, anxiety, and poor social functioning (see Lanctôt, Émond, & Leblanc). This seems particularly the case for females, although research is too preliminary for us to know which girls will continue along which specific pathways as they move forward to adulthood. This work clearly illustrates two fundamental concepts of developmental psychopathology: multifinality—the notion that similar risk factors can result in diverse outcomes; and, equafinality—the notion that different risk factors can produce the similar outcome. As research progresses, it is our hope that we will better understand what determines how development unfolds for each individual child so that intervention can target specific points of risk, as well as windows of opportunity, to better support healthy development.

Admittedly, the study of individual level factors has dominated the majority of research on aggression and violence to date. The examination of aggression among girls throughout this volume, however, emphasizes the importance of developing a more comprehensive understanding of the impact of socio-cultural and gender role factors on the initiation, development, and contextual precursors of aggressive behavior, and understanding how these same factors can play a role in the victimization of girls (see Jackson; Artz). Contributors to this volume also provide a gendered analysis of the application of law and social policy to girls who become enmeshed in various systems due to their antisocial and aggressive behavior (see Connolly, Wayte, & Lee; Reitsma-Street; Woolard). This multi-level ecological approach is essential to an integrated multi-disciplinary understanding and an ecologically tailored and effective response to aggression for girls, and boys as well.

Finally, various chapters in this book address the issue of intervention (see Geiger, Zimmerman-Gembeck, & Crick; Levene, Walsh, & Augimeri; Moretti, Da Silva, & Holland; Pepler, Walsh, & Levene). The challenge of developing effective interventions for girls at different stages of development is sizeable. There are many important points to be gleaned from the research presented in this volume that we hope will inform those who are involved in the treatment of girls with aggressive and violent behavior problems. In particular, the importance of relationships in girls' psychological development stands out as a salient factor to keep in the forefront of intervention (see Downey, Irwin, Ramsay, & Ayduk; Moretti, DaSilva, & Holland; Pepler, Walsh & Levene). At the same time, we must keep in mind that many risk factors for aggression and violence influence girls and boys similarly. Therefore, building girls' programs on lessons we have learned from intervention trials with boys, while keeping in mind unique gender issues, is likely to be more productive than ignoring past research. For example, the chapter by Levene, Walsh, and Augimeri illustrates how programming can be tailored for pre-adolescent girls, yet inclusive of intervention components with demonstrated efficacy.

The work presented in this book reflects a point of departure in research on aggression, from a focus on boys to an examination of the etiology and developmental course of aggression in girls. We anticipate that the next decade will bring many insights into risk and protective factors, and models of intervention that target the social-psychological conditions that hamper healthy development in girls (see Underwood). Such advances are only possible with the support of granting agencies and institutions. In this respect, we wish to acknowledge the support of the Canadian Institutes of Health Research, Institute of Gender and Health, in partnership with the Institute of Human Development, Child and Youth Health, which provided funding for a New Emerging Team grant directed by Dr. Marlene Moretti. Their support has been instrumental in the publication of this book, and their vision of interdisciplinary partnership, in collaboration with community and government agencies, will stimulate innovative and rapid knowledge development in the field. Similarly, we would like to extend our appreciation to a number of agencies for their support of the Vancouver Conference on Aggressive and Violent Girls, namely: the Ministry for Child and Family Development; Department of Justice Canada, Youth Justice Policy; National Strategy on Community Safety and Crime Prevention; Vancouver Gonzaga Foundation; Simon Fraser University Centre for the Advancement of Child Health in conjunction with the Institute for Health, Research and Education; and, the Simon Fraser University Mental Health, Law and Policy Institute. We also wish to extend our appreciation to Simon Fraser University for their provision of a publication grant, and to Monique Layton for her superb editorial assistance.

REFERENCES

Puzzanchera, C., Stahl, A. L., Finnegan, T. A., Tierney, N., & Snyder, H. N. (2003). *Juvenile Court Statistics 1998*. Washington, DC: Office of Juvenile Justice and Delinquency Prevention.

Statistics Canada. (2001). *Canadian dimensions: Youth and adult crime rates*. Online. Available: *http://www.statcan.ca/english/Pgdb/legal14a.htm* .

U. S. Department of Health and Human Services. (2001). *Youth violence: A report of the Surgeon General*. Rockville, MD: U. S. Department of Health and Human Services, Centers for Disease Control and Prevention, National Center for Injury Prevention and Control; Substance Abuse and Mental Health Services Administration, Center for Mental Health Services; and National Institutes of Health, National Institute of Mental Health.

2

Rejection Sensitivity and Girls' Aggression

GERALDINE DOWNEY, LAUREN IRWIN, MELISSA RAMSAY, AND OZLEM AYDUK

Studies of maladaptive behavior in women have traditionally focused on difficulties that are self-destructive in nature, such as suicidal behavior, eating disorders, and self-mutilation (e.g., Canetto & Lester, 1995; Cross, 1993; Nolen-Hoeksema, 1987). However, in the last several years, there has been a shift toward seeking to understand women's maladjustment in its aggressive and socially harmful forms (Ayduk, Downey, Testa, Ying Yen, & Shoda, 1999). This shift has, in part, been the result of a greater awareness of the existence and prevalence of women's harmful acts. For example, between 1988 and 1997, the rate of criminal activity rose more dramatically for female (69%) than for male (26%) adolescents, as measured by court referrals (Bureau of Justice Statistics, 1999). Finally, interest in female aggressive behavior has also been encouraged by studies on close relationships that find women use strategies such as direct physical aggression (e.g., Archer & Ray, 1989; Arias, Samios, & O'Leary, 1987; Ben-David, 1993; Deal & Wampler, 1986; Plass & Gessner, 1983), verbal aggression (e.g., Billingham & Sack, 1987; deWeerth & Kalma, 1992), and the undermining of others' social relationships (e.g., Bjorkqvist, Osterman, & Lagerspetz, 1992; Cairns & Cairns, 1994; Crick & Grotpeter, 1995) to inflict intentional harm (Ayduk et al., 1999).

GERALDINE DOWNEY, LAUREN IRWIN, and MELISSA RAMSAY • Department of Psychology, Columbia University, New York City, New York, United States, 10027. OZLEM AYDUK • Psychology Department, University of California, Berkeley, California, United States, 94720.

A lack of consensus on how to define and assess female antisocial behavior has spurred researchers to further investigate the development, course, and consequences of female maladaptive aggressive behavior (Hipwell, Loeber, Stouthamer-Loeber, Keenan, White, & Kroneman, 2002). Such research is beginning to clarify the specific situations and contexts that trigger female aggression, the form that women's hostility takes, and the function (both intrapersonal and interpersonal) it serves. First, female hostility is often expressed as relational aggression, particularly in private contexts and towards significant others, especially romantic partners (see Ben-David, 1993). Second, conditions that trigger female aggression occur when interpersonal relationships are deemed threatened or devalued (Harris, 1993). Third, female hostility takes the form of both verbal and direct physical aggression. For example, women have been found to engage in physical aggression toward significant others more often than once thought, and to do so more frequently than men (Archer, 2000). Fourth, women's anger appears to serve an expressive function and follows situations that elicit overwhelming feelings of despair and helplessness (Ayduk et al., 1999; Ben-David, 1993; Eskin & Kravitz, 1980). Thus, it has been suggested that women's expression of aggression and hostility reflects a loss of self-control and is therefore more reactive than reflective or instrumental in nature (Campbell, Muncer, & Coyle, 1992). In addition, women's aggressive behavior (whether relational or physical) consistently displays a stronger link with depression than is true for men.

Given the central importance of close relationships in women's lives (Gilligan, 1982; see Cross & Madson, 1997, for review), issues of acceptance and rejection appear to play a particularly salient role in women's interpersonal interactions (Purdie & Downey, 2000). It has been posited that maintaining harmonious intimate relationships is integral to women's self-concept (Baumeister & Sommer, 1997; Cross & Madson, 1997). Yet, some women react aggressively towards important others when the threat of rejection is perceived. Such reactions threaten the security and stability of the relationship, and, in turn, the woman's self-concept. What cognitive-affective processes might account for this distinctive pattern of female hostility?

Our efforts to address this question have focused on the role that Rejection Sensitivity (RS) may play in helping explain why some women show high levels of relational, and even physical, aggression against the very people they care about most. Our model also takes into account a resilience-generating process (i.e., self-regulation) that may play a potentially crucial role in breaking the link between RS and maladaptive behavior. Self-regulatory competency appears to protect RS women from the maladaptive consequences of the RS disposition. However, women who show a combination of both high RS and poor self-regulatory abilities appear to be particularly vulnerable to aggressive behavior toward significant others, as well as other personal and interpersonal difficulties. Although the mechanisms of the RS model hold true for both male and female populations, we have found that the context and resultant behavior can differ for women and men. In this chapter, our theoretical interpretation of RS and aggression, as well as our findings, refer to women. However, we want to clarify at the outset that most of these results also apply to men, but we have found that the results for men have generally been weaker and less consistent than for women.

In this chapter, we first describe the RS model and the evidence that we have in support of the links in the model. We next describe the role of self-regulatory competency in moderating the maladaptive effects of RS. Whereas our focus is primarily on the links between RS and aggression, we also discuss how RS may place women at risk for other forms of harmful behavior. Specifically, we propose that, whereas the perception of the occurrence of rejection may unleash hostile retaliation, the threat of rejection may also prompt behavior that is intended to prevent rejection but instead puts the self or others in harm's way. For example, women may put themselves at risk for personal harm, as when they tolerate abusive behavior or engage in unprotected sex in order to maintain a relationship (Purdie & Downey, 2000). Furthermore, women may engage in antisocial behavior to maintain a relationship, such as concealing weapons or drugs for a romantic partner (Bedell, 1999).

THE REJECTION SENSITIVITY MODEL

The RS model (see Figure 1) has been conceptualized as a cognitive-affective processing system to anxiously expect, readily perceive, and overreact to rejection. Reflecting the influence of attachment theory (Bowlby, 1969, 1973, 1980; Erikson, 1950; Horney, 1937; Sullivan, 1953), the RS model proposes that severe, prolonged rejection leads people to develop defensive (i.e. anxious or angry) expectations that others will reject them. When rejection cues are subsequently encountered, they activate a defensive motivational system (Link 1). In this state of threat, high RS (HRS) individuals are ready to interpret ambiguous or even slightly negative, interpersonal information as evidence of rejection expectations fulfilled (Link 2). Hostile thoughts and actions are likely to result (Link 3), and overreactions, especially those involving hostility and aggression, are likely to elicit actual rejection by others (Link 4). Consequently, rejection expectations, whatever their origin, become reality and are thus reinforced,

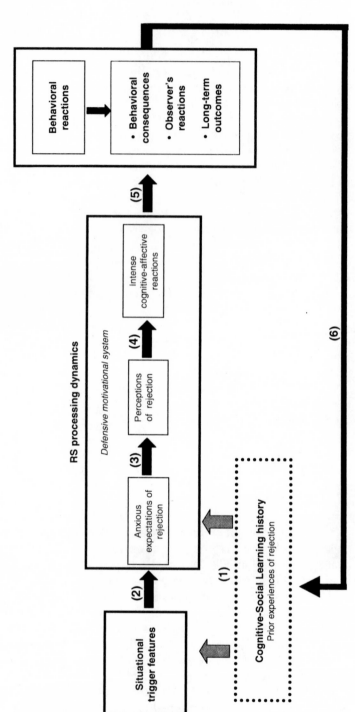

Figure 1. Theoretical model of Rejection Sensitivity.

perpetuating the RS cycle (Link 5) (Downey, Freitas, Michaelis, & Khouri, 1998).

OPERATIONALIZING RS

According to a cognitive-affective processing system approach to personality, a particular personality disposition (i.e., anxious rejection expectations) should be most evident in an individual's thoughts, feelings and behaviors in situations pertinent to the given disposition (Mischel & Shoda, 1995). Applying this concept to the RS model, measurable differences in RS should be particularly apparent in situations where an individual is vulnerable to rejection, such as when they request the support of a significant other. This assumption is reflected in the Rejection Sensitivity Questionnaire (RSQ), which assesses anxious rejection expectations through a series of hypothetical situations involving the possibility of rejection (Downey & Feldman, 1996, Study 1)[1].

RS—THE DEFENSIVE MOTIVATIONAL SYSTEM

In this section, we review evidence in support of the RS model focusing on the defensive expectations of rejection, perceptions of rejection, and reactions to rejection.

DEFENSIVE EXPECTATIONS OF REJECTION (LINK 2)

Given our assumption that defensive expectations of rejection form the core of RS, we have posited that in children, defensive expectations of rejection develop due to messages of rejection communicated to them through potential behavior that is emotionally or physically abusive or neglectful. Such painful and distressing rejection then generates defensive expectations in new situations where rejection seems possible, with implications for long-term personal and interpersonal adjustment.

Indeed, rejection by parents or peers is linked to the formation and continuation of defensive expectations for rejection in adolescents and early adults (Levy, Ayduk, & Downey, 2001). Two longitudinal studies of middle-school students revealed that over time, actual experiences of rejection increased defensive expectations of rejection. Specifically, over a one-year period, parents' reports of harsh parenting practices predicted an increase

---

[1] For more information on the measure and for references to studies describing its psychometric properties, please refer to our website, *www.columbia.edu/cu/psychology/socialrelations*.

in their children's defensive expectations of rejection (Downey, Khouri, & Feldman, 1997). Over a 4-month period, reports of rejection by peers predicted an increase in students' defensive expectations of peer rejection (Downey, Bonica, London, & Paltin, in press). In addition, cross-sectional studies of college and high-school students showed that defensive expectations of rejection were associated with childhood experiences of parental emotional neglect (Downey et al., 1997) and family violence (Downey, Lebolt, & O'Shea-Lauber, 1995; Feldman & Downey, 1994).

PERCEPTIONS OF REJECTION (LINK 3)

When in the presence of rejection cues, do HRS women more readily perceive rejection than those low in RS (LRS)? Empirical support for the third link in the RS model has been found in both experimental and field studies (Downey & Feldman, 1996; Downey, Lebolt, Rincon, & Freitas, 1998). In a laboratory experiment ostensibly about first impressions, students who anxiously expected rejection (based on their RSQ scores) felt more rejected than those low in anxious rejection expectations when told that a stranger (who was actually a confederate) with whom they had just finished a friendly conversation, had declined to continue with the study (which involved meeting with them a second time) (Downey & Feldman, 1996, Study 2). No differences emerged when an explicit explanation (constraints in experimenter's time) was given for the early termination. At study onset, all women had reported high levels of enthusiasm for interacting with the potential dating partner, yet the experimental manipulation induced rejection perceptions above baseline *uniquely* in the HRS women. HRS women in the experimental condition also tended to attribute the stranger's ambiguously intentioned rejection to something they themselves had said or done, whereas LRS women tended to explain the same behavior in impersonal terms.

In a laboratory study of middle-school children, those high in RS felt more rejected and became more distressed than those low in RS when told that a friend whom they had selected as a study partner, did not want to leave class to do so (Downey, Lebolt, et al., 1998, Study 2). As in the previous study, no differences were found when a situational explanation (teacher would not give permission) was given for the friend not leaving class. Thus, defensive expectations of rejection also appear to prime HRS children to more readily perceive potential signs of rejection.

To further establish whether anxious expectations of rejection predicted the perception of intentional rejection, Downey and Feldman undertook a prospective longitudinal examination of college students in romantic relationships (1996, Study 3). The study tested whether rejection expectations (assessed before the beginning of a new romantic relationship) predicted perceptions of harmful intent in a new partner's insensitive behavior (e.g. being inattentive or distant). For HRS women, only the results showed that anxious expectations of rejection predicted a readiness to attribute hurtful intent to a new romantic partner's ambiguous or insensitive actions. The prospective relationship between RS and attributions of hurtful intent did not change when other relevant personality dispositions (e.g. introversion, neuroticism, self-esteem, general attachment style, social anxiety, and social avoidance) were statistically controlled.

REACTIONS TO PERCEIVED REJECTION (LINK 4)

Having documented that anxious expectations of rejection prompt a readiness to perceive rejection, we sought to examine the link between perceptions of rejection and hostile reactions in HRS women. We hypothesized that given HRS women's tendency to perceive intentional rejection in innocuous or ambiguous rejection cues, they may be likely to respond with hostile behavior when rejection is perceived. Their hostile behavior might in turn elicit actual rejection, which could eventually erode even committed relationships. In a study of dating couples, we investigated whether feelings of rejection triggered hostility in ongoing relationships to a greater extent in HRS than LRS individuals (Downey, Freitas, et al., 1998, Study 1). Specifically, we examined HRS and LRS women's hostility toward romantic partners as a function of day-to-day variation in feelings of rejection in their ongoing romantic relationships. A longitudinal daily diary design was selected to capitalize on the naturally occurring relationship conflict situations that can trigger rejection expectations (Downey, Freitas, et al., 1998). As predicted, HRS women showed a higher probability of reporting conflicts than did LRS women on days after they felt rejected, but not otherwise. HRS women's, but not HRS men's, resulting hostility also significantly accounted for their partners' relationship dissatisfaction. Multilevel modeling (Bolger & Zuckerman, 1995; Kenny, Kashy, & Bolger, 1998) revealed that on days proceeded by naturally occurring conflict, HRS women's partners were more likely than LRS women's partners to experience relationship dissatisfaction and to think of ending the relationship. RS also predicted a greater frequency of relationship breakup for women, even when controlling for partners' initial level of RS, relationship satisfaction, and commitment. The effect was similar, but weaker, for men. These findings were not attributable to the effect of stable partner background characteristics or to the contaminating effect of prior day's dissatisfaction and thoughts of ending the relationship. Finally, the reported differential impact of conflict on partners of HRS and LRS women was also evident to the women themselves: on the days proceeded by conflict, partners were perceived to be less accepting and more withdrawn by HRS than by LRS women.

To further explore the assumption that the negative behavior of HRS women during conflicts mediated their partners' post-conflict negativity, we videotaped couples discussing a self-selected unresolved relationship issue using a paradigm developed by Gottman (1979) for studying marital conflict (Downey, Freitas, et al., 1998, Study 2). In support of our daily diary study findings, women high in RS engaged in more hostile behavior during the discussion than did LRS women. Further analyses indicated that HRS women's hostility explained the relatively higher post-conflict anger and resentment about the relationship experienced by the partners of HRS women. Therefore, hostile behaviors actually elicit rejection from others, confirming initial expectations about the likelihood of rejection. Even controlling for partner's pre-conflict anger, relationship commitment, and satisfaction did not change this relationship. Thus for HRS women, their expectations influence, rather than merely reflect, the reality of their ongoing relationships. We believe this self-fulfilling prophecy is one reason why it may be difficult to intervene in the RS cycle; HRS women's tendency to expect, perceive, and overreact to rejection increases their likelihood of being rejected. Finally, a prospective study of young women further showed that RS predicted heightened levels of both physical and verbal hostility in adolescent girls during relationship conflicts. Although rates of actual physical fights were relatively low (10%), their occurrence significantly associated with expectations of rejection. These findings suggest that RS is a risk factor for the early onset of violence and dysfunction in young women's romantic relationships (Purdie & Downey, 2000).

Does the relationship between RS and relational difficulties extend beyond romantic relationships? In a longitudinal study of early adolescents, we found that it does (Downey, Lebolt, et al., 1998, Study 3). We tested whether early adolescents, who expected and perceived rejection from peers and teachers, engaged in more disruptive behavior (e.g. getting into fights), and experienced increased interpersonal difficulties over time. Fifth, sixth, and seventh grade children's self-reports of RS, acts of aggression, and feelings of victimization were compared with teacher reports of aggression, social competence, and RS, and with the Dean of Students' reports of fights with peers and conflict with school personnel. Our analysis revealed that RS predicted differences in aggression, antisocial behavior, and being victimized. Over a one-year period, HRS children became more aggressive towards their peers, showed a decline in positive classroom behavior, and became more sensitive and reactive to negative interpersonal events. Specifically, defensive rejection expectations undermined the peer and teacher relationships in ways that were likely to elicit rejection and erode wellbeing. Consequently, these children were more frequently punished for misbehavior and were at a greater risk for suspension from school.

WHY DO ANXIOUS EXPECTATIONS OF REJECTION LEAD TO HOSTILITY?

The studies described in this chapter, while depicting the links involved in the RS-hostility cycle, do not explain *why* women who fearfully expect rejection engage in the type of hostile behaviors likely to elicit rejection. To unpack the perceptual processes that may give rise to this outcome, we sought to specifically address why thoughts of rejection frequently lead to hostility. One possible explanation is that when HRS women perceive even mild rejection, they may view it as signifying the irreversible loss of a relationship. Their subsequent desire to take revenge may therefore be an outward expression of hurt and hopelessness (Ayduk et al., 1999). In order to test the hypothesis that HRS women respond aggressively only when rejection is perceived, rather than across situations, we compared HRS and LRS women's reactions in two contexts.

First, using a sequential priming-pronunciation paradigm, Ayduk et al. (1999, Study 1) tested whether specifically priming thoughts of rejection facilitated thoughts of hostility to a greater extent in HRS than LRS women, rather than being more chronically accessible in HRS than LRS women. In this paradigm, participants' speed in beginning to pronounce a target word (preceded by the presentation of a prime word) reliably measures the strength of mental associations between the prime and the target constructs (see Bargh, Raymond, Pryor, & Strack, 1995; Bargh, Chaiken, Raymond, & Hymes, 1996). The results showed that HRS women begin pronouncing hostility words (e.g., hit) faster than LRS women *uniquely* when the words were preceded by rejection words (e.g., abandon). When other negative words (e.g., vomit) served as the prime, HRS and LRS women did not differ in onset of their pronunciation of hostile words. These findings provide experimental evidence that rejection automatically activates hostility to a greater extent in HRS than in LRS women, and that HRS and LRS women do not differ in the chronic accessibility of hostile thoughts. Whereas the initial studies in this series focused on women, we have recently replicated the findings in men (Ayduk & Downey, 2003).

Second, we established that hostile thoughts, activated by rejection expectations, translate into hostile behaviors to a greater extent in HRS than in LRS women. In a laboratory experiment, Ayduk et al. (1999, Study 2) recruited women to participate in a study of how people form impressions in an internet-based "dating chat-room." To facilitate their on-line discussion, participants were asked to write a biosketch that would be exchanged with a "partner" (all participants actually received the same biosketch). Participants were then told that the interaction would not occur either because the partner did not want to continue with the on-line interaction portion of the study and had departed (experimental condition) or due to equipment failure (control condition). All participants then evaluated their assigned partner's biosketch. In support of our hypothesis, HRS women expressed indirect retaliatory rejecting behavior (in the form of more negative evaluations of their partner) in direct response to perceived rejection by this potential partner. In the absence of rejection cues (i.e., the broken equipment explanation), HRS and LRS women evaluated their partner similarly, again confirming the idea that HRS women are not more dispositionally hostile but instead are subject to psychological processes that are triggered within particularly salient contexts (Mischel & Shoda, 1995). When we repeated this experiment for men, we found that rejection by a potential chat-room partner elicited retaliatory indirect aggression only when it occurred in front of an audience of peers (Ayduk & Downey, 2003).

Several explanations as to why rejection elicits retaliatory behavior in HRS women can be drawn from these results. Perhaps HRS women perceived more subtle negativity in the confederate's behavior during the initial interaction than did LRS women, and then used this information to disambiguate the partner's ambiguous behavior. If so, HRS women may have perceived more negativity during the initial interaction because more existed, or because they were more attentive to their partner's negative behavior than were LRS women. It is also possible that HRS women tended to personalize ambiguously intentioned negative outcomes, whereas those low in RS tended not to. We are currently testing these possibilities.

MOTIVATED EFFORTS TO PREVENT REJECTION

As we have shown, the combination of high investment in close relationships coupled with anxious expectations and a heightened propensity to perceive and overreact to minor or ambiguous cues of rejection, leads HRS women to engage in hostile acts if security is perceived to be threatened. Therefore, destructive aggression may actually arise from feelings of disconnection and separateness, and may be an effort on the part of HRS women to attempt to regain some sense of control in a situation in which they feel powerless (Jack, 1999). Our data suggest that these patterns of reactive behavior are likely to perpetuate the RS cycle and put HRS women, and others close to them, at risk for relationship difficulties. We propose that the aggressive behavior of HRS women is engaged in when their worst fears, i.e., rejection, are realized. This explanation implies that HRS women should be likely to engage in strenuous, and perhaps excessive (and ultimately self-defeating) efforts to prevent rejection.

Evidence from a number of our studies support this claim by showing that HRS women exhibit a heightened propensity to engage in risky acts or in behaviors that make them uncomfortable in order to maintain a romantic relationship. In a prospective study, young women in sixth and seventh grade who were high in RS reported a greater willingness, two years later, to do things that they knew were wrong in order to maintain their current dating relationship (Purdie & Downey, 2000). Similarly, in a study of college-aged women, RS predicted a heightened likelihood of having done things that felt wrong or uncomfortable in order to maintain a relationship (Downey, Ayduk, Irwin, & Ramsay, under review).These findings suggest that their desire to maintain their relationship goals may motivate HRS women to engage in antisocial or delinquent behavior if they believe such activity will prevent rejection by a significant other. The threat of rejection may also prompt women to make great efforts to comply with a partner's wishes at the expense of their own goals (Cross & Madson, 1997), including being ingratiating, overly agreeable, and overly revealing of intimate information. Compliance may also place women in troubled relationships at risk for future victimization (Ayduk et al., 1999), as well as in dangerous situations, such as not speaking up and remaining in abusive relationships. We have also repeatedly found a link between RS and self-silencing in women (e.g., Ayduk et al. 2003). HRS women, when attempting to retain a desired level of intimacy, may attempt to suppress their emotionally driven cognitions and behaviors (Jack, 1991 & 1999; Jack & Dill, 1992) to avert rejection outcomes. Although this more reflective (as opposed to reactive) behavior may be positive in that it averts overt aggression and repercussions of hostility, such strategies carry their own dangers. In response to perceived rejection from romantic partners, self-defeating efforts, such as self-blame, self-silencing, and compliance strategies, may be self-damaging avenues through which HRS women experience and express their hurt and distress. Self-silencing, in particular, is viewed as a risk factor for depression (Gratch, Bassett, & Attra, 1995; Jack & Dill, 1992). Patterns of internalizing reactions may put HRS women at a greater risk for self-harming behaviors, such as substance abuse and/or eating disorders. For example, loss of self-esteem following rejection may also take the form of dysregulated eating behavior in which HRS women use eating to regain love and acceptance.

Together these findings suggest that HRS women are vulnerable to engaging in potentially self-damaging reactions in their efforts to avoid rejection and in order to gain acceptance. Thus, the same cognitive-affective processing dynamic, RS, that increases risk for aggression in women may also account for the traditional described pattern of self-harmful behavior displayed by some women.

SUPPORT FOR RS-AGGRESSION LINK IN INCARCERATED FEMALES

The evidence we have presented concerning RS and aggression is based on data from college students and from a demographically high-risk sample of early adolescents. However, a critical test of the RS model is its applicability to women who have engaged in seriously aggressive and/or antisocial behavior. Bedell (1999) addressed this question in a study of women incarcerated in a maximum-security prison, using a measure of RS developed specifically for this population. In a sample of 63 women, RS was found to be associated with childhood exposure to rejection as well as with depression, substance abuse, and involvement in violent relationships. The female inmates reported high levels of involvement in violent romantic relationships (60%), substance abuse (73%), and moderate to high levels of depression. Anxiety about rejection was also significantly related to being the victim of physical aggression, and expectations of rejection were significantly associated with being the perpetrator of physical aggression.

These findings suggest that for female offenders, chronic rejecting experiences and the rejection concerns to which such experiences give rise, may contribute to depression and interpersonal difficulties. Involvement in drugs may be an effort to numb experiences of traumatic memories of childhood abuse, violence, depression, and feelings of rejection. Bedell proposes that living and growing up in a violent and rejecting environment may lead some women to adopt violence and aggression as the only available and viable option for resolving disputes and for dealing with relationship difficulties. As suggested by Jack (1999), women who have been severely abused as children may resort to physical aggression as a familiar means of maintaining intimacy, and as a way of sustaining their attachment to others. Applied to female inmates, exposure to violent and traumatic childhood and adult experiences may lead to expectations of familiar patterns of violence and aggression. Consequently, in new romantic relationships, relational violence and abuse may be accepted as a way of life, and feelings of powerlessness may stand in the way of positive change.

RS MODERATORS: SELF-REGULATION ABILITY
AND ATTENTIONAL CONTROL

Despite the link between RS and aggression, and other maladaptive outcomes, there is reason to believe that not all women who fear and expect rejection show such maladaptive behaviors. A theoretically relevant factor related to creating more adaptive functioning in vulnerable women is how well they are able to regulate themselves under conditions of stress. Effective self-regulation when in a state of heightened arousal—whether positively or negatively valenced—should enable the inhibition of undesired, impulsive behaviors, and may facilitate the enactment of effective problem-solving strategies. Based on this rationale, we have undertaken a set of studies to investigate the prediction that self-regulatory ability, and strategic attention deployment in particular, protect women high in anxious expectations of rejection from the negative consequences associated with their expectations.

EVIDENCE OF THE PROTECTIVE ROLE OF
SELF-REGULATORY ABILITY

In two studies, self-regulatory ability was assessed in the classic self-imposed delay of gratification (DG) paradigm (Mischel, 1974; Mischel, Shoda, & Rodriguez, 1989). In this paradigm, children are presented with a choice between an immediate or smaller reward and a delayed but larger reward. Shortly after the child selects the option of the larger reward, delay becomes increasingly difficult. Mischel's original research demonstrated that individual differences in the amount of time that a child could delay gratification reflected whether the child could shift his or her attention away from "hot" consummatory features of the delay situation to "cooler" features, in an effort to attenuate their frustrative arousal. Mischel demonstrated that children who use purposeful self-distraction and cognitive reframing are more successful at delay, and that delay time is a predictor of both short-term and long-term adjustment.

Does DG protect HRS women against aggressive behaviors and low-self-esteem (Ayduk et al., 2000)? Our findings indicate that it does. Ayduk et al. (2000) showed that those HRS women from the original Mischel study who had exhibited low delay ability, reported lower self-esteem and used more crack/cocaine, as compared to their high delay or LRS counterparts. Additionally, the HRS-low delay group was more easily stressed and had more troubled relationships (Ayduk, Downey, & Mischel, 2003, unpublished data). This pattern of findings was replicated and extended to aggressive behaviors in a one-year prospective study with middle-school children. HRS children who were low in delay ability, reported lower self-worth and showed higher levels of aggression and peer rejection than either the high delay or LRS groups (Ayduk et al., 2000).

These findings concerning the interactive effect of RS and poor self-regulatory skills have led us to further explore this potentially troubling combination. Of particular interest was whether this combination of processing dispositions might contribute to increased risk for a personality disorder, Borderline Personality Disorder (BPD), that is disproportionately found in women. Its symptomatology encompasses difficulties that our data suggest characterize those high in RS and low in delay. A core symptom of BPD is intense anger. BPD is also marked by a pervasive pattern of highly unstable and volatile interpersonal relationships, lack of self-identity or sense of self, feelings of emptiness, impulsivity, and extreme instability of affect (i.e. reactive mood swings) (American Psychiatric Association, 2000). Self-harmful behavior associated with BPD includes bulimia and substance abuse. BPD individuals have a desperate fear of abandonment, and may go to great lengths to maintain their relationships (American Psychiatric Association, 2000; Paris, 2003). Thus, not surprisingly, extreme sensitivity to rejection is a characteristic of many people with BPD. The perception of rejection can trigger overreactions that include aggressive or hostile behavior, inevitably leading to partner conflict. Thus the combination of intensive reactivity to interpersonal stress, combined with poor emotional self-regulation, can lead to stormy and chaotic interpersonal relationships.

We found support for the hypothesis that HRS and low DG (assessed with a self-report questionnaire) would predict clinically significant levels of BPD in a sample of 350 college students. Moreover, BPD and RS interacted in this sample such that those who evidenced combined HRS and low self-regulation showed borderline symptoms : low self-worth, aggression, victimization, bulimia, depression, and substance abuse (Downey et al., under review).

INTERVENTIONS TO DECREASE THE RS–AGGRESSION LINK, AND OTHER FORMS OF MALADJUSTMENT

Research indicates that flexible and strategic attentional deployment is essential for distress- and impulse-inhibition (Derryberry & Rothbart, 1997; Field, 1981; Gerardi, Rothbart, Posner, & Kepler, 1996; Rothbart & Ahadi, 1994; Sethi, Mischel, Aber, Shoda, & Rodriguez, 2000). In other words, being able to attenuate arousal by "cooling" impulse-eliciting features of a situation, may help explain why some HRS women cope more rationally and reflectively, in accordance with their long-term relationship goals. Conversely, the prototypical "hot" RS-hostility dynamic primarily characterizes those HRS women with poor self-regulatory ability. Therefore, self-regulatory competency can be thought of as serving a moderating role for the negative interpersonal and personal consequences of anxious expectations of rejection in HRS women.

The findings described in this chapter led us to begin to examine whether interventions intended to increase the flexible and strategic deployment of attention under stress might reduce the ill-effects of RS. The first step in this goal has been to conduct a laboratory-based intervention with the goal of replacing the apparently automatic affectively-mediated "hot" response to rejection with a more instrumental, reflective, and cognitively mediated "cool" response. The characteristic "hot" system reaction of HRS women who perceive rejection is thought to occur when, in a state of distress, access to "cooling" processes and strategies (i.e. the ability to think rationally and reflect on the situation) is inhibited. The result of this inhibition is that informational processing becomes rapidly driven by emotional impulses (Davis, 1992; Fanselow, 1994; LeDoux, 1995; Metcalfe & Mischel, 1999; Zillmann, 1993). Thus, under conditions of rejection, HRS women are unable to access and utilize self-regulatory strategies that foster "cool" system processing that attenuates reactive hostility (Ayduk et al., 1999).

Does activating "cool-abstract" (i.e., reflective, rational focus) thought processes lead to less anger following rejection? In research involving college students, we manipulated attentional focus by asking participants to recall interpersonal experiences involving anger. Those individuals in the "hot" ideation condition were asked to focus on their emotional experience of the memory, whereas those in the "cool" condition focused on cognitive aspects of their memory, designed to activate the abstract processes that characterize the "cool" system. The "hot" ideation group demonstrated shorter reaction times to hostility words during a lexical decision task, than did the "cool" condition group. These results indicate a stronger mental link between rejection and anger. Rejection and anger were countered against by a focus away from emotional and visceral aspects of a recalled situation in the "cool" condition. Relative to participants in the "cool" condition, "hot" participants also evidenced greater explicit anger, as reported through their ratings and coded essay data. Therefore, across implicit and explicit measures, the activation of a "hot" emotional attentional focus acts as a catalyst for hostile reactions, whereas employment of a "cool" focus seems to protect against dysregulated behavior, particularly in the case of HRS people. This intervention worked equally well for men and women.

In summary, one of the great challenges facing HRS women in rejection-related situations is their ability to overcome automatic "hot" system processing (Ayduk & Mischel, 2002). The ability to employ self-control strategies appears to buffer HRS women against overreactions to rejection, thereby reducing the risk of negative outcomes for which HRS women are vulnerable. By learning to employ self- and attentional-control strategies, HRS women with low self-control may be able to focus more on contextual cues that offer possible alternative explanations to perceived rejection thus preventing behavioral overreactions.

SUMMARY

Throughout this chapter, we have described research that expands our knowledge regarding situations that elicit women's hostility and aggression, and what function this behavior serves. We have posited that the RS model sheds light on some of the dynamics involved in female hostility. Our results illustrate that a more complete understanding of women's hostility and aggression in close relationships requires taking into account the significance of interpersonal acceptance and rejection for women, as well as the broader constellation of maladaptive behavior in which women's aggression is embedded—depression, eating disorders, and dependency. It appears that RS negatively influences how women think, feel, and behave in different kinds of relationships. RS also leads to a self-fulfilling prophecy where women's fears and expectations of rejection get confirmed, influencing current and future behavioral patterns and relationship health.

However, we posit that the RS-hostility cycle may be interrupted by the successful employment of self-control and attentional strategies. Intercepting HRS women's harmful attributional biases and self-defeating reactive behaviors, by replacing them with alternative explanations and self-regulation tools, may permit women to respond more adaptively in situations when they feel threatened. HRS women who are encouraged to believe that they have control in a situation where they had previously felt none, may thus be able to diffuse their anxiety and break the self-fulfilling effect of the RS-hostility link.

REFERENCES

American Psychiatric Association (2000). *Diagnostic and statistical manual of mental disorders* (4th ed.) Washington, DC: Author.

Archer, J. (2000). Sex differences in aggression between heterosexual partners: A meta-analytic review. *Psychological Bulletin, 126*, 651–680.

Archer, J., & Ray, N. (1989). Dating violence in the United Kingdom: A preliminary study. *Aggressive Behavior, 15*, 337–343.

Arias, I., Samios, M., & O'Leary, K. D. (1987). Prevalence and correlates of physical aggression during courtship. *Journal of Interpersonal Violence, 2*, 82–90.

Ayduk, O., & Downey, G. (in preparation, 2003). *Gender differences and similarities in the dynamics of rejection sensitivity.*

Ayduk, O., & Mischel, W. (2002). When smart people behave stupidly: Reconciling inconsistencies in social–emotional intelligence. In R. J. Sternberg (Ed.), *Why smart people can be so stupid* (pp. 86–105). New Haven, CT: Yale University Press.

Ayduk, O., & Velilla, E. (2003). Implications of rejection sensitivity and self-control for relational vulnerabilities. Paper presented at the Biennial Meetings of the Society for Research in Child Development, Tampa, Florida.

Ayduk, O., Downey, G., Testa, A., Yen, Y., & Shoda, Y. (1999). Does rejection elicit hostility in rejection sensitive women? *Social Cognition, 17*, 245–271.

Ayduk, O., Mendoza-Denton, R., Mischel, W., Downey, G., Peake, P., & Rodriguez, M. (2000). Regulating the interpersonal self: Strategic self-regulation for coping with rejection sensitivity. *Journal of Personality and Social Psychology, 79*, 776–792.

Ayduk, O., Downey, G., & Mischel, W. (unpublished data, 2003). Columbia University, NY.

Bargh, J. A., Raymond, P., Pryor, J. B., & Strack, F. (1995). Attractiveness of the underling: An automatic power-sex association and its consequences for sexual harassment and aggression. *Journal of Personality and Social Psychology, 68*, 768–781.

Bargh, J. A., Chaiken, S., Raymond, P., & Hymes, C. (1996). The automatic evaluation effect: Unconditional automatic attitude activation with a pronunciation task. *Journal of Experimental Social psychology, 32*, 104–128.

Baumeister, R., & Sommer, K. L. (1997). What do men want? Gender differences and two spheres of belongingness: Comments on Cross and Madson (1997). *Psychological Bulletin, 122*, 38–44.

Bedell, P. (1999). Fostering resilience in women in prison. Columbia University, NY.

Ben-David, S. (1993). The two facets of female violence: The public and the domestic domains. *Journal of Family Violence, 8*, 345–359.

Billingham, R. E., & Sack, A. R. (1987). Conflict tactics and the level of emotional commitment among unmarrieds. *Human Relations, 40*, 50–74.

Bjorkqvist, K., Osterman, K., & Lagerspetz, M. J. (1992). Indirect aggression: Conceptions and misconceptions. In K. Bjorkqvist, & P. Niemela (Eds.), *Of mice and women: Aspects of female aggression* (pp. 51–53). San Diego, CA: Academic Press.

Bolger, N., & Zuckerman, A. (1995). A framework for studying personality in the stress process. *Journal of Personality and Social Psychology, 69*, 890–902.

Bowlby, J. (1969). *Attachment and loss: Vol 1. Attachment.* NY: Basic.

Bowlby, J. (1973). *Attachment and loss: Vol 2. Separation.* NY: Basic.

Bowlby, J. (1980). *Attachment and loss: Vol 3. Loss, sadness, and depression.* NY: Basic.

Bureau of Justice Statistics. (1999). *Special report: Women offenders.* (NCJ 175688). Washington, DC: Greenfeld & Snell.

Cairns, R. B., & Cairns, B. D. (1994). *Lifelines and risks: Pathways of youth in our time.* Cambridge, England: Cambridge University Press.

Campbell, A., Muncer, S., & Coyle, E. (1992). Social representation of aggression as an explanation of gender differences: A preliminary study. *Aggressive Behavior, 18*, 95–108.

Canetto, S. S., & Lester, D. (Eds.). (1995). *Women and suicidal behavior.* NY: Springer.

Crick, N. R., & Grotpeter, J. K. (1995). Relational aggression, gender, and social-psychological adjustment. *Child Development, 66*, 710–722.

Cross, L. W. (1993). Body and self in feminine development: Implications for eating disorders and delicate self-mutilation. *Bulletin of the Menninger Clinic, 57*, 41–68.

Cross, S. E., & Madson, L. (1997). Models of the self: Self-construals and gender. *Psychological Bulletin, 122*, 5–37.

Davis, M. (1992). The role of the amygdala in fear and anxiety. *Annual review of Neuroscience, 15*, 353–375.

Deal, J. E., & Wampler, K. S. (1986). Dating violence: The primacy of previous experience. *Journal of Personal and Social Relationships, 3*, 457–471.

Derryberry, D., & Rothbart, M. (1997). Reactive and effortful processes in the organization of temperament. *Development and Psychopathology, 9*, 633–652.

deWeerth, C., & Kalma, A. P. (1992). Female aggression as a response to sexual jealousy: A sex role reversal? *Aggressive Behavior, 19*, 265–279.

Downey, G., Bonica, C., London, B. E., & Paltin, I. (in press). Causes and consequences of rejection sensitivity. *Journal of Research in Adolescence.*

Downey, G., & Feldman, S. (1996). Implications of rejection sensitivity for intimate relationships. *Journal of Personality and Social Psychology, 70*, 1327–1343.

Downey, G., Lebolt, A., & O'Shea-Lauber, K. (1995, March). Implications of rejection sensitivity for adolescent peer and dating relationships. Paper presented at the Society for Research on Adolescence Conference, Indianapolis, IN.

Downey, G., Khouri, H., & Feldman, S. (1997). Early interpersonal trauma and adult adjustment: The mediational role of rejection sensitivity. In D. Cicchetti & S. Toth (Eds.), *Rochester Symposium on Developmental Psychopathology, Volume VIII: The effects of trauma on the developmental process* (pp. 85–114). Rochester, NY: University of Rochester Press.

Downey, G. Freitas, A. L. Michealis, B, & Khouri, H. (1998). The self-fulfilling prophecy in close relationships: Do rejection sensitive women get rejected by their partners? *Journal of Personality and Social Psychology, 75*, 545–560.

Downey, G., Lebolt, A., Rincon, C., & Freitas, A. L. (1998). Rejection sensitivity and adolescent interpersonal difficulties. *Child Development, 69*, 1072–1089.

Downey, G., Ayduk, O., Irwin, L., & Ramsay, M. (under review). *A CAPS approach to Borderline Personality Disorder.*

Erikson, E. (1950). *Childhood and society.* NY: Norton.

Eskin, M., & Kravitz, M. (1980). *Child abuse and neglect.* Washington, DC: U.S. Department of Justice.

Fanselow, M. S. (1994). Neural organization of the defensive behavior system responsible for fear. *Psychometric Bulletin & Review, 1*, 429–438.

Feldman, S., & Downey, G. (1994). Rejection sensitivity as a mediator of the impact of childhood exposure to family violence on adult attachment behavior. *Development and Psychopathology, 6*, 231–247.

Field, T. (1981). Infant gaze aversion and heart rate during face-to-face interactions. *Infant Behavior and Development, 4*, 307–215.

Gerardi, G., Rothbart, M. K., Posner, M. I., & Kepler, S. (1996, April). *The development of attentional control: Performance on a spatial Stroop-like task at 24, 30, and 36–39 months of age.* Poster session presented at the annual meeting of the International Society for Infant Studies, Providence, RI.

Gilligan, C. (1982). *In a different voice: Psychological theory and women's development.* Cambridge, MA: Harvard University Press.

Gottman, J. M. (1979). *Marital interaction: Experimental investigations.* NY: Academic Press.

Gratch, L. V., Bassett, M. E., & Attra, S. L. (1995). The relationship of gender and ethnicity to self-silencing and depression among college students. *Psychology of Women Quarterly, 19*, 509–515.

Harris, M. B. (1993). How provoking! What makes men and women angry. *Aggressive Behavior, 19*, 199–213.

Hipwell, A. E., Loeber, R., Stouthamer-Loeber, M., Keenan, K., White, H. R., & Kroneman, L. (2002). Characteristics of girls with early onset disruptive and antisocial behaviour. *Criminal Behaviour and Mental Health, 12*, 99–118

Horney, K. (1937). *The neurotic personality of our time*. NY: Norton.

Jack, D. C. (1991). *Silencing the self: Women and depression*. Cambridge, MA: Harvard University Press.

Jack, D. C. (1999). *Behind the mask: Destruction and creativity in women's aggression*. Cambridge, MA: Harvard University Press.

Jack, D. C., & Dill, D. (1992). The Silencing the Self Scale: Schemas of intimacy associated with depression in women. *Psychology of Women Quarterly, 16*, 97–106.

Kenny, D. A., Kashy, D., & Bolger, N., (1998). Data analysis in social psychology. In D. Gilbert, S. Fiske, & G. Lindzey (Eds.), *Handbook of social psychology* (4th ed., pp. 233–268). NY: McGraw Hill.

LeDoux, J. E. (1995). Setting "stress" into motion: Brain mechanisms of stimulus evaluation. In M. J. Friedman, D.S. Charney, & A. Y. Deutch (Eds.), *Neurobiological and clinical consequences of stress: From normal adaptation to post-traumatic stress disorder* (pp. 125–134). PA: Lippincott-Raven Publishers.

Levy, S., Ayduk, O., & Downey, G. (2001). Implications of rejection for relations with significant others and social groups. In M. Leary (Ed.), *Interpersonal rejection* (pp. 251–290). NY: Oxford University Press.

Metcalfe, J., & Mischel, W. (1999). A hot/cool-system analysis of delay of gratification: Dynamics of willpower. *Psychological Review, 106*, 3–19.

Mischel, W. (1974). Cognitive appraisals and transformations in self-control. In B. Weiner (Ed.), *Cognitive views of human motivation* (pp. 33–49). New York: Academic Press.

Mischel, W., & Shoda, Y. (1995). A cognitive-affective system theory of personality: Reconceptualizing situations, dispositions, dynamics and invariance in personality structure. *Psychological Review, 102*, 246–268.

Mischel, W., Shoda, Y., & Rodriguez, M. L. (1989). Delay of gratification in children. *Science, 244*, 933–938.

Nolen-Hoeksema, S. (1987). Sex differences in unipolar depression: Evidence and theory. *Psychological Bulletin, 101*, 259–282.

Paris, J. (2003). *Personality disorders over time: Precursors, course, and outcome*. Washington, DC: American Psychiatric Publishing.

Plass, M. S., & Gessner, J. C. (1983). Violence in courtship relations: A southern sample. *Free Inquiry in Creative Sociology, 11*, 198–202.

Purdie, V., & Downey, G. (2000). Rejection sensitivity and adolescent girls' vulnerability to relationship-centered difficulties. *Child Maltreatment, 5*, 338–350.

Rothbart, M. K., & Ahadi, S. A. (1994). Temperament and the development of personality. *Journal of Abnormal Psychology, 103*, 55–66.

Sethi, A., Mischel, W., Aber, J. L., Shoda, Y., & Rodriguez, M. L. (2000). The role of strategic attention deployment of self-regulation: Predicting preschoolers' delay of gratification from mother-toddler interactions. *Developmental Psychology, 36*, 767–777.

Sullivan, H. S. (1953). *The interpersonal theory of psychiatry*. NY: Norton.

Zillmann, D. (1993). Mental control of angry aggression. In D. M. Wegner & J. W. Pennebaker (Eds.), *Handbook of mental control* (pp. 370–392). Englewood Cliffs, NJ: Prentice Hall.

The Science of Relational Aggression
Can We Guide Intervention?

TASHA C. GEIGER, MELANIE J. ZIMMER-GEMBECK, AND NICKI R. CRICK*

A preventive intervention research cycle is often necessary when attempting to moderate a complex problem such as aggression (Heller, 1996; Poulin, Dishion, & Burraston, 2001). The first step in this cycle includes defining the problem, developing measures for accurate assessment, and documenting prevalence. Ideally, these studies are at first moderate in size, but later include epidemiological studies with large, population-based samples. This step also examines subpopulations to identify those with the highest rates of the behavior. The second step should include developmental research to determine who is most likely to engage in high levels of the behavior during which period(s) of life, who is at risk of continuing or escalating the behavior, and how detrimental effects of the problem behavior vary by age.

The third part of the preventive intervention research cycle involves examining the precursors and correlates of the behavior so that interventions can also be targeted toward the *processes* that lead to problem behavior,

* Preparation of this manuscript was supported by grants to the third author from the National Institute of Mental Health and the National Science Foundation.

TASHA C. GEIGER AND NICKI R. CRICK • Institute of Child Development, University of Minnesota, Minneapolis, Minnesota, United States, 55455 • MELANIE J. ZIMMER-GEMBECK • School of Applied Psychology, Griffith University, Gold Coast, Queensland, Australia, 9726.

in addition to the behavior of interest (Catalano, Hawkins, Berglund, Pollard, & Arthur, 2002). Concurrent with these efforts, the development of comprehensive models and other theoretical insights often take place. Once these research tasks provide substantial explanation of the targeted problem, interventions developed from this foundation have the greatest potential to be effective. Next, evaluations of these interventions determine effectiveness and, in turn, inform theory and future empirical research, completing a first cycle.

Frequently, however, once a problem is recognized and publicized, community members, government and nongovernmental agencies, policymakers, and concerned individuals find the problem too great and deserving of intervention to wait for some of these important research tasks to be conducted before implementing programs. In fact, evaluation of programs becomes difficult because, for example, schools may deem the problem so important that being in a control group is not acceptable. Relational aggression and victimization among youths and adults has recently received this attention in the U.S., Canada, Australia, and other countries. Relational aggression is defined as "behaviors that harm others through damage (or threat of damage) to relationships or feelings of acceptance, friendship, or group inclusion" (Crick et al., 1999, p. 77). Relational aggression includes, for example, social exclusion or spreading rumors with the intent to harm others, or as a form of retaliation (Crick & Grotpeter, 1995). In contrast to physical aggression in which the agent of harm is actual or threatened physical damage, relational aggression involves actual or threatened damage to relationships as the vehicle of harm.

Many U.S. television programs and other media outlets (e.g., *The Oprah Winfrey Show, The New York Times*) and more than 10 popular books (e.g., Simmons, 2002) have concentrated on aggressive females and relational forms of aggression since the year 2000. These accounts have attributed many social and psychological problems to relational aggression and victimization, particularly among females. This recent media coverage has contributed to the growing interest in campaigns to increase awareness of relational aggression and victimization, and to implement interventions, especially among females. Given this interest, it is time to consider the state of more rigorous, empirically-based information on relational aggression and victimization within the context of the preventive intervention research cycle.

As a first step toward addressing this issue, we address four topics in this chapter. Consistent with the first goal of a preventative research cycle, we focus on the definition and nature of relational, social, and indirect forms of aggression. Part of the difficulty in understanding the popular media's presentation of relational aggression stems from differing opinions about what constitutes a normative level of gossiping and exclusion, and what is inappropriate and candidate for intervention. Hence, we describe what differentiates normal levels of nonphysical forms of aggression from problematic levels, and we describe the prevalence of these behaviors. We also consider that these forms of aggression can be covert in nature, thus hampering their assessment.

Next, we focus on whether intervention for relationally aggressive behaviors is a necessary endeavor and highlight some of the controversy surrounding this issue. The controversy primarily involves the second step of the research cycle in which the detrimental effects of the problem behaviors should be documented before intervention is warranted. To address the third step of the preventive intervention research cycle, we review studies of the correlates and potential contributing factors to nonphysical forms of aggression. Our concluding topic concerns whether there is a research base on which to develop interventions for relational aggression that can, at best, reduce problem behaviors and, at least, do not harm.

DEFINITION, MEASUREMENT, AND PREVALENCE OF RELATIONAL AGGRESSION AND VICTIMIZATION

According to Crick and colleagues (e.g., Crick & Grotpeter, 1995), relational aggression involves both direct behaviors (e.g., telling someone "you can't come to my birthday party unless you give me that sandwich") and indirect acts (e.g., getting even with someone by giving them the silent treatment). Although this definition has been used widely, a brief review of studies of nonphysical forms of aggression reveals some lack of consensus in terminology and definitions of the phenomenon. Other commonly used terms include indirect aggression (e.g., Bjorkqvist, Lagerspetz, & Kaukiainen, 1992) and social aggression (e.g., Galen & Underwood, 1997). As the term implies, indirect aggression involves hostile acts that are nonconfrontational in nature. Thus, it involves some covert behaviors that overlap with relational aggression (e.g., spreading rumors); however, it does not capture relationally aggressive acts that are more direct (e.g., saying "I won't be your friend if you don't share that ice cream with me"). Further, in contrast to relational aggression, indirect aggression can include covert behaviors that do not involve manipulation of relationships (e.g., putting sugar in someone's gas tank). Relational aggression can also be differentiated from social aggression. Although definitions of social aggression have been offered by a number of investigators, including Patterson (Patterson, Reid, & Dishion, 1982) who considered the term to refer to physical acts of hostility, Galen and Underwood (1997) proposed that social aggression refers to behaviors that attack another's self esteem or social status. Hence, verbal insults (calling someone mean names) could be considered social aggression because insults are likely to damage self-esteem; however, these acts would not be considered relational aggression because relationships were not the agent of harm.

Given the different definitions and the number of researchers investigating the topic, it is not surprising that a range of measurement techniques have been used to assess relational, and related forms of, aggression. The majority of researchers have utilized peer nomination techniques in which classmates identify those who are relationally aggressive or victimized by using a list of behaviors such as social exclusion, ignoring, and threatening to end friendships (Crick & Grotpeter, 1995). Others use observational methods (e.g., Ostrov & Keating, in press); focus groups or interviews (e.g., Owens, Shute, & Slee, 2000a), self-report measures (e.g., Lagerspetz, Bjorkqvist, & Peltonen, 1988), or teacher reports (e.g., Crick, Casas, & Mosher, 1997). Regardless of the method used, the data gathered all tend to have some limitations that can affect findings and lead to inconsistent descriptions of the nature of relational aggression. For example, highly skewed distributions can result because only a minority of individuals is identified as victimized or as engaging in moderate to high levels of relational aggression. The source of information may also impact our understanding of relational aggression. Different reporters may have differential access to the observation of the targeted behaviors and, if so, this may introduce bias into reports. Overall, the variety of definitions and measurement techniques may be one reason for varying prevalence rates and differing conclusions about populations most likely to engage in relationally aggressive behaviors and most likely to be victims.

Lack of attention to developmental differences may be another cause of differing conclusions regarding prevalence and consequences of relational aggression. Often findings related to relational aggression differ according to the age group studied, and researchers have noted these inconsistent findings. That relational aggression is associated with maladjustment during early and middle childhood (e.g., Crick, 1996), but associated, in some cases, with increased acceptance or popularity among adolescents (e.g., Salmivalli, Kaukiainen, & Lagerspetz, 2000), does not necessarily indicate poor construct validity. Rather, these investigations point to a developmental phenomenon potentially worthy of additional exploration. Specifically, the impact of socially manipulative behaviors may change as the nature and relevance of friendships, cliques, and same and opposite sex peer groups changes. It appears that processes involved in relational aggression unfold over time.

There have also been many different evidence-based conclusions regarding which relationally aggressive behaviors and what level of behaviors are normative, rather than deviant or problematic. It has been argued that, at low or moderate levels, relationally aggressive behavior is common and normative. At some point, most people have gossiped, ignored, or intentionally excluded someone. Further, these behaviors have been found to have some beneficial purposes, such as an opportunity for discussing an interpersonal conflict with a third party or letting a peer know, through gossiping, that a child may need some assistance (Underwood, Galen, & Paquette, 2001). However, gossiping to be helpful to a peer does not appear to be consistent with the construct of nonphysical aggression and can contribute to continued difficulty defining this construct. Gossiping can be used to gain assistance for a peer, to build rapport (i.e., feelings of group inclusion), or to harm another's reputation and relationships. Importantly, however, definitions of aggression typically are based on either the intent to harm (a focus on the intent of the behavior) and/or the actual delivery of harm (a focus on the consequences of the behavior). These criteria are not met when the goal is to assist a friend. To facilitate a consensus on the nature of relational aggression, behaviors included in the definition and in assessments should include only those acts that involve the intent and/or actual delivery of harm.

The difficulty of differentiating normal from problem behavior is not unique to the study of relational aggression. Problem behaviors are often best described along a continuum (e.g., Caron & Rutter, 1991). Maladaptive behaviors or symptoms of psychological disorders are observed, to some degree, in normal populations. A degree of physical aggression is common among young children (Coie & Dodge, 1998); mild depressed mood may be expected at times of high stress and during important life transitions; symptoms of anxiety disorders, particularly phobias and separation anxiety (Malcarne & Hansdottir, 2001), are commonly exhibited among children. Thus, professionals have criteria for determining when a pattern of behavior is pathological or deviant. These criteria include a meaningful cluster of maladaptive behaviors that are present at a clinically significant level, cause significant distress and/or impairment in functioning (American Psychiatric Association, 1994), and interfere with the successful accomplishment of necessary developmental tasks (Cicchetti & Cohen, 1995). Although generally well-adjusted individuals may use tactics similar to relational aggression, research has demonstrated that engagement in a variety of these behaviors at relatively high levels is often pathological. Specifically, these behaviors have been associated with maladjustment (Crick, 1996) and they interfere with developmental tasks such as peer relations and friendships (Grotpeter & Crick, 1996).

Few studies have reported the proportion of youths who engage in moderate or high levels of relational aggression or experience this level of relational victimization. Further, studies in which this issue has been addressed often use assessment methods that are less than ideal for evaluating prevalence (e.g., children's narratives; Xie, Swift, Cairns, & Cairns, 2002). Most existing investigations have included average aggression scores or group comparisons (e.g., males vs. females) of average levels of aggression. This is not the most useful information when the task is to estimate the size of the population that will benefit and to develop interventions to aid this group. Estimates become more difficult to obtain when age- and gender-specific prevalence rates are required to develop interventions for a particular subgroup. In sum, it is time for a review of the literature to estimate prevalence of relational aggression within gender and age groups, and to identify gaps in our knowledge of prevalence. The need and impact of an intervention at a population level is difficult to estimate without this epidemiological information.

IS RELATIONAL AGGRESSION A PROBLEM?

Relational aggression can interfere with succeeding at an essential developmental task of middle childhood, that of forming and maintaining intimate, close relationships with peers, and this is true for the victims and the aggressors (Crick, Casas, & Nelson, 2002). Researchers have reported associations between relational aggression and peer rejection among preschoolers (Crick et al., 1997), elementary school children (Rys & Bear, 1997), and college students (Werner & Crick, 1999). Relationally aggressive children are also more lonely than nonrelationally aggressive children (Prinstein, Boergers, & Vernberg, 2001). Similarly, victims of relational aggression exhibit increased levels of a number of social difficulties including peer rejection, social avoidance, social anxiety, and loneliness (Craig, 1998; Crick & Bigbee, 1998). In addition to difficulties with social relationships, other forms of maladjustment are elevated among aggressors and victims of relational aggression, namely externalizing and internalizing problems (Crick & Bigbee, 1998; Prinstein et al., 2001).

Although engagement in relational aggression has been associated with children's adjustment problems, some behaviors that fall within the domain of relational aggression also accompany positive functioning at some ages and in some contexts (e.g., Salmivalli et al., 2000). Others have reported no association between social aggression and maladjustment including academic competence, popularity and affiliation (Xie et al., 2002). A recent study, however, illustrates that these findings may not be contradictory. Using a combination of reports of who is "popular" and who is "liked", girls who were popular but not as well-liked were more relationally aggressive (Lease, Kennedy, & Axelrod, 2002). It may be that relationally aggressive girls can be centrally located in the peer group and accepted by some, but not as well-liked as others who are not relationally aggressive. Consistent with this hypothesis, Crick and Grotpeter (1995) showed that relationally aggressive children are significantly more likely than nonrelationally aggressive peers to be categorized as controversial in sociometric status. That is, they are both highly liked (probably by friends) and highly disliked (probably by victims) by their agemates.

If relationally aggressive behaviors (which are, by definition, done with the intent to harm) are associated with some aspects of positive functioning, these data partly explain why individuals continue to aggress and why it is difficult to persuade youths to discontinue these behaviors. However, the same relationally aggressive episodes that may result in a "positive" outcome (e.g., keeping a peer in an exclusive relationship) may at the same time lead to aversive consequences (e.g., making the targeted peer resentful; making the actor less desirable as friend in the eyes of other children). Nevertheless, although a few studies point to some personal advantages of involvement in relational aggression for the perpetrators, the numerous studies of adjustment and relational aggression described previously clearly demonstrate that relational aggression is clearly dysfunctional at times or at certain levels, as is relational victimization. Thus, a complete understanding of the nature of aggression and its positive and negative features is a worthwhile task. However, researchers must be concise in their interpretations of this data and clearly indicate the contexts in which particular aspects of aggression are linked with psychosocial functioning. This precise explication of findings will prevent misinterpretation or over-generalization of results.

RELATIONAL AGGRESSION, GENDER, AND AGE

One quick search of the Internet reveals that the popular media emphasize the participation of girls in relational aggression to the neglect of boys. It is clear that boys are more physically aggressive than girls, and when levels of physical and relational aggression are compared, girls are more likely to use relational aggression only, whereas boys often use both physical and relational aggression (Coie & Dodge, 1998; Crick, 1997). Girls are found to be more relationally or indirectly aggressive than boys in most studies; however, some have found that boys are more relationally aggressive than girls (David & Kistner, 2000). Also, girls and boys may, at particular ages, engage in relational aggression to the same degree (e.g., Rys & Bear, 1997). These discrepancies may be largely due to methodological variations in assessment. Researchers have used approaches that are likely to involve biases (e.g., teacher report, self report), however, those using more objective approaches (e.g., naturalistic observations) have consistently found girls to be significantly more relationally aggressive than boys for children as young as the preschool years (e.g., Ostrov & Keating, in press).

THE STATE OF THE EVIDENCE: ARE WE READY TO INTERVENE?

We next consider whether we have enough information about the prevalence, effects, and antecedents of relational aggression to launch effective intervention efforts. After more than 40 years of developmental studies of physical aggression and antisocial behavior, beginning even before the pioneering studies of Glueck and Glueck (1968), Robins (1978), and Patterson (Patterson et al., 1982), some within the field have only recently converged on theories and intervention programs that are documenting effectiveness. Some of the most promising models for preventing antisocial behavior require a multi-faceted approach. Dodge (1993) reviews the literature in this area and explains how this approach focuses on processes leading to problem behaviors and promotes positive youth development by addressing the quality of the parent-child relationship, parenting skills, children's social cognitions, peer group relationships (e.g., deviancy training), academic problems, and low quality neighborhoods.

In comparison to the history of research on physical aggression and related problems, the study of nonphysical forms of aggression is new, with increased attention to the phenomenon occurring only in the late 1980s and early 1990s. Thus, this is a young field of research and it is difficult to be entirely comfortable with the application of this limited knowledge base in order to develop comprehensive and effective interventions for relationally aggressive children. Yet, the explosion of media coverage regarding aggressive girls has led to the implementation of programs that target these behaviors. However, care and caution is advised. As others have found in the area of physical aggression (Poulin et al., 2001), some approaches to intervention that appear reasonable on the surface have been found to cause harm when rigorously evaluated.

An example of a possibly premature intervention strategy comes from a school-based effort designed to decrease the use of relational aggression among girls that was recently described in the *New York Times Magazine* (Talbot, 2002). Students attended classes to learn how to be friendlier with each other. This intervention seemed to promote awareness of relational aggression and allowed the girls to discuss peer difficulties with an adult. The nature of the intervention, however, raises a number of potential concerns which highlight the need for both research-based programs and outcome evaluation. First, the intervention targeted only females, whereas studies show that a significant number of males also engage in relational aggression (e.g., Rys & Bear, 1997). Second, aggressors and victims interacted in groups, creating potential for revictimization. This was particularly likely when girls were instructed to write anonymous apology notes that were read aloud by instructors to the groups. One letter included the following: "I'm sorry that I talked about you behind your back. I once even compared your forehead/face to a minefield... I'm really sorry I said these things even though I might still believe them." (Talbot, 2002, p. 26). This repetition of the comments made may have resulted in further damage to at least one member of the group. A research based approach to relational aggression may have led these interventionists in a different direction — one which may be potentially less harmful and more effective. Specifically, group forms of intervention for aggressive children have often been contra-indicated because children share deviant experiences and can encourage each other's continued aggressive behavior (Poulin et al., 2001). Researchers have also noted that, to avoid having a negative impact and further ostracizing victims of relational aggression, teachers often try to surreptitiously assist victims. Teachers may facilitate a child's integration into a peer group without drawing attention to the child (Owens, Slee, & Shute, 2000b). Thus, interventionists are again cautioned to base their programs on existing research, and are reminded of the importance of determining the effectiveness of their efforts.

We believe we do have a sufficient knowledge base from which to draw information to begin small-scale intervention and experimental research studies directed at curbing the excessive use of nonphysical forms of aggression. Relatively few studies have examined antecedents of relational aggression and none of the available investigations have employed designs that illuminate direction of effect. Keeping in mind these limitations, however, we describe the relevant findings and comment on their potential usefulness for developing interventions.

Children who are relationally aggressive tend to have friendships marked by certain characteristics. They have elevated anxiety about maintaining relationships and place a great importance on having close, exclusive relationships. Relationally aggression children maintain friendships that are high in intimacy, and in exclusivity or jealousy (Grotpeter & Crick, 1996). Children who are sensitive to loss or abandonment and feel their friendships are precarious may use relationally aggressive strategies in an attempt to intensify their relationships. They may exclude those who will potentially threaten their friendships, and may use aggressive strategies to control and manipulate their friends to maintain relationships. Recent theory has also proposed that relational victimization may lead to high sensitivity to rejection by others, and future problems in relationships (Downey, Bonica, & Rincon, 1999).

There is some evidence that the family relationships of relationally aggressive children have a number of characteristics in common with their friendships. Specifically, the parent-child relationships of relationally aggressive children have been shown to involve relatively high levels of desire for exclusivity as well as jealousy exhibited toward the child by the parent (e.g., mother may convey that she wants more exclusive interaction with her daughter and seek to exclude other family members or friends). In addition, relationally aggressive children have been shown to play the role of peacemaker when their parents fight (Crick et al., 1999). Taken together, these findings suggest that relationally aggressive children may develop a relatively high level of perceived control over relationships or the perceived *need* to control relationships as a result of their interactions with family and friends. If so, these issues may be an important focus of future intervention efforts. Further, interviews and discussion groups of adolescent girls and their teachers revealed that girls use some indirect forms of relational aggression in an attempt to maintain close relationships and to be a part of their group (Owens et al., 2000a). These findings point toward teaching social problem solving skills and encouraging proactive attempts at social inclusion such as engaging in school activities, clubs, or sports.

Social-information processing research also highlights a possible avenue for intervention. Several studies have shown that, relative to peers, relationally aggressive children exhibit hostile attributional biases when confronted with relational conflicts (Crick, Grotpeter, & Bigbee, 2002). That is, they are more likely than peers to perceive that relational slights have occurred for hostile reasons when that is not necessarily the case. These types of processing biases may increase the likelihood of future engagement in aggression (i.e., relational aggression may be used as retaliation); however, empirical verification of this idea awaits future research.

Similar to physical aggression, relational aggression is often linked with peer rejection (Crick & Grotpeter, 1995). However, some studies find that relational aggression may increase one's status among some peers, especially during adolescence (Salmivalli et al., 2000). Hence, social skill training may be warranted for some provocateurs at some ages, but interventions in middle school might be more effective if they are targeted at school climate or peer groups and acceptance of, and support for, these behaviors. To further protect victims from additional negative interactions with peers, separate intervention efforts for aggressors and victims might be warranted. In fact, research indicates that aggressors need to learn more appropriate social skills and self-control strategies and parent involvement is often warranted (Coie & Dodge, 1998), whereas victims may require activities to improve self-worth and feelings of competence or assertiveness training (Juvonen & Graham, 2001; Olweus, 1994).

Overall, there are challenges to enacting interventions against indirect (or relational) aggression. Consideration of the form of the intervention must also depend on age, gender, and past behavior or participants. Often the idea of implementing a comprehensive intervention can be very daunting and expensive. Not only can the high cost of such efforts serve as an obstacle to successful implementation, but schools can often be overwhelmed with programs ranging from friendship groups to substance use prevention. Schools may have difficulty making priorities or are more convinced by strong advocates than evidence of need.

Fortunately, a simple and relatively inexpensive intervention that focuses on awareness of the problem has shown to be an effective first step toward reducing aggression. Olweus (1994) informed teachers and parents that physical aggression and victimization are serious problems plaguing schools. This increased education was effective in reducing bully and victim problems. Although Olweus' campaign was primarily targeted toward physical forms of aggression, such an approach might be particularly important for reducing relational aggression. As discussed above, although parents and teachers are likely aware of the presence of relational aggression and victimization among children, they may not be aware of the prevalence of the problem and the potential deleterious effects of such behavior, namely, maladjustment among perpetrators and, especially, victims. Further, relational aggression and victimization may not be as easily detected as physical forms. To address this difficulty, teachers and parents might be instructed to take children's reports of relationally aggressive attacks seriously, and to intervene, particularly when these reports are repeated. Increased monitoring during unstructured time (e.g., recess, hallways) has been recommended to prevent physical aggression (Olweus, 1994), and it will also likely reduce the occurrence of relational aggression and facilitate its detection.

To implement these recommendations, an appropriate first step should be to undertake a campaign to promote awareness of the problem among parents and teachers, and the effects of such campaigns on children's behaviors should be evaluated. Olweus (1994) comments on the importance of intervening at the level of the community, school, classroom, and the individual. Thus, a more involved intervention strategy would include instructing parents and teachers on how to manage aggressive children and how to assist victims of aggression.

Programs might include teaching children to identify relational aggression and instructing them on how to respond (e.g., by trying to include the victim or refusing to participate in group exclusion). Less research addresses this aspect of intervention, but it seems that a useful strategy would be to add a focus on relational aggression to existing programs on bullying and physical aggression that have some evidence of effectiveness, and to assess the effects of these programs on relational aggression and victimization (e.g., Leff, Power, Manz, Costigan, & Nabors, 2001).

Of course, the overall form of the intervention may also vary according to the goals of the program (e.g., reduced aggression, increased assertiveness for victims, increased social skills, reduced distress/maladjustment). Interventionists should also be cognizant of our limited evidence regarding age-related differences in the nature and impact of relational aggression, and be careful not to apply the same intervention strategies for both younger and older children. Similarly, boys and girls may benefit from intervention to reduce relational aggression, but the strategies that may be most effective for girls may differ from those used for boys. It is crucial for interventionists to be aware that our knowledge of the antecedents of relational aggression is limited at this point. This will significantly reduce the scope of intervention approaches until the necessary empirical information is available.

In sum, intervention approaches to address relational aggression are currently being implemented. We are now at a point where the research can begin to direct the design, implementation, and evaluation of small-scale intensive interventions or larger information campaigns. However, some current efforts may be premature. It seems more productive to first expand existing well-designed school-based interventions for bullying and physical aggression to include a focus on relational aggression (i.e., adapt them to be appropriate for targeting relational aggression, if possible). Future evaluation of these programs should also include an assessment of relational aggression (e.g., attitudes, intended behaviors, and actual behaviors). These outcome studies will, in turn, lead to revisions in the theories of relational aggression, and ultimately to a better explication of the nature and impact of relational aggression on children and adults.

REFERENCES

American Psychiatric Association. (1994). *Diagnostic and statistical manual of mental disorders* (4th ed.). Washington, DC: Author.

Bjorkqvist, K., Lagerspetz, K. M. J., & Kaukiainen, A. (1992). The development of direct and indirect aggressive strategies in males and females. In K. Bjorkqvist & P. Niemela

(Eds.), *Of mice and women: Aspects of female aggression*. San Diego, CA: Academic Press.

Caron, C., & Rutter, M. (1991). Comorbidity in child psychopathology: Concepts, issues and research strategies. *Journal of Child Psychology and Psychiatry, 32*, 1063–1080.

Catalano, R. F., Hawkins, J. D., Berglund, L., Pollard, J. A., & Arthur, M. W. (2002). Prevention science and positive youth development: Competitive or cooperative frameworks. *Journal of Adolescent Health, 31*, 230–239.

Cicchetti, D., & Cohen, D.J. (1995). Perspectives on developmental psychopathology. In D. Cicchetti & D.J. Cohen (Eds.), *Developmental psychopathology: Theory and methods* (vol. 1, pp. 3–20). New York: Wiley.

Coie, J. D., & Dodge, K. A. (1998). Aggression and antisocial behavior. In W. Damon (Series Ed.) & N. Eisenberg (Vol. Ed.), *Handbook of child psychology: Vol. 3. Social, emotional, and personality development* (5th ed., pp. 779–862). New York: Wiley.

Craig, W. M. (1998). The relationship among bullying, victimization, depression, anxiety, and aggression in elementary school children. *Personality and Individual Differences, 1*, 123–130.

Crick, N. R. (1996). The role of overt aggression, relational aggression, and prosocial behavior in the prediction of children's future social adjustment. *Child Development, 67*, 2317–2327.

Crick, N. R. (1997). Engagement in gender normative versus gender nonnormative forms of aggression: Links to social-psychological adjustment. *Developmental Psychology, 33*, 610–617.

Crick, N. R., & Bigbee, M. A. (1998). Relational and overt forms of peer victimization: A multi-informant approach. *Journal of Consulting and Clinical Psychology, 66*, 337–347.

Crick, N. R., Casas, J. F., & Mosher, M. (1997). Relational and overt aggression in preschool. *Developmental Psychology, 33*, 589–600.

Crick, N. R., Casas, J. F., & Nelson, D. A. (2002). Toward a more comprehensive understanding of peer maltreatment: Studies of relational victimization. *Current Directions in Psychological Science, 11*, 98–101.

Crick, N. R., & Grotpeter, J. K. (1995). Relational aggression, gender, and social-psychological adjustment. *Child Development, 66*, 710–722.

Crick, N. R., Grotpeter, J. K., & Bigbee, M. A. (2002). Relationally and physically aggressive children's intent attributions and feelings of distress for relational and instrumental peer provocations. *Child Development, 73*, 1134–1142.

Crick, N. R., Werner, N. E., Casas, J. F., O'Brein, K. M., Nelson, D. A., Grotpeter, J., & Markon, K. (1999). Childhood aggression and gender: A new look at an old problem. In D. Bernstein (Ed.), *Nebraska symposium on motivation* (pp. 75–141). Lincoln, NE: University of Nebraska Press.

David, C. F., & Kistner, J. A. (2000). Do positive self-perceptions have a "dark side"? Examination of the link between perceptual bias and aggression. *Journal of Abnormal Child Psychology, 28*, 327–337.

Dodge, K. A. (1993). The future of research on the treatment of conduct disorder. *Development and Psychopathology, 5*, 311–319.

Downey, G., Bonica, C., & Rincon, C. (1999). Rejection sensitivity and adolescent romantic relationships. In W. Furman, B. B. Brown, & C. Feiring (Eds.), *The development of romantic relationships in adolescence* (pp. 148–174). New York: Cambridge University Press.

Galen, B. R., & Underwood, M. K. (1997). A developmental investigation of social aggression in children. *Developmental Psychology, 33*, 589–600.

Glueck, S., & Glueck, E. (1968). *Delinquents and non-delinquents in perspective*. Cambridge, MA: Harvard University Press.

Grotpeter, J. K., & Crick, N. R. (1996). Relational aggression, overt aggression, and friendship. *Child Development, 67*, 2328–2338.

Heller, K. (1996). Coming of age of prevention science: Comments on the 1994 National Institute of Mental Health-Institute of Medicine prevention reports. *American Psychologist*, *51*, 1123–1127.

Juvonen, J., & Graham, S. (Eds.). (2001). *Peer harassment in school: The plight of the vulnerable and victimized.* New York: Guilford Press.

Lagerspetz, K. M. J., Bjorkqvist, K., & Peltonen, T. (1988). Is indirect aggression typical of females? Gender differences in aggressiveness in 11- to 12-year-old children. *Aggressive Behavior*, *14*, 403–414.

Lease, A. M., Kennedy, C. A., & Axelrod, J. L. (2002). Children's social constructions of popularity. *Social Development*, *11*, 87–109.

Leff, S. S., Power, T. J., Manz, P. H., Costigan, T. E., & Nabors, L. A. (2001). School-based aggression prevention programs for young children: Current status and implications for violence prevention. *School Psychology Review*, *30*, 344–362.

Malcarne, V. L., & Hansdottir, I. (2001). Vulnerability to anxiety disorders in childhood and adolescence. In J. Price & R. Ingram (Eds.), *Vulnerability to psychopathology: Risk across the lifespan.* (pp. 271–303). New York: Guilford Press.

Olweus, D. (1994). *Bullying at school.* Cambridge, UK: Longman.

Ostrov, J. M., & Keating, C. F. (in press). Gender differences in preschool aggression during free play and structured interactions: An observational study. *Social Development.*

Owens, L., Shute, R., & Slee, P. (2000a). 'Guess what I just heard!': Indirect aggression among teenage girls in Australia. *Aggressive Behavior*, *26*, 67–83.

Owens, L., Slee, P., & Shute, R. (2000b). 'It hurts a hell of a lot...': The effects of indirect aggression on teenage girls. *School Psychology International*, *21*, 359–376.

Patterson, G. R., Reid, J. B., & Dishion, T. J. (1982). *Antisocial boys.* Eugene, OR: Castalia.

Poulin, F., Dishion, T. D., & Barraston, B. (2001). 3-Year iatrogenic effects associated with aggregating high-risk adolescents in cognitive-behavioral preventive interventions. *Applied Developmental Science*, *5*, 214–224.

Prinstein, M. J., Boergers, J., & Vernberg, E. M. (2001). Overt and relational aggression in adolescents: Social-psychological adjustment of aggressors and victims. *Journal of Clinical Child Psychology*, *30*, 479–491.

Robins, L. N. (1978). Study childhood predictors of adult antisocial behavior: Replications from longitudinal studies. *Psychological Medicine*, *8*, 611–622.

Rys, G. S., & Bear, G. G. (1997). Relational aggression and peer relations: Gender and developmental issues. *Merrill-Palmer Quarterly*, *43*, 87–106.

Salmivalli, C., Kaukiainen, A., & Lagerspetz, K. (2000). Aggression and sociometric status among peers: Do gender and type of aggression matter? *Scandinavian Journal of Psychology*, *41*, 17–24.

Simmons, R. (2002). *Odd girl out: The hidden culture of aggression in girls.* New York: Harcourt.

Talbot, M. (2002, February 24). Girls just want to be mean. *New York Times Magazine*, 24–65.

Underwood, M. K., Galen, B. R., & Paquette, J. A. (2001). Top ten challenges for understanding gender and aggression in children: Why can't we all just get along? *Social Development*, *10*, 248–266.

Werner, N. E., & Crick, N. R. (1999). Relational aggression and social-psychological adjustment in a college sample. *Journal of Abnormal Psychology*, *108*, 615–623.

Xie, H., Swift, D. J., Cairns, B. D., & Cairns, R. B. (2002). Aggressive behavior in social interaction and developmental adaptation: A narrative analysis of interpersonal conflicts during early adolescence. *Social Development*, *11*, 205–224.

4

Aggression from an Attachment Perspective

Gender Issues and Therapeutic Implications

MARLENE M. MORETTI, KIMBERLEY DASILVA, AND ROY HOLLAND*

Aggressive behavior in girls and women typically occurs within the context of close interpersonal relationships. The purpose of this chapter is to provide an overview of research on the relationship between attachment and aggression and to discuss the function that aggressive behavior may play in close relationships. Clearly, not all aggressive and violent behavior can be explained in terms of attachment. We argue, however, that many aggressive acts in intimate relationships can be understood from this perspective. Furthermore, we propose that identifying the attachment function of aggressive behavior can help to delineate meaningful subgroups of individuals who differ in the function that their aggressive behavior serves, the targets of their aggressive acts, and in their therapeutic needs.

Specifically, we propose that from an attachment perspective, aggressive behavior can be understood: 1) a coercive attempt to provoke others

* Preparation of this chapter was supported through grants to the first author from the Canadian Institutes of Health Research and the Human Early Learning Partnership (HELP). We wish to express our appreciation to the staff, families and youth of the Maples Adolescent Treatment Centre, Burnaby, British Columbia for their support and participation in this research.

MARLENE M. MORETTI AND KIMBERLEY DASILVA • Department of Psychology, Simon Fraser University, Burnaby, British Columbia, Canada, V5A 1S6. ROY HOLLAND • Maples Adolescent Treatment Centre, Burnaby, British Columbia, Canada, V5G 3H4.

into engagements; 2) a reaction to perceived rejection or threat of loss of close relationships; or 3) an instrumental act to gain power, control, or some other desired outcome.

We suggest that aggressive behavior in girls, compared to boys, more frequently reflects a coercive strategy to engage others and maintain their availability and responsiveness. Furthermore, girls are less likely than boys to engage in instrumental aggressive acts. We present empirical findings to support this view, illustrated by excerpts from attachment interviews with high-risk adolescent girls who speak about the situations that provoke their aggressive behavior and what they hope to achieve through it. Implications for therapeutic intervention are briefly reviewed, and cautionary notes regarding the limits of an attachment perspective are stated.

ATTACHMENT THEORY: FUNDAMENTALS

At the heart of Bowlby's (1969, 1973, 1980) classic theory of attachment is the primacy of the human inclination for emotional bonds with others. Bowlby proposed that the attachment system is biologically based and essential for survival and well being across the life span. Bowlby's theory went further than simply explicating attachment as a fundamental human drive. Drawing on the principle of physiological homeostasis, he characterized attachment as a control system that serves to balance proximity to attachment figures during periods of distress, with exploration during periods of safety. To account for the goal-directed quality of interactions and continuity of attachment related behaviors over the life span, Bowlby proposed the notion of "internal working models", cognitive-affective structures that develop through experiences in care-giving relationships and guide future interpersonal expectations, behaviors, and responses. Internal working models provide mental maps of the key features of past experiences and procedural knowledge which guide behavior to ensure that attachment needs are met to the fullest extent possible in any given context.

The quality of interactions with attachment figures corresponds to the content of internal working models and the development of corresponding behavioral strategies. It is this aspect of Bowlby's model that speaks to the relationship of attachment to psychological well being versus pathology and formed the basis of initial classification systems in the field (Ainsworth, Blehar, Waters, & Wall, 1978). The initial three category classification system identified three basic attachment patterns. Children who experienced their primary caregivers as consistently available and responsive to their signals of distress were identified as having a fundamentally "secure pattern" of attachment. When distressed, secure children actively seek support; their exploration of the world is not hampered by heightened vigilance or concern about the whereabouts or reactions of their caregiver. The internal working model of the secure child encompasses a view of others as competent and caring and a view of the self as worthy of care and attention.

In contrast, children who experience their caregiver as *inconsistently* available and *inappropriately* or *inadequately* responsive were identified as having an "anxious-ambivalent" pattern of attachment. These children cannot be certain of their caregivers' availability or responsiveness, and therefore remain hyper-vigilant and preoccupied with securing their attention. The internal working model of the anxious-ambivalent child encompasses a view of others as unreliable, but at times responsive, and a view of the self as inadequate or lacking in characteristics that consistently attract care from others. Because these children are preoccupied with their caregivers' availability, their exploration of the environment is suppressed. Behaviorally, anxious-ambivalent children are frequently aggressive with their caregivers, demanding their attention yet unable to derive solace from their comfort. Displays of need are often exaggerated in a bid to "capture" the attention of their attachment figure. The term "preoccupied" is used to describe the attachment pattern of these individuals as adults (Main, Kaplan, & Cassidy, 1985). They express strong interpersonal needs, establish relationships quickly, and their interpersonal behavior is described as intense and demanding (Shaver & Hazan, 1993).

The third classic attachment pattern is that of the children who experience their parents as consistently rejecting of their needs (Ainsworth et al., 1978). These "anxious-avoidant" children learn early in their lives to disguise and/or diminish their attachment needs, even in the presence of their caregiver, for fear of rejection and punishment. Yet their apparent calm merely masks their true level of distress (Dozier & Kobak, 1992). The internal working model of the anxious-avoidant child encapsulates a view of others as rejecting and punishing of attachment needs, and a view of themselves as unacceptable and repulsive. Behaviorally these children avoid contact with their caregivers, focusing instead on peripheral features of their environment to distract their attention.

The term "dismissing" is used to describe the attachment patterns of avoidant children as adults (Main et al., 1985; Shaver & Hazan, 1993). Dismissing adults minimize the importance of attachment relationships and are reluctant to express interpersonal needs. During the last decade, two forms of avoidant-dismissing attachment have been differentiated in adults and adolescents: avoidant-dismissing versus avoidant-fearful (Bartholomew & Horowitz, 1991). Avoidant-dismissing attachment refers to the classic avoidant pattern of disengagement from attachment figures and denigration of the importance of attachment needs and associated feelings. In contrast, avoidant-fearful attachment is characterised by the tendency to avoid attachment figures due to fear of rejection coupled with the desire to pursue relationships. These two forms of avoidant attachment have distinctive correlates in adults and differ in the contexts that give rise to aggression, as we will later discuss.

ATTACHMENT AND AGGRESSION

Does attachment theory offer insight into the roots of aggression and violence? Bowlby (1973) believed so. He reasoned that although anger—at appropriate times and in appropriate amounts—is functional in preserving attachment relationships because it is an effective signal to attachment figure of distress, extreme anger, aggression, and violence are not. Bowlby (1973) noted that "the most violently angry and dysfunctional responses of all, it seems probable, are elicited in children and adolescents who not only experience repeated separations but are constantly subjected to the threat of being abandoned" (p. 288). He underscored the importance of threats to attachment as a determinant of aggressive behavior by drawing on Burnham's (1965) observations of violent adolescents: one adolescent who murdered his mother exclaimed afterwards "I couldn't stand to have her leave me". Another, a youth who placed a bomb in his mother's luggage prior to her departure on an airplane, explained "I decided that she would never leave me again" (p. 290, cited in Bowlby, 1973).

These case examples are powerful, but is there empirical support for a relationship between attachment and aggression? There is little question that attachment is an important determinant of general emotional and behavioral adjustment in both children and adolescents (Doyle & Moretti, 2001; Schneider, Atkinson, & Tardiff, 2001). In normative samples, youths who are securely attached to their mothers engage in more pro-social behavior, are perceived as more socially competent, are rated by adults as more empathic and compliant, and demonstrate higher positive and lower negative affect in social interactions than do insecure children (Allen & Land, 1999). In contrast, insecurely attached children show poor emotional regulation; are defiant, hostile, and aggressive toward mothers and peers; and suffer rejection from their peers (Allen & Land, 1999). Similarly in late adolescence, securely attached youths are better able to regulate uncomfortable affective states, particularly feelings of anger, and are perceived as less hostile by their peers. They appropriately seek support from others in times of stress and more successfully manage the transition to high school (Allen et al., 2002; Florian, Mikulincer, & Bucholtz, 1995; Papini & Roggman, 1992). In contrast, insecure attachment in adolescence is associated with a range of mental health problems (Allen, Hauser, & Borman-Spurrell, 1996), including suicidality (Lessard & Moretti, 1998), and drug use (Lessard, 1994).

Turning to studies specifically examining aggression, research provides clear empirical support for the relationship between insecure attachment and aggression, both concurrently and prospectively: children and adolescents with insecure attachment patterns have significantly more behavior problems, including aggressive behavior, than are those with secure attachment (Allen, Moore, Kuperminc, & Bell, 1998; Doyle & Moretti, 2001; Lyons-Ruth, 1996). What *form* of insecure attachment is associated with aggressive behavior is less clear. Early studies identified higher levels of aggressive and noncompliant behavior in children with anxious-avoidant versus all other attachment patterns (Renken, Egeland, Marvinney, Mangelsdorf, & Sroufe, 1989). For example, anxious-avoidant attachment in infancy was found to predict negativity, noncompliance, and hyperactivity at 3.5 years of age, and higher ratings of problem behavior in grades one to three.

Studies of adolescents have also supported a relationship between avoidant attachment and delinquency or deviance. Rosenstein and Horowitz (1996) found that the diagnosis of conduct disorder in adolescent in-patients was associated with the avoidant-dismissing attachment pattern. Results also showed that dismissing attachment was associated with antisocial, narcissistic, and paranoid personality characteristics. Similarly, Allen et al. (1996) found that derogation of attachment, characteristic of the avoidant dismissing style, was associated with concurrent criminal behavior and drug use in adulthood among individuals who had been hospitalized for psychopathology during adolescence. These results mirror those found with children showing an association between avoidant attachment, behavior problems, and non-compliance. In contrast, more recent research suggests a relationship between "disorganized" attachment, characterized by the lack of a consistent behavioral strategy to meet attachment needs, and aggressive behavior in children. (Lyons-Ruth & Jacobvitz, 1999).

To add to the complexity, recent studies of adolescents suggest a relationship between preoccupied attachment and aggressive behavior. Based on attachment interviews with at-risk adolescents, Allen et al., (1998) found that preoccupied teens were more likely to engage in delinquent activities, including getting into physical fights and assaulting people than were secure teens. Similarly, Allen et al., (2002) found that anxious-preoccupied attachment at age 16 in moderately at-risk adolescents predicted increasing delinquent behavior between the ages of 16 to 18 years.

How can *different* patterns of attachment organization be similarly related to aggressive behavior? We believe the answer lies not simply in conceptualizing a relationship between insecure attachment and the *amount* of aggressive behavior, but in understanding how types of insecure attachment relate to the form, function, and the target of aggressive behavior. Recall that the anxious-preoccupied individual is unable to anticipate whether their attachment figure will consistently respond, and if they do, whether their continued availability can be depended upon. An effective means to eliciting the attention of an attachment figure, and maintaining engagement once it is established, is to display heightened expressions of need which may include, but are not limited to, extreme anger, threats, and acts of aggression and violence. Because the function of aggressive behavior from a preoccupied standpoint is to increase and maintain engagement within close relationships, targets of aggressive acts are most likely limited to established or potential attachment partners (i.e., parent, romantic partner, or close friend). Furthermore, we can predict that aggressive behavior will be elicited in contexts where the preoccupied individual perceives cues of potential abandonment. Greater depth of preoccupation will be associated with greater vigilance of abandonment and greater susceptibility to interpret ambiguous cues as indicative of this intent by others.

In contrast to the preoccupied individual who experiences at least intermittent reinforcement of attachment needs within close relationships, the fearful-avoidant individual has experienced consistent rejection. Longing for acceptance and closeness, but fearing rejection, the fearful-avoidant individual is also vigilant to perceptions of threat of rejection, loss, or abandonment. This is particularly acute in situations where the fearful-avoidant individual is, or potentially could become, dependent on others. Recall, however, that individuals with avoidant attachment tend *not* to express anger in close relationships because of fear of further rejection. Yet, evidence shows that avoidant individuals display clear signs of physiological agitation at separation (Dozier & Kobak, 1992). Hence, because anger cannot be expressed to the attachment figure, it may be displaced on other aspects of the environment (Ainsworth et al., 1978), including the self.

In sum, while preoccupied individuals typically direct aggression toward those they are close to, the fearful individual is reluctant to aggress in close relationships. There is one exception to this general rule. Mayseless (1991) theorized that fearful-avoidant individuals may engage in aggressive and violent acts within close relationships when they feel pressured into intimacy. On the surface this seems paradoxical—why would an individual who longs for acceptance and connection respond with anger and aggression when these are offered? If we keep in mind, however, that fearful-avoidant individuals fundamentally believe that others will ultimately reject them, it becomes clear that the opportunity for connection provokes intense anxiety, particularly when it is experienced as intrusive. This analysis is consistent with Dutton's (1999) observation that spousal abuse was observed most frequently in men characterized with fearful-avoidant attachment who perceived their partners as demanding and intrusive. Indeed, Dutton (1999) has theorized that the most volatile relationships involve the pairing of an anxious-preoccupied female, who demands engagement, and a fearful-avoidant male who wishes to be engaged but is unable to tolerate intimacy.

What about the dismissing-avoidant individual? In contrast to preoccupied and fearful attachment, which is characterized by over-activation of the attachment system, dismissing attachment is characterized by under-activation or suppression (Bartholomew, 1990). These individuals seem uninterested in attachment relationships with others, satisfied with their sense of self-worth and competency to manage in the world, and somewhat oblivious to the feelings and needs of others. It is therefore unlikely that aggression and violence have an interpersonal function or precipitate in the dismissing individual. Nonetheless, it quite possible that dismissing individuals may aggress against others in order to meet instrumental goals, and to do so in such a way as to seriously fail to consider the rights and welfare of their victims. Thus, in contrast to both the preoccupied and fearful individual, the targets of aggression for the dismissing individual may not necessarily be restricted to individuals with whom they have close relationships. Instead, dismissing individuals may aggress against strangers and acquaintances alike. Furthermore, the function of their aggression may ultimately be to achieve an instrumental rather than interpersonal goal, and thus be unrelated to needs for connection and closeness with others. On the other hand, the need to achieve dominance and control over resources may figure strongly in their motivations for aggression.

In sum, an attachment model of aggression and violence may help us to differentiate the function and target of aggression across individuals who are frequently described as a homogeneous group (see Table 1). In the next section of this chapter we briefly consider the importance of gender in this analysis.

TABLE 1. ATTACHMENT PATTERNS IN RELATION TO THE FUNCTION AND TARGET OF AGGRESSIVE BEHAVIOR

Attachment Pattern	Function of Aggression	Target of Aggression
Preoccupied	To coerce and maintain engagement.	Intimate others perceived as existing or potential attachment figures.
Fearful Avoidant	Displaced expression of anger at caregiver; to distance others who demand intimacy.	Aggression shifted away from attachment figures and sometimes to self; Aggression targeted at attachment figures only under pressure for intimacy.
Dismissing Avoidant	To achieve instrumental goals.	Aggression targeted at intimate partners and strangers alike.

GENDER AND ATTACHMENT

Although research has not identified gender differences in the percentage of children, adolescents, or adults with secure attachment patterns (Ijzendoorn et al., 2000), there are gender differences in the distribution of insecure attachment patterns. In a study of young adults, Bartholomew and Horowitz (1991) report that the distribution of insecure attachment patterns disproportionately represents females in the preoccupied quadrant and males in the dismissing quadrant. Why might females be more likely to develop anxious-preoccupied attachment patterns and males to develop dismissing-avoidant attachment?

Research on parental socialization practices indicates that girls, in comparison to boys, are more frequently socialized to attend to the needs and well being of others and to judge their self-worth in terms of others opinion of them (Cross & Madson, 1997; Moretti & Higgins, 1999). In a recent study (Moretti, Rein, & Wiebe, 1998), we examined the degree to which young women and men perceived themselves to fall short of the standards that they held for themselves versus the standards that their parents and peers held for them, and how this was in turn related to symptoms of depression. As predicted, women but not men suffered from symptoms of depression when they perceived themselves to fall short of the standards that they believed their parents and peers held for them. That is, others' expectations were more important to young women than to young men in determining their emotional well-being. Our recent study (Moretti, Holland, & McKay, 2001) examining the relationship between self-perceptions and assaultive behavior in high-risk adolescents confirmed these findings. It is possible that in conditions that give rise to the development of insecure attachment, socialization of girls to regulate in terms of close relationships—that is, to engage in "relational self-regulation"—can result in preoccupied attachment.

In contrast to girls, boys are more commonly socialized toward independence and autonomy in decision making (Baumeister & Sommer, 1997). An interesting line of research by Pomerantz and Ruble (1998) illustrates the subtle nature of these gender-typed socialization practices. This work showed that while mothers were equally likely to be "controlling" with their daughters and their sons, they were more likely to employ control without granting autonomy with their daughters than their sons. She also found that the use of control without granting autonomy increased the extent to which children accepted responsibility for failure. Although socialization toward independence may have many beneficial consequences, in the extreme it may result in a disregard for the wishes and welfare of others. Such an outcome would be consistent with the development of dismissing attachment, and may occur more frequently in males than females who are exposed to conditions giving rise to the development of insecure attachment.

In sum, gender-typed socialization practices, particularly in adverse conditions which undermine attachment security, may result in different types of insecure attachment patterns for girls and boys. Girls may be more likely to develop preoccupied attachment; in contrast, boys may be more inclined to move toward dismissing attachment.

GENDER, ATTACHMENT, AND AGGRESSION: PRELIMINARY FINDINGS

A recent analysis of data from our study of high-risk adolescents offered the opportunity to examine the specificity of relationships between insecure attachment patterns and engagement in aggressive behavior (Obsuth, Luedemann, Peled, & Moretti, 2002). Participants were 105 boys and 65 girls, with a mean age of 14 years ($SD = 1.5$) who were provided family and community services at a provincial centre for youths with severe behavioral problems. Youths completed the Family Attachment Interview (FAI; Bartholomew & Horowitz, 1991), a semi-structured interview modeled after the Adult Attachment Interview (AAI; Main & Goldwyn, 1998). The interview contains questions and coding dimensions that are virtually identical to those included in the AAI, however raters using the FAI assess the extent to which the interview corresponds to each of four attachment prototypes (secure, preoccupied, fearful, dismissing) by assigning a rating on a 1 to 9 point scale, where 1 represents no correspondence and

9 represents an excellent fit. This procedure allows researchers to derive both categorical and dimensional ratings for each participant. Reliability and validity of the interview with high-risk adolescents have been established (Scharfe, 2002).

Not surprisingly, and consistent with previous studies of clinical populations, our findings showed that the vast majority of youths were predominantly insecure in their attachment pattern. Significant gender differences emerged in the distribution of insecure attachment patterns. As predicted, girls were more likely to be classified as preoccupied in their attachment organization (40%) than were boys (15%), whereas boys were significantly more likely to be classified as dismissing (31%) than girls (6%). No difference was detected in the proportion of girls and boys classified as fearful (42% and 35% respectively).

Youths also completed the Youth Self-Report (Achenbach, 1995), a commonly used and well validated measure of emotional and behavioral functioning, and the Beck Depression Inventory (Beck, Steer, & Garbin, 1988). Of interest to the current analysis were items that tapped aggression to *others* (e.g., "I physically attack others") versus aggression to *self* (e.g., "I deliberately try to hurt or kill myself"). Two scales were formed, each comprised of four items, to tap these two focal points of aggressive behavior. To assess the specificity of attachment to aggressive behavior, aggression scale scores were regressed onto dimensional scores representing each of the three attachment prototypes. With respect to aggression directed toward others, results confirmed that increases in preoccupied attachment were uniquely associated with higher levels of aggression toward others, $\beta = .18$, $p = .03$; neither fearful nor dismissing attachment ratings were significant predictors. Gender did not moderate the relationship between preoccupied attachment and aggression toward others, suggesting that preoccupied attachment functions similarly for boys and girls. With respect to aggression toward self, findings also confirmed that higher ratings of fearful attachment were associated with higher levels of self-directed aggression, $\beta = .25$, $p = .001$. Again, fearful attachment was similarly associated with self-directed aggression for girls and boys.

The unique relationships we found between preoccupied attachment and aggression toward others, and fearful attachment and aggression toward self, were reflected in the way that girls spoke about what provoked their behavior and what they hoped to achieve through it. For example, Anna, age 16, had been in 18 different placements since she was first placed into care at age 11. She was extremely demanding, aggressive, and sometimes violent to her foster parents. Anna described how her last placement finally broke down when a new foster child was placed in the same home. Unable to tolerate her foster mother's attention to this new child, Anna threatened to kill them both. Anna stated, "My mom (foster mom) doesn't even notice me anymore! I love my mom so much! Why is she doing this to me?" Jacki, age 13, was expelled from school for harassing male peers. Eventually she was charged when she threatened to kill a boy who would not reciprocate her interests. Jacki stated, "I can't sleep because I think about him all the time." Not surprisingly, Jacki was easily lured into situations that placed her at risk because of her strong needs for acceptance and connection. Both Anna and Jacki were deeply preoccupied in their attachment organization. Unable to trust that others would meet their attachment needs, they engaged in persistent coercive behavior that they hoped would capture the attention of others, but which ultimately undermined their relationships.

In contrast, Susan's interview illustrated features of fearful attachment. By age 15, she had dropped out of school, hung around with delinquent peers, and frequently ran away from home. Although angry with her parents for placing her in care, Susan stated, "I'm homesick. I look forward to seeing my parents on visits but I don't think they miss me because they hate me. They're not proud of me. I don't think they would even miss me if I were dead. I'm not the little girl they wanted."

While these findings should be viewed as preliminary, they are consistent with the findings of Allen et al. (1998) and offer support for the specificity of relationships between attachment organization and aggressive behavior. The fact that preoccupied and fearful attachment had similar associations with aggressive behavior for both girls and boys is consistent with the fundamental assumptions of attachment theory: that attachment organization, rather than gender, explains whether aggression is likely to be directed externally toward others. Unfortunately this study did not lend itself to a careful analysis of the function and target of aggression as it relates to dismissing attachment. Further research using methods that differentiate the *form* in which aggressive behavior is expressed (e.g., overt versus relational), the *function* or goal it is intended to achieve (interpersonal versus instrumental), and the *target* to whom it is directed (others in close relationships, the self, strangers) is required to fully test the specificity of relationships between attachment and aggression that we have presented.

THERAPEUTIC IMPLICATIONS

Theoretical models that provide a general understanding of the etiology of clinical problems are useful in guiding intervention; those that offer a framework for understanding which individuals are likely to suffer from *what types of problems*, and under *which conditions*, are far better. Attachment theory has the potential of informing intervention at this highly differentiated level, and thus is an important framework for organizing interventions targeted at problems of aggression. We have argued that aggression in girls, compared to boys, is most frequently an expression of coercive attempts to engage others. If this is the case, interventions are most likely to be effective when they assist girls to better meet their needs for interpersonal connectedness in ways that are neither hurtful to themselves or others. It is essential to support girls to develop a sense of healthy autonomy that allows them to remain connected in their relationships with others, but also to feel competent, worthy, and comfortable with their autonomy. Attachment is a developmental construct that reaches beyond the simple *content* of internal working models of self and others; other developmental processes, such as affect regulation and cognitive information processing, develop hand-in-hand with the emergence of attachment patterns. For this reason, it is important that interventions for aggressive girls address clinical needs related to the hyperactivation of the attachment system, including heightened vigilance to potential rejection and abandonment, reduced capacity to modulate affective responses, limited social skill issues related to managing interpersonal relationships, and poor integration between affective and cognitive experience. In this regard, it is essential that interventions take into consideration the fact that many girls who show severe aggressive and violent behavior have themselves been subjected to victimization, often of a severe and chronic nature (e.g., Moretti & Odgers, 2001; Reebye, Moretti, Wiebe, & Lessard, 2001).

Perhaps the most significant implication of an attachment perspective, however, is the importance of directing intervention strategies beyond the aggressive behavior of girls to the relational context in which they are embedded. Attachment is inherently a relational construct which demands a systemic focus beyond the individual (Moretti & Holland, 2003). Understanding attachment related behavior from a systemic perspective entails an appreciation for how individuals reinforce each other's perceptions and reactions within relationships. For example, as girls become more coercive of others' engagement with them, it is likely that their attachment figures retreat and reject them. This can only escalate their perceptions of abandonment and rejection and propel them into further and more extreme coercive measures. Interventions that help girls and caregivers to exit this coercive cycle are essential. The inclusion of interventions that target important relationships—such as Earlscourt's Girls Connection focus on mother-daughter relationships—are likely an important component of programming for girls.

Attachment theory is at the heart of a variety of intervention strategies, many of which have been empirically validated (Johnson & Whiffen, 2003). Our own work using attachment focused, multisystemic intervention strategies for girls and boys with severe conduct disorders has provided promising results that point to the critical importance of supporting families in finding new strategies to support greater attunement to, and support of, adolescent attachment needs (Moore, Moretti, & Holland, 1998; Moretti & Holland, 2003; Moretti, Holland, & Moore, 2002). We cannot review various approaches in the space of this chapter, but they should be given careful attention in the development of gender tailored interventions for girls.

STRENGTHS AND WEAKNESSES OF AN ATTACHMENT PERSPECTIVE

Perhaps the most distinctive advantages to understanding aggression from an attachment perspective are the developmental framework that it provides and the functional analyses that it provides for understanding behavior. Attachment theory helps us to understand how and why particular behavioral strategies develop, the function that they serve, and to whom behaviour is targeted. In doing so, it allows us to make sense of heterogeneity within populations of aggressive individuals, whether they are children, adolescents, or adults.

Attachment theory also holds the promise of integrating theories about aggression and violence that appear to diverge in very fundamental ways. For example, while some models of aggression hold that oversensitivity to rejection and low self-esteem give rise to aggression, others contend that the lack of regard for others and narcissistic high self-esteem is at the core of aggressive behavior (Bushman & Baumeister, 2002). How can two fundamentally different views of aggression be equally valid?

An attachment perspective provides compelling explanations of distinctive patterns of aggressive behavior and elucidates how each can develop from attachment related experiences. Furthermore, it gives rise to specific, testable hypotheses that can be assessed across a range of developmental periods. Importantly, attachment theory carries our perspective from individual to social context and back again, making us aware of the social embeddedness quality of human behavior. Finally, attachment theory provides clear direction about the development of interventions for individuals. In the case of girls, interventions must take the form of addressing their interpersonal needs, behaviors, and the interpersonal relationships that they seek to maintain.

No theory is without limitations, and attachment theory is no exception. Of high relevance to the field of aggression is the question of the relative importance of attachment insecurity in predicting negative developmental outcomes in "normative" versus high-risk contexts. Although similar *patterns* of outcomes are present in normative and clinical samples (Allen & Land, 1999), research shows that the relation between attachment and adjustment is *stronger* among children in high-risk contexts (e.g., poverty, low social support, parental psychopathology; Lyons-Ruth, 1996). How particular contextual factors and modeling of aggressive behavior influence the expression of aggression relative to attachment status remains unknown. Other issues, particularly significant to the adolescent developmental period, are also open to debate. For example, although recent studies show that parents continue to rank at the top as important attachment figures well into early adulthood (Trinke & Bartholomew, 1997), we do not fully understand how adolescents negotiate the transition in attachment figures from parents to peers, and finally to romantic partners. Future research investigating these issues will do much to further our understanding of normative and atypical development of attachment and its significance for understanding aggression and violence.

REFERENCES

Achenbach, T. M. (1995). Youth self-report. Burlington: University of Vermont, Department of Psychiatry.

Ainsworth, M. S., Blehar, M. C., Waters, E., & Wall, S. (1978). *Patterns of attachment: A psychological study of the strange situation.* Hillsdale, NJ: Erlbaum.

Allen, J. P., Hauser, S. T., & Borman-Spurrell, E. (1996). Attachment theory as a framework for understanding sequelae of severe adolescent psychopathology: An 11-year follow-up study. *Journal of Consulting and Clinical Psychology, 64,* 254–263.

Allen, J. P., & Land, D. (1999). Attachment in adolescence. In J. Cassidy & P. R. Shaver (Eds.), *Handbook of attachment: Theory, research, and clinical applications* (pp. 319–355). New York: Guildford.

Allen, J. P., Marsh, P., McFarland, C., Boykin, K., Land, D. J., Jodl, K. M., & Peck, S. (2002). Attachment and autonomy as predictors of the development of social skills and delinquency during midadolescence. *Journal of Consulting and Clinical Psychology, 70,* 55–66.

Allen, J. P., Moore, C., Kuperminc, G., & Bell, K. (1998). Attachment and adolescent functioning. *Child Development, 69,* 1406–1419.

Bartholomew, K. (1990). Avoidance of intimacy: An attachment perspective. *Journal of Social and Personal Relationships, 7,* 147–178.

Bartholomew, K, & Horowitz, L. M. (1991). Attachment styles among young adults: A test of a four-category model. *Journal of Personality and Social Psychology, 61,* 226–244.

Baumeister, R. F., & Sommer, K. L. (1997). What do men want?: Gender differences and two spheres of belongingness: Comment on Cross and Madson (1997). *Psychological Bulletin, 122,* 38–44.

Beck, A. T., Steer, R. A., & Garbin, M. M. (1988). Psychometric properties of the Beck Depression Inventory: Twenty-five years of evaluation. *Clinical Psychology Review, 8,* 77–100.

Bowlby, J. (1969). *Attachment and loss: Vol. 1. Attachment.* New York: Hogarth Press.

Bowlby, J. (1973). *Attachment and loss: Vol. 2. Separation.* New York: Basic.

Bowlby, J. (1980). *Attachment and loss. Vol. 3 Loss, sadness and depression.* NY: Basic Books.

Bushman, B. J., & Baumeister, R. F. (2002). Does self-love or self-hatred lead to violence? *Journal of Research in Personality, 36,* 543–545.

Cross, S. E., & Madson, L. (1997). Models of the self: Self-construals and gender. *Psychological Bulletin, 122,* 5–37.

Doyle, A. B., & Moretti, M. M. (2001). *Attachment to parents and adjustment in adolescence: Literature review and policy implications* [Report]. Ottawa: Health Canada. File number 032ss.H5219-9-CYH7/001/SS.

Dozier, M., & Kobak. R. R. (1992). Psychophysiology in attachment interviews: Converging evidence for deactivating strategies. *Child Development, 63,* 1473–1480.

Dutton, D. G. (1999). The traumatic origins of intimate rage. *Aggression and Violent Behavior, 4,* 431–448.

Florian, V., Mikulincer, M., & Bucholtz, I. (1995). Effects of adult attachment style on the perception and search for social support. *Journal of Psychology, 129,* 665–676.

Ijzendoorn, M., Moran, G., Belsky, J., Pederson, D., Bakersman-Kranenburg, M. J., & Kneppers, K. (2000). The similarity of siblings' attachment to their mother. *Child Development, 71,* 1086–1098.

Johnson, S., & Whiffen, V. (2003) *Clinical applications of attachment theory.* NY: Guildford.

Lessard, J. C. (1994) *The role of psychological distress and attachment in adolescent substance use.* Unpublished Master's Thesis. Simon Fraser University.

Lessard, J. C., & Moretti, M. M. (1998). Suicidal ideation in an adolescent clinical sample: Attachment patterns and clinical implications. *Journal of Adolescence, 21,* 383–395.

Lyons-Ruth, K. (1996). Attachment relationships among children with aggressive behavior problems: The role of disorganized early attachment patterns. *Journal of Consulting and Clinical Psychology, 64,* 64–73.

Lyons-Ruth, K., & Jacobvitz, D. (1999). Attachment disorganization: Unresolved loss, relational violence, and lapses in behavioral and attentional strategies. In J. Cassidy & P. R. Shaver (Eds.), *Handbook of attachment: Theory, research, and clinical applications* (pp. 520–554). New York: Guildford Press.

Main, M., & Goldwyn, R. (1998). *Adult attachment scoring and classification system.* Unpublished manuscript. University of California at Berkeley.

Main, M., Kaplan, N., & Cassidy, J. (1985). Security in infancy, childhood, and adulthood: A move to the level of representation, *Monographs of the Society for Research in Child-Development, 50,* 66–104.

Mayseless, O. (1991). Adult attachment violence and courtship violence. *Family Relations, 40,* 21–28.

Moore, K., Moretti, M. M., & Holland, R. (1998). A new perspective on youth care programs: Using attachment theory to guide interventions for troubled youth. *Residential Treatment for Children and Youth, 15,* 1–24.

Moretti, M. M., & Higgins, E. T. (1999). Own versus other standpoints in self-regulation: Developmental antecedents and functional consequences. *Review of General Psychology, 3,* 188–223.

Moretti, M. M., & Holland, R. (2003). Navigating the journey of adolescence: Parental attachment and the self from a systemic perspective. In S. Johnson & V. Whiffen (Eds.), *Clinical Applications of Attachment Theory.* NY: Guildford.

Moretti, M. M., Holland, R., & McKay, S. (2001). Self-other representations and relational and overt aggression in adolescent girls and boys. *Behavioral Sciences and the Law, 19,* 109–126.

Moretti, M. M., Holland, R., & Moore, K. (2002). Youth at risk: Systemic intervention from an attachment perspective. In M. V. Hayes & L. T. Foster (Eds.), *Too small to see, too big to ignore* (pp. 233–252). Victoria: Western Geographic Series, University of Victoria.

Moretti, M. M., Rein, A. S., & Wiebe, V. J. (1998). Relational self-regulation: Gender differences in risk for dysphoria. *Canadian Journal of Behavioural Science, 30,* 243–252.

Odgers, C., & Moretti, M. M. (2002). Aggressive and antisocial girls: Research update and challenges. *International Journal of Forensic Mental Health, 1,* 103–119.

Osbuth, I., Luedemann, M., Peled, M., & Moretti, M. M. (2002). *Attachment and aggression in a clinical adolescent sample.* Paper presented at the Vancouver Conference on Aggressive and Violent Girls, Vancouver, Canada.

Papini, D. R., & Roggman, L. A. (1992). Adolescent P\perceived Attachment to parents in relation to competence, depression, and anxiety: A longitudinal study. *Journal of Early Adolescence, 12,* 420–440.

Pomerantz, E. M., & Ruble, D. N. (1998). The role of maternal control in the development of sex differences in self-evaluative factors. *Child Development, 69,* 458–478.

Reebye, P., Moretti, M. M., Wiebe, V. J., & Lessard, J. C. (2001). Symptoms of posttraumatic stress disorder in adolescents with conduct disorder: Sex differences and onset patterns. *Canadian Journal of Psychiatry, 45,* 746–751.

Renken, B., Egeland, B., Marvinney, D., Mangelsdorf, S., & Sroufe, L. A. (1989). Early childhood antecedents of aggression and passive-withdrawal in early elementary school. *Journal of Personality, 57,* 257–281.

Rosenstein, D. S., & Horowitz, H. A. (1996). Adolescent attachment and psychopathology. *Journal of Consulting and Clinical Psychology, 64,* 244–253.

Scharfe, E. (2002). Reliability and validity of an interview assessment of attachment representations in a clinical sample of adolescents. *Journal of Adolescent Research, 17,* 532–551.

Schneider, B. H., Atkinson, L., & Tardif, C. (2001). Child-parent attachment and children's peer relationships: A quantitative review. *Child Development, 37,* 86–100.

Shaver, P. R., & Hazan, C. (1993). Adult romantic relationships: Theory and evidence. In D. Perlman & W. Jones (Eds.), *Advances in personal relationships* (Vol. 4, pp. 29–70). London: Kingsley.

Trinke, S. J., & Bartholomew, K. (1997). Hierarchies of attachment relationships in young adulthood. *Journal of Social and Personal Relationships, 14,* 603–625.

5

The Social Context of Children's Aggression

TRACY VAILLANCOURT AND SHELLEY HYMEL

Researchers and philosophers have long pondered the nature and origins of aggression among humans, but it is only recently that we have begun to understand the diverse forms that aggressive behavior can take as well as the complexity of its development. The goal of this chapter is to review current conceptualizations of aggression, with particular interest in how aggression varies as a function of both gender and development. Against this backdrop, we argue for a broader perspective on the socialization of aggression, which more fully considers the social context in which it develops and the influence of peers.

THE MANY FACES OF AGGRESSION

Historically, studies have focused primarily on overt, physical, and verbal aggression, which is more characteristic of boys than girls (e.g., Maccoby & Jacklin, 1974). Pioneering studies of "indirect aggression" by Feshbach (1969, 1971), however, lead to consideration of psychological forms of aggression, including social exclusion, isolation, gossip, rumor spreading, and public humiliation, that may more accurately capture the way that aggression is expressed by girls (see Crick, this volume;

TRACY VAILLANCOURT • Department of Psychology, McMaster University, Hamilton, Ontario, Canada, L8S 4L8. SHELLEY HYMEL • Faculty of Education, University of British Columbia, Vancouver, British Columbia, Canada, V6T 1Z4.

1, 2003). Although debates continue regarding definitional jorkqvist, 2001; Underwood, Galen, & Paquette, 2001; Vaillan- ress), a growing body of research addressing "social aggression" Cairns, Neckerman, Ferguson, & Gariepy, 1989; Galen & Under- wood, 1997), "indirect aggression" (Bjorkqvist, Lagerspetz, & Kaukiainen, 1992; Lagerspetz, Bjorkqvist, & Peltonen, 1988), and "relational aggression" (Crick, 1995; Crick & Grotpeter, 1995) represents an important new direc- tion in this area that emphasizes the interpersonal nature of such behavior and gender differences in its expression.

The importance of distinguishing various forms of aggression is un- derscored by the fact that physical, verbal, and social (relational, indirect) aggression each follows distinct developmental trajectories, suggesting the possibility of unique socialization processes. Longitudinal studies have shown that *physical aggression* increases during the first years of life, as children acquire control of their limbs, reaching a peak at about 30 months of age and declining thereafter (e.g., Broidy et al., 2003; Cote et al., 2003). Most preschoolers display some physical aggression, but the majority learn to regulate their use of physical aggression by middle childhood (see Coie & Dodge, 1998; Tremblay, 2000, in press), with rates of physical aggression decreasing with age (e.g., Brame, Nagin, & Tremblay, 2001; Broidy et al., 2003; Cote et al., 2003). By adolescence, physical aggression and fighting become quite rare (Coie & Dodge, 1998), even among chronically aggres- sive youths (Tremblay, 2001), although there are a few who increase in violent behavior during adolescence (Moffit, 1993). Given evidence that physical aggression is normative during preschool and declines thereafter, Tremblay (2000, in press) argues that the critical question is not how one learns to be physically aggressive, but how one learns *not* to be aggressive, and why some children fail to regulate their aggressive behavior.

Verbal aggression has been more difficult to operationally define (see Underwood, 2003). Nevertheless, research to date indicates that, in contrast to physical aggression, verbal aggression increases normatively across the preschool years, as children acquire language skills, stabilizing thereafter (e.g., Coie & Dodge, 1998). Other, often more recent, studies suggest that the use of verbal aggression (e.g., name calling) continues to increase with age (Bjorkqvist, Lagerspetz, et al., 1992).

Finally, cross-sectional (e.g., Bjorkqvist, Lagerspetz, et al., 1992; Trem- blay, 1999) and longitudinal studies (Cairns et al., 1989; Vaillancourt, Cote, Farhat, LeBlanc, Boivin, & Tremblay, 2003) have shown that children's use of indirect and social forms of aggression increases from early to mid- dle childhood and into adolescence and is quite normative during child- hood and preadolescence (see Underwood, 2003). Some (e.g., Bjorkqvist, Lagerspetz, et al., 1992; Bjorkqvist, Osterman, Kaukiainen, 1992) suggest that social aggression reaches a peak during early adolescence and declines thereafter but research by Owens (1996) suggests that social aggression continues to rise into high school for girls. Increases in indirect/social aggression across childhood coincide with the development of advanced verbal and cognitive skills that are necessary for such social manipulation (Bjorkqvist, Lagerspetz, et al., 1992; Bjorkqvist, Osterman, et al., 1992) and use of such behavior is associated with higher social intelligence (Kaukiainen et al., 1999).

Taken together, research on developmental changes in aggression suggests that there may be heterotypic continuity in aggression, meaning that the face of aggression changes over time. Bjorkqvist et al. (Bjorkqvist, Lagerspetz, et al., 1992; Bjorkqvist, Osterman, et al., 1992) suggest that, as children mature, their use of aggression changes from physical to verbal to indirect, commensurate with maturational changes that take place in the developing system (e.g., advanced verbal and social-cognitive skills). Several cross-sectional (e.g., Bjorkqvist, Lagerspetz, et al., 1992; Tremblay, 1999) and longitudinal (e.g., Brame, et al., 2001; Broidy et al., 2003; Cote et al., 2003; 2001; Vaillancourt et al., 2003) studies of aggression support this claim. However, in a recent longitudinal study of over 3000 children aged 4 to 11, Vaillancourt, Brendgren, et al. (in press) found no evidence to support the hypothesis that as children mature their way of aggressing becomes more refined (i.e., from physical to indirect). Rather, these authors found that children were rather consistent in the type of aggression they employed with stability rate of $r =.55$ for physical aggression and $r =.45$ for indirect aggression reported across a four-year period.

Research to date, then, shows that physical aggression is normative in the preschool years, then declines, while verbal and social forms of aggression emerge later, but become increasingly normative with age. Developmental trajectories, however, differ for boys and girls. One of the most enduring sex differences documented is that boys engage in more physical aggression than girls (e.g., Hyde, 1984; Maccoby & Jacklin, 1974), although this gender difference emerges gradually. Sex differences in physical aggression are not evident among toddlers (e.g., Loeber & Hay, 1997; Hay, Castel, & Davies, 2000), and are sometimes, but not always found among preschoolers (see Underwood, 2003). By the elementary years, however, girls become less physically aggressive than boys, with increasing sex differences in virtually all indices of physical aggression throughout childhood and adolescence (Underwood, 2003).

Gender differences in *verbal aggression* have not been consistently documented (Underwood, 2003), although when reported, boys are found to engage in more verbal aggression than girls (Maccoby & Jacklin, 1974; McCabe & Lipscomb, 1988). Underwood (2003) emphasizes that one noteworthy exception here is observational research by Archer, Pearson, and Westeman (1988) who found greater verbal aggression among elementary school girls. Nevertheless, boys are viewed by peers as more verbally aggressive across cultural groups (Osterman et al., 1994) and into adolescence (Salmivalli, Kaukiainen, & Lagerspetz, 2000).

With regard to more *psychological* forms of aggression, research indicates that children as young as 3–4 years of age engage in indirect/social aggression (e.g., Crick, Casas, & Mosher, 1997; Vaillancourt et al., 2003; in press), although gender differences in social (relational, indirect) aggression have not been consistently reported. Some studies indicate higher levels of relational aggression among girls (e.g., Crick & Grotpeter, 1995; Crick, et al., 1997; Lagerspetz, et al., 1988; Vaillancourt, et al., 2003); others demonstrate differences in favor of boys (e.g., Hennington, Hughes, Cavell, & Thompson, 1998; Tomada & Schneider, 1997), or no sex differences at all (e.g., Crick, et al., 1997 for peer evaluations; Rys & Bear, 1997; Willoughby, Kupersmidt, & Bryant, 2001). In her comprehensive review, Underwood (2003) concludes that boys engage in more physical aggression than girls, and perhaps more verbal aggression, and that girls are more likely to engage in social than physical aggression. It is not clear, however, that girls engage in more social/indirect/relational aggression than boys.

In sum, research to date has considered three very different forms of aggression, with evidence that the frequency of each form varies considerably as a function of age and gender. Of interest, then, are the factors that underlie the development and maintenance of such behavior. Although research on the origins of aggression has not systematically considered variations as a function of the form that aggressive behavior takes, studies to date do reflect our current knowledge regarding the underpinnings of aggression.

ORIGINS OF AGGRESSION

In an attempt to understand the emergence of aggression, developmental research has investigated a wide range of potential causes and risk factors (see Coie & Dodge, 1998; Tremblay, in press for reviews). Childhood aggression has been linked to individual characteristics, both biological and psychological, including hyperactivity (e.g., Lahey, McBurnett, & Loeber, 2000), difficult temperament (Plomin, 1983), lower resting heart rate and skin conductance (Fowles, 1988), lower serotonin metabolite 5-HIAA (Moore, Scarpa, & Raine, 2002), and lower levels of testosterone (Schaal, Tremblay, Soussignan, & Susman, 1996), to name a few. Youth aggression has also been associated with early environmental factors, including obstetrical complications (Arseneault, Tremblay, Boulerice, & Saucier, 2002), maternal smoking (Fergusson, Woodward, & Horwood, 1998; Raine, 2002), and prenatal drug exposure (Olofsson, Buckley, Andersen, & Friis-Hansen, 1983). Family characteristics have been extensively examined, with greater aggression found in children from lone parent families (Lykken, 2001), low socioeconomic status families (see Tremblay, 1999), and in families with a history of criminality (Keenan & Shaw, 1994). Aggression has also been linked to parent-child relationships, with greater aggression associated with parental hostility (vs. warmth), particular attachment and coercive interaction patterns, use of physical punishment and discipline practices, and abuse, although the links are often complex (see Coie & Dodge, 1998). Finally, an extensive literature has considered links between aggressive behavior and exposure to violent television and video games (e.g., Huesmann, Moise-Titus, Podolski & Eron, 2003).

At first glance, this list of risk factors seems striking in its diversity, consistent with long-held assumptions that aggression is the result of a continual interaction between biology and environment. However, upon closer inspection, the correlates may also reflect somewhat of a unifying bias in which researchers have prioritized individual and family characteristics over other socialization factors such as the peer group. The lack of attention to peers is especially curious in that children spend a significant portion of their day with peers, and that peer-directed aggression has been a primary outcome within this literature. In the paragraphs that follow, we provide an overview of a growing body of research on the social context of children's aggression, in which peer influences play a critical role in the development and maintenance of aggressive behaviors.

Research on the origins of aggression has historically been guided by two contrasting theoretical views, situated within the longstanding nature-nurture debate (Coie & Dodge, 1998). Philosophers such as Hobbes and James, psychoanalysts such as Freud, and ethologists such as Conrad Lorenz have viewed aggression as biologically inevitable, an instinctive and largely innate human behavior. In contrast, philosophers like Rousseau who viewed the newborn as innately good and Locke who viewed the infant as a *tabula rasa* (blank slate) have lead to theories that consider aggression to be primarily the result of socialization processes and societal/cultural influences. Within the latter tradition, Bandura's (1973) social learning theory has dominated psychological inquiry on the development of aggression. More recently, social information processing theories (e.g., Crick & Dodge, 1996) have extended this work by considering the cognitive processes that an individual engages in to determine the likelihood of aggression, but social learning theory has remained the primary guiding force in research on the *socialization* of aggression.

The central tenet of Bandura's (1973) theory is that aggression is learned through direct or vicarious rewards and/or through the imitation of powerful or revered models that are perceived to be similar to the self. This perspective has generated three major research foci with regard to the socialization of aggression. An extensive body of research has examined links between aggression and parental behavior (e.g., lack of warmth, inconsistent discipline, physical abuse, see Coie & Dodge, 1998 for a review). Links between observed television violence and aggressive behavior have also garnered considerable research attention (e.g., Anderson & Bushman, 2002; Huesmann et al., 2003). The third major research focus has considered the impact of peers, but has been limited to an examination of the influence of deviant peers and delinquent gangs on aggression, studied almost exclusively during adolescence. Association with deviant peers and gangs has been clearly linked to increased delinquent and antisocial behavior, both concurrently and predictively (e.g., Battin, Hill, Abbott, Catalano, & Hawkins, 1998; Thornberry, Krohn, Lizotte, & Chard-Wierschem, 1993). It is not clear, however, whether affiliation with deviant peers reflects *homophily* (like seeking like) or the fact that aggressive youths have limited alternatives for more positive peer contacts (see Coie & Dodge, 1998).

More recent research has begun to specify the *processes* through which peer influences operate. For example, Dishion (e.g., Dishion, McCord, & Poulin, 1999) has documented the operation of peer "deviancy training" using relatively straightforward operant and social learning principles (Bandura, 1973). They argue that aggressive and antisocial behaviors are directly encouraged through within-group reinforcement (attention, laughter, general interest in negative behavior) and punishment for adhering to mainstream social norms. In addition, motivation to engage in deviant behavior is enhanced through the values and meanings provided for such behavior by deviant peers. Association with deviant peers has also been linked to increased aggressive behavior through social cognitive processes like moral disengagement (Bandura, 1999), where the negative impact of behavior is gradually minimized through a number of self-regulatory mechanisms (e.g., justification of negative acts, blaming and dehumanizing the victim, etc.) that serve to disinhibit, reduce guilt, and make negative acts more palatable. Several studies have shown that aggressive (as compared with non-aggressive) children express more positive and normative beliefs about aggression, viewing such behavior as less "bad" or "wrong" and, importantly, more acceptable (see Coie & Dodge, 1998; Guerra, Huesmann, & Hanish, 1995), leading to increases in delinquent behavior over time (Thornberry, Lizotte, Krohn, Farnworth, & Jang, 1994). Similarly, students who admit to bullying others are more likely to view victims as deserving and/or different, and more likely to see bullying as acceptable either generally or within their own peer sub-group (Hymel, Bonanno, Rocke Henderson, & McCreith, 2002). These findings are consistent with social learning theory, as even Bandura (1973) recognized the potential for aggression to serve a utilitarian purpose in "many social groups" in terms of gaining approval and admiration from peers, and in maintaining and acquiring social status within "deviant group(s)" (p. 3). Studies of the influence of deviant peers, however, reflect a rather narrow perspective on how aggression is socialized within the peer group, and has been limited primarily to consideration of overt physical (not social) forms of aggression. A much broader view of peer socialization is required, considering how the larger peer group responds to aggression.

AGGRESSION AS A SOCIAL ENTERPRISE

Bjorkqvist (2001) argues that, in all the forms it takes, aggression is social, not only in the sense that such behavior typically involves a perpetrator and a victim, but also in light of evidence that peers are frequently present as observers of such behavior. For example, observational studies of schoolyard bullying indicate that bystanders were present in 85% to 88% of bullying episodes (Craig & Pepler, 1995; Hawkins, Pepler, & Craig, 2001). The social quality of aggression may be especially true of social/indirect/relational aggression in which social liaisons are often the source of attack as well as the vehicle used to inflict harm on others. One would hope that aggressive behavior, regardless of the form it takes, would not be tolerated by the larger peer group; that aggressive children would be negatively reinforced or punished by the peer group and in time become less aggressive. And, in fact, it is well documented that aggressive children are generally disliked and hence "rejected" within the larger peer group (see Coie & Dodge, 1998). This may not be the case for all forms of aggression. When links between relational (social) aggression and peer rejection have been examined, it is *controversial* students (those who are both liked and disliked) rather than *rejected* students who peers view as the most relationally aggressive (e.g., Crick & Grotpeter, 1995; Tomada & Schneider, 1997).

Although links between (physical) aggression and peer rejection are well established, they do not tell the whole story. Contradictory findings have also been reported. Over 25 years ago, Olweus (1977) found that male adolescent aggressors were *average* (not rejected) in peer acceptance. Dodge, Coie, Petit, and Price (1990) found that aggression was *positively* related to peer acceptance among first grade boys. Both Dodge et al. (1990)

and Olweus (1994) suggested that, with age, aggressive children would become less well accepted, as peers become less willing to tolerate such behavior. Consistent with this notion, Humphreys and Smith (1987) found that bullying behavior was mostly carried on by high status boys in grade 1, but was primarily associated with lower peer status in grade 3. In stark contrast, studies have also shown that children's admiration for, and approval of, aggressive peers increases with age (e.g., Bukowski, Sippola, & Newcomb, 2000; Huesmann & Guerra, 1997). In light of these findings, it is not surprising to learn that, even though overt aggression is one of the strongest correlates of peer rejection (Coie & Dodge, 1998), it is also true that only about half of aggressive children are actually rejected within their peer group (e.g., Cillessen, van Ijzendoorn, van Lieshout, & Hartup, 1992).

Coie and Dodge (1998) offer several possible explanations for why some aggressive children are not rejected within the peer group. First, this may reflect distinctions that peers make about particular types of aggressive behaviors, with some forms of aggression, particularly aggression in response to direct peer provocation, being viewed positively by peers, with perpetrators seen as able to "stand up for themselves" (e.g., Lancelotta & Vaughn, 1989; Olweus, 1977). Second, links between aggression and rejection may depend on peer group norms, with aggressive children being more rejected/disliked in subgroups where such behavior is infrequent or non-normative (e.g., Boivin, Dodge, & Coie, 1995; Wright, Giammarino, & Parad, 1986). In this regard, it is noteworthy that levels of aggressive behavior vary considerably across schools and classrooms (Kellam, 1990) and that the correlation between rejection and (physical) aggression is stronger for girls (for whom such behavior is less likely) than for boys (for whom such behavior is more typical; Lancelotta & Vaughn, 1989). Third, Coie and Dodge cite research by Bierman (1986; Bierman, Smoot, & Aumiller, 1993) that shows that aggressive children who are rejected display more additional negative behaviors than those who are not rejected. Relatedly, they review several studies of victimization that suggest that "ineffectual" aggressive children (e.g., those who are both bullies and victims) may be more likely to be rejected by their peers.

Although Coie and Dodge (1998) provide a thought-provoking and plausible discussion of why some aggressive children might not be rejected by peers, recent research suggests several further possibilities in which aggressive behavior is actively encouraged within the mainstream peer group. Over the past decade, a growing body of research on children's social networks shows that (physically) aggressive youths do have friends and are often central members of their social clique, although they may be rejected or unpopular/disliked at the *group* level (e.g., Cairns, Cairns,

Neckerman, Gest, & Gariepy, 1988; Vandell & Hembree, 1994). Gender differences may also be important here, with physically aggressive girls found to be lower in network centrality than physically aggressive boys (e.g., Estell, Cairns, Farmer, & Cairns, 2002; Farmer & Rodkin, 1996). In one of the few studies to consider the social networks of relationally/indirectly/socially aggressive children, Xie and colleagues (Xie, Cairns, & Cairns, 2002; Xie, Swift, Cairns, & Cairns, 2002) found that social aggression was associated with high network centrality, whereas physically aggression was not, a finding that held true for both girls and boys. Further research is needed to clarify the relationship between network indices and various forms of aggression as a function of gender and age, as well as other potentially relevant group characteristics. It is clear, however, that at least some aggressive youth actually enjoy fairly high social status within the group (e.g., Estell et al., 2002; Dodge et al., 1990; Luthar & McMahon, 1996; Rodkin, Farmer, Pearl, & Van Acker, 2000). Positive associations between aggression and perceived popularity have been demonstrated for physical as well as social forms of aggression (e.g., Lease, Kennedy, & Axelrod, 2002; Prinstein & Cillessen, in press). As well, in a study investigating the relationship between bullying and social power among adolescents (grades 6 to 10), Vaillancourt, Hymel, and McDougall (in press) found that over 50% of peer nominated bullies were viewed by peers as powerful and popular.

At first glance, the results of these studies may appear to contradict previous findings regarding links between aggression and peer rejection. This is not the case. Instead, they point to a need to carefully consider how one's social status within a group is assessed (e.g., sociometric evaluations of likeability, peer assessments of popularity or power, indices of network centrality). Ethnographic research has long suggested the distinction between popularity (status) and liking, at least among girls. For example, Eder (1985) followed a large sample of adolescent girls over the transition to junior high school (grades 6–8). In what she called the "cycle of popularity", Eder found that some students achieved high levels of status or popularity as a function of such things as attractiveness, social skills, or participation in peer-valued activities such as cheerleading. Initially, these girls were viewed positively by their classmates, who recognized that alliances with these popular girls could enhance their own status. Over time, however, these popular girls engaged in a variety of negative behaviors which eventually contributed to peer perceptions of these girls as popular but not necessarily likeable. Similarly, Merten (1997) described the behaviors of a group of girls (the "dirty dozen") who were perceived by peers as both popular and powerful but as socially aggressive in their behavior.

Parkhurst and Hopmeyer (1998) also distinguished between liking/disliking (as assessed by traditional sociometric measures) and peer perceptions of status, popularity, and power. They reported a positive association between peer reports of "starts fights" and peer perceptions of popularity which referred to visibility and influence within the peer group and not peer liking per se. Similarly, Vaillancourt and Hymel (in press) found that both relationally and physically aggressive students were viewed by schoolmates as both popular and powerful, although they were simultaneously rejected (disliked) by peers. Research by Cillessen and Mayeux (2002), however, underscores the importance of examining these links across time and for distinct forms of aggression. They found that, during the middle school and high school years, use of *relational* aggression became increasingly negatively associated with peer liking but increasingly positively related to perceived popularity for both boys and girls. Interestingly, as children aged, the use of *physical* aggression was associated with greater peer liking for both boys and girls.

REINFORCING AGGRESSION

Within children's peer groups, aggression often "works". Years ago, Patterson, Littman, & Bricker (1967) demonstrated that victimized children who were successful in reducing peer aggression through counter-aggression were more likely to become aggressive subsequently. In considering the implication of this finding, Coie and Dodge (1998) suggest that "environments that allow children to be exposed to aggression, to try out aggression, and to experience its positive instrumental consequences are likely to have children who develop aggressively" (p. 797). The research reviewed herein demonstrates, not only that childhood and adolescent aggression is social (Bjorkqvist, 2001), but that it may be sanctioned by the larger peer network, who afford perpetrators considerable status and power. This seems to be especially true of relational aggression for both girls and boys (e.g., Cillessen & Mayeux, 2002; Vaillancourt & Hymel, in press) and for physical aggression for boys only (e.g., Bukowski et al., 2000; Cillessen & Mayeux, 2002).

Returning to social learning theories of aggression, these findings certainly suggest that, at least for some children, such behavior is "rewarded" within youth peer groups and, as Bandura (1973) himself suggested, can serve a utilitarian purpose in "many social groups" in terms of gaining approval and admiration from peers, and in terms of maintaining and acquiring social status, not only within "deviant group(s)" (p. 3), but also in mainstream peer groups. Consistent with social learning theory, children's peer groups may indeed be training grounds for aggression, with high status aggressive individuals providing models of aggressive behavior that are powerful, revered, and perceived as similar to the self, effectively countering more adult-based sanctions against aggressive behavior. As Cairns et al. (1988) suggest, "aggressive coalitions of students can devastate the authority of adults" (p. 822). This may be particularly true for social/indirect/relational aggression for which there are less clear adult-based prohibitions or "zero-tolerance" policies. Indeed, recent research by Goldstein, Tisak, and Boxer (2002) has shown that even preschool children (both boys and girls) judged relationally aggressive behavior to be more acceptable than physical and verbal aggression, although girls viewed relationally aggressive behavior as less acceptable than did boys.

Additional support for the idea that peers often encourage aggression comes from research on bullying, a subcategory of aggressive behavior (Olweus, 1999). For instance, O'Connell, Pepler, and Craig (1999) found that, on average, four children were present as observers during bullying episodes (range 2 to 14 peers), and that bystanders reinforced the bully 54% of the time by passively watching and 21% of the time by actively modeling the bully. Moreover, bullies were seldom punished for their hurtful behavior. In fact, peers intervened on behalf of the victim only 11% of the time, while teachers did so only 4% of the time (Craig & Pepler, 1995). Although disturbing, these findings are consistent with research by Salmivalli and colleagues demonstrating that bullying is a group affair with many bully-supporting roles that are maintained and reinforced over time (Salmivalli, Lagerspetz, Bjorkqvist, Osterman, & Kaukiainen, 1996).

CONCLUSIONS

Thirty years ago, Bandura (1973) stated that "a complete theory of aggression, whatever its orientation, must explain how aggressive patterns of behavior are developed, what provokes people to behave aggressively, and what maintains their aggressive actions" (p. 43). Traditionally, research on the development and maintenance of aggression has prioritized family and individual characteristics, both biological and psychological, in attempting to understand the etiology of aggression. This focus is highly appropriate and has proved quite fruitful. However, it is clear that outcomes such as aggression emerge as a result of a number of different factors, not just one or two, with dynamic interactions between biological and environmental characteristics. Greater attention to the role of the peer group in the development and maintenance of aggression can enhance our understanding of the phenomenon, but only if we are open to a broader consideration of the socialization influence of peers (e.g., Harris, 1995, 1998). To date, research examining peer influences on aggression has emphasized the role of deviant peers, delinquent gangs and peer rejection, implicitly highlighting a negative view of peer contributions to socialization. Our goal in the present chapter was to review recent research suggesting a far more complex set of processes through which the mainstream peer culture can encourage and support the maintenance of aggressive behavior. Future research must consider the processes through which various forms of aggressive behavior are socialized within children's peer groups, in addition to families. As this area of research unfolds, it is likely that peers can function as both risk and protective factors in the development and maintenance of aggression, suggesting new possibilities for intervention. We hope that the present chapter is successful in stimulating such work.

REFERENCES

Anderson, C. A., & Bushman, B. J. (2002). The effects of media violence on society. *Science*, 295, 2377–2379.

Archer, J., Pearson, M. A., & Westeman, K. E. (1988). Aggressive behavior of children aged 6–11: Gender differences and their magnitude. *British Journal of Social Psychology, 27*, 371–384.

Arseneault, L., Tremblay, R. E., Boulerice, B., & Saucier, J-F. (2002). Obstetrical complications and violent delinquency: Testing two developmental pathways. *Child Development, 73*, 496–508.

Bandura, A. (1973). *Aggression—A social learning analysis.* New Jersey: Prentice-Hall.

Bandura, A. (1999). Moral disengagement in the perpetration of inhumanities. *Personality and Social Psychology Review, 3*, 193–209.

Battin, S. R., Hill, K. G., Abbott, R. D., Catalano, R. F., & Hawkins, J. D. (1998). The contribution of gang membership to delinquency beyond delinquent friends. *Criminology, 36*, 93–115.

Bierman, K. L. (1986). The relation between social aggression and peer rejection in middle childhood. In R. J. Prinz (Ed.), *Advances in behavioral assessment of children and families* (vol. 2, pp. 151–178). Greenwich, CT: JAI.

Bierman, K. L., Smoot, D. L., & Aumiller, K. (1993). Characteristics of aggressive-rejected, aggressive (non-rejected), and rejected (non-aggressive) status. *Development and Psychopathology, 7*, 669–682.

Bjorkqvist, K. (2001). Comments to "Top ten challenges for understanding gender and aggression in children: Why can't we all just get along?": Different names, same issues. *Social Development, 10*, 272–274.

Bjorkqvist, K., Lagerspetz, K. M. J., & Kaukiainen, A. (1992). Do girls manipulate and boys fight?: Developmental trends in regard to direct and indirect aggression. *Aggressive Behavior, 18*, 117–127.

Bjorkqvist, K., Osterman, K., & Kaukiainen, A. (1992). The development of direct and indirect aggressive strategies in males and females. In K. Bjorkqvist & P. Niemela (Eds.), *Of mice and women: Aspects of female aggression* (pp. 51–64). San Diego, CA: Academic Press.

Boivin, M., Dodge, K. A., & Coie, J. D. (1995). Individual-group behavioral similarity and peer status in experimental play groups of boys: The social misfit revisited. *Journal of Personality and Social Psychology, 69,* 269–279.

Brame, B., Nagin, D. S., & Tremblay, R. E. (2001). Developmental trajectories of physical aggression from school entry to late adolescence. *The Journal of Child Psychology and Psychiatry, 58,* 389–394.

Broidy, L. M., Nagin, D. S., Tremblay, R. E., Brame, B., Dodge, K., Fergusson, D., Horwood, J., Loeber, R., Laird, R., Lynam, D., Moffitt, T., Bates, J. E., Pettit, G. S., & Vitaro, F. (2003). Developmental trajectories of childhood disruptive behaviors and adolescent delinquency: A six site, cross-national study. *Developmental Psychology, 39,* 222–245.

Bukowski, W. M., Sippola, L. K., & Newcomb, A. F. (2000). Variations in patterns of attraction to same- and other-sex peers during early adolescence. *Developmental Psychology, 36,* 147–154.

Cairns, R. B., Cairns, B. D., Neckerman, H., Ferguson, L. L., & Gariepy, J. (1989). Growth and aggression: 1. Childhood to early adolescence. *Developmental Psychology, 25,* 320–330.

Cairns, R. B., Cairns, B. D., Neckerman, H., Gest, S., & Gariepy, J. (1988). Social networks and aggressive behavior: Peer support or peer rejection? *Developmental Psychology, 24,* 815–823.

Cillessen, A. H. N., & Mayeux, L. (2002). From censure to reinforcement: Developmental changes in the role of aggression in peer relations. In T. Vaillancourt & P. C. Rodkin symposium, *Functions of aggression in children's peer relations,* for the XV Meeting of the International Society for Research in Aggression, Montreal, Canada.

Cillessen, A. H. N., van Ijzendoorn, H. W., van Lieshout, C. F. M., & Hartup, W. W. (1992). Heterogeneity among peer-rejected boys: Subtypes and stabilities. *Child Development 63,* 893–905.

Coie, J. D., & Dodge, K. A. (1998). Aggression and antisocial behavior. In William Damon (Series Ed.) and Nancy Eisenberg (Volume Ed.), *Handbook of Child Psychology,* Fifth Edition, Vol. 3: *Social, Emotional and Personality Development* (pp. 779–862). New York: Wiley.

Cote, S., Vaillancourt, T., Farhat, A., LeBlanc, J. C., Nagin, D., & Tremblay, R. (2003). Developmental Trajectories of Physical Aggression during Childhood: A Nation Wide Longitudinal Study of Canadian Children. Manuscript submitted for publication.

Craig, W. M., & Pepler, D. J. (1995). Peer processes in bullying and victimization: An observational study. *Exceptionality Education Canada, 5,* 81–95.

Crick, N. R. (1995). Relational aggression: The role of intent attributions, feelings of distress, and provocation type. *Development and Psychopathology, 7,* 313–322.

Crick, N. R., Casas, J. F., & Mosher, M. (1997). Relational and over aggression in preschool. *Developmental Psychology, 33,* 589–600.

Crick, N. R., & Dodge, K. (1996). Social information-processing mechanisms in reactive and proactive aggression. *Child Development, 67,* 993–1002.

Crick, N. R., & Grotpeter, J. K. (1995). Relational aggression, gender, and social-psychological adjustment. *Child Development, 66,* 710–722.

Dishion, T. J., McCord, J., & Poulin, F. (1999). When interventions harm: Peer groups and problem behavior. *American Psychologist, 54,* 755–764.

Dishion, T. J., Patterson G. R., Stoolmiller, M., & Skinner, M. L. (1991). Family, school, and behavioral antecedents to early adolescent involvement with antisocial peers. *Developmental Psychology, 27,* 172–180.

Dodge, K. A. , Coie, J. D., Pettit, G., & Price, J. (1990). Peer status and aggression in boys' groups: Developmental and contextual analyses. *Child Development, 61,* 1289–1309.

Eder, D. (1985). The cycle of popularity: Interpersonal relations among female adolescents. *Sociology of Education, 58,* 154–165.

Estell, D. B., Cairns, R. B., Farmer, T. W., & Cairns, B. D. (2002). Aggression in inner-city early elementary classrooms: Individual and peer-group configurations. *Merrill-Palmer Quarterly, 48*, 52–76.

Farmer, T. W., & Rodkin, P. C. (1996). Antisocial and prosocial correlates of social positions: The social network centrality perspective. *Social Development, 5*, 174–188.

Fergusson, D. M., Woodward, L. J., & Horwood, L. J. (1998). Maternal smoking during pregnancy and psychiatric adjustment in late adolescence. *Archives of General Psychiatry, 55*, 721–727.

Feshbach, N. D. (1969). Sex differences in children's modes of aggressive responses toward outsiders. *Merrill-Palmer-Quarterly, 15*, 249–258.

Feshbach, N. D. (1971). Sex differences in adolescent reactions toward newcomers. *Developmental Psychology, 4*, 381–386.

Fowles, D. C. (1988). Psychophysiology and psychopathy: A motivational approach. *Psychophysiology, 25*, 373–391.

Galen, B. R., & Underwood, M. K., (1997). A developmental investigation of social aggression among children. *Developmental Psychology, 33*, 589–600.

Goldstein, S. E., Tisak, M. S., & Boxer, P. (2002). Preschoolers' normative and prescriptive judgments about relational and overt aggression. *Early Education and Development, 13*, 23–39.

Guerra, N. G., Huesmann, L. R., & Hanish, L. (1995). The role of normative beliefs in children's social behavior. In N., Eisenberg (Ed.) *Review of personality, development, and social psychology: The interface* (pp. 140–158). Thousand Oaks, CA: Sage.

Harris, J. R. (1995). Where is the child's environment? A group socialization theory of development. *Psychological Review, 102*, 458–489.

Harris, J. R. (1998). *The nurture assumption: Why children turn out the way they do.* New York: Free Press.

Hawkins, D. L., Pepler, D. J., & Craig, W. M. (2001). Naturalistic observations of peer interventions in bullying. *Social Development, 10*, 512–527.

Hay D. F., Castel J., & Davies L. (2000). Toddlers's use of force against familiar peers: A precursor of serious aggression? *Child Development, 71*, 457–467.

Hennington, C., Hughes, J. N., Cavell, T. A., & Thompson, B. (1998). The role of relational aggression in identifying boys and girls. *Journal of School Psychology, 36*, 457–477.

Huesmann, L. R., & Guerra, N. G. (1997). Children's normative beliefs about aggression and aggressive behavior. *Journal of Personality and Social Psychology, 72*, 408–419.

Huesmann, L. R., Moise-Titus, J., Podolski, C., & Eron, L. (2003). Longitudinal relations between children's exposure to TV violence and their aggressive and violent behavior in young adulthood: 1977–1992. *Developmental Psychology, 39*.

Humphreys, A. P., & Smith, P. K. (1987). Rough-and-tumble play, friendship, and dominance in school children: Evidence for continuity and change with age. *Child Development, 58*, 201–212.

Hyde, J. S. (1984). How large are gender differences in aggression: A developmental meta-analysis. *Developmental Psychology, 20*, 722–736.

Hymel, S., Bonanno, R. A., Rocke Henderson, N., & McCreith, T. (2002). Moral disengagement and school bullying: An investigation of student attitudes and beliefs. In J. LeBlanc (Chair), *Aggression in school*, International Society for Research on Aggression, July 2002, Montreal, PQ.

Johnson, J. G., Cohen, P., Smailes, E. M., Kasen, S., & Brook, J. S. (2002). Television viewing and aggressive behavior during adolescence and adulthood. *Science, 295*, 2468–2471.

Kaukiainen, A., Bjorkqvist, K., Lagerspetz, K., Osterman, K., Salmivalli, C., Rothberg, S., & Ahlbo, A. (1999). The relationship between social intelligence, empathy and three types of aggression. *Aggressive Behavior, 25*, 81–89.

Keenan, K., & Shaw, D. S. (1994). The development of aggression in toddlers: A study of low-income families. *Journal of Abnormal Child Psychology, 22*, 53–77.

Kellam, S. G. (1990). Developmental epidemiological framework for family research on depression and aggression . In G. R. Patterson (Ed.), *Depression and aggression in family interaction* (pp. 11–48). Hillsdale, NJ: Erlbaum.

Lagerspetz, K. M., Bjorkqvist, K., & Peltonen, T. (1988). Is indirect aggression typical of females? Gender differences in aggressiveness in 11- to 12-year old children. *Aggressive Behavior, 14*, 403–414.

Lahey, B. B., McBurnett, K., & Loeber, R. (2000). Are attention-deficit hyperactivity disorder and oppositional defiant disorder developmental precursors to conduct disorder? In A. Sameroff, M. Lewis, & S. Miller (Eds.), *Handbook of developmental psychopathology* (pp. 431–446). New York: Plenum.

Lancelotta, G. X., & Vaughn, S. (1989). Relation between types of aggression and sociometric status: Peer and teacher perceptions. *Journal of Educational Psychology, 81*, 86–90.

Lease, A. M., Kennedy, C. A., & Axelrod, J. L. (2002). Children's social constructions of popularity. *Social Development, 11*, 87–109.

Loeber, R., & Hay, D. (1997). Key issues in the development of aggression and violence from childhood to early adulthood. *Annual Review of Psychology, 48*, 371–410.

Lorenz, K. (1966). *On aggression.* New York: Harcourt, Brace and World.

Luthar, S. S., & McMahon, T. J. (1996). Peer reputation among inner-city adolescents: Structure and correlates. *Journal of Research on Adolescence, 6*, 581–603.

Lykken, D. T. (2001). Parental licensure. *American Psychologist, 56*, 885–894.

Newcomb, A. F., Bukowski, W. M., & Pattee, L. (1993). Children's peer relations: A meta-analytic review of popular, rejected, neglected, controversial, and average sociometric status. *Psychological Bulletin, 113*, 99–128.

Maccoby, E. E., & Jacklin, C. N. (1974). *The psychology of gender differences.* Stanford, CA: Stanford University Press.

McCabe, A., & Lipscomb, T. (1988). Sex differences in children's verbal aggression. *Merrill Palmer Quarterly, 34*, 389–401.

Merten, D. E. (1997). The meaning of meanness: Popularity, competition, and conflict among junior high school girls. *Sociology of Education, 40*, 175–191.

Moffitt, T. E. (1993). Adolescence-limited and life-course-persistent antisocial behavior: A developmental taxonomy. *Psychological Review, 100*, 674–701.

Moore, T. M., Scarpa, A., & Raine, A. (2002). A meta-analysis of serotonin metabolite 5-HIAA and antisocial behavior. *Aggressive Behavior, 28*, 299–316.

Nagin, D., & Tremblay, R. E. (2001). Parental and early childhood predictors of persistent physical aggression in boys from kindergarten to high school. *Archives of General Psychiatry, 58*, 389–394.

O'Connell, P., Pepler, D., & Craig, W. (1999). Peer involvement in bullying: Insights and challenges for intervention. *Journal of Adolescence, 22*, 437–452.

Olofsson, M., Buckley, W., Andersen, G. E., & Friis-Hansen, B. (1983). Investigation of 89 children bory by drug-dependent mothers. *Acta Psychiatrica Scandinavica, 72*, 407–410.

Olweus, D. (1977). Aggression and peer acceptance in adolescent boys: Two short-term longitudinal studies of ratings. *Child Development, 48*, 1301–1313.

Olweus, D. (1994). Bullying at schools: Basic facts and effects of a school based intervention program. *Journal of Child Psychology and Psychiatry and Allied Disciplines, 35*, 1171–1190.

Olweus, D. (1999). Sweden. In P. K. Smith, Y. Morita, J. Junger-Tas, D. Olweus, R. Catalano, & P. Slee (Eds.), *The nature of school bullying* (pp. 7–27). New York: Routledge

Osterman, K., Bjorkqvist, K., Lagerspetz, K., Kaukiainen, A., Huesmann, L. R., & Fraczek, A. (1994). Peer and self-estimated aggression and victimization in 8-year-old children from five ethnic groups. *Aggressive Behavior, 20,* 411–428.

Osterman, K., Bjorkqvist, K., Lagerspetz, K. M. J., Kaukiainen, A., Landau, S. F., Fraczek, A., & Caprara, G. V. (1998). Cross-cultural evidence of female indirect aggression. *Aggressive Behavior, 24,* 1–8.

Owens, L. D. (1996). Sticks and stones and sugar and spice: Girls' and boys' aggression in schools. *Australian Journal of Guidance and Counseling, 6,* 45–55.

Parkhurst, J. T., & Hopmeyer, A. (1998). Sociometric popularity and peer-perceived popularity: Two distinct dimensions of peer status. *Journal of Early Adolescence, 18,* 125–144.

Patterson, G. R., Littman, R. W., & Bricker, W. (1967). Assertive behavior in children: A step toward a theory of Aggression. *Monographs of the Society for Research in Child Development, 32* (5, Serial No. 113).

Plomin, R. (1983). Childhood temperament. In B. B. Lahey & A. E. Kazdin (Eds.), *Advances in clinical child psychology* (Vol. 6, pp. 45–92) New York: Plenum.

Prinstein, M. J., & Cillessen, A. H. N. (in press). Forms and functions of adolescent peer aggression associated with high levels of peer status. *Merrill-Palmer Quarterly.*

Raine, A. (2002). Annotation: The role of prefrontal deficits, low automatic arousal, and early health factors in the development of antisocial and aggressive behavior in children. *Journal of Child Psychology and Psychiatry, 43,* 417–434.

Rys, G. S., & Bear, G. G., (1997). Relational aggression and peer relations: Gender and developmental issues. *Merrill-Palmer Quarterly, 43,* 87–106.

Rodkin, P. C., Farmer, T. W., Pearl, R., & Van Acker, R. (2000). Heterogeneity of popular boys: Antisocial and prosocial configurations. *Developmental Psychology, 36,* 14–24.

Salmivalli, C., Kaukiainen, A., & Lagerspetz, K. (2000). Aggression and sociometric status among peers : Do Gender and type of aggression matter ? *Scandinavian Journal of Psychology, 41,* 17–24.

Salmivalli, C., Lagerspetz, K., Bjorkqvist, K., Osterman, K., & Kaukiainen, A. (1996). Bullying as a group process: Participant roles and their relations to social status within the group. *Aggressive Behavior, 22,* 1–15.

Schaal, B., Tremblay, R. E., Soussignan, R., & Susman, E. J. (1996). Male testosterone linked to high school dominance but low physical aggression in early adolescence. *Journal of the American Academy of Child and Adolescent Psychiatry, 35*(10), 1322–1330.

Thornberry, T. P., Krohn, M. D., Lizotte, A. J., & Chard-Wierschem, D. (1993). The role of juvenile gangs in facilitating delinquent behavior. *Journal of Research in Crime and Delinquency, 30,* 55–87.

Thornberry, T. P., Lizotte, A. J., Krohn, M. D., Farnworth, M., & Jang, S. J. (1994). Delinquent peers beliefs and delinquent behavior: A longitudinal test of interaction theory. *Criminology, 32,* 47–83.

Tomada, G., & Schneider, B. H. (1997). Relational aggression, gender, and peer acceptance: Invariance across culture, stability over time and concordance among informants. *Developmental Psychology, 33,* 601–609.

Tremblay, R. E. (1999). When children's social development fails. In D. P. Keating & C. Hertzman (Eds.), *Developmental health and the wealth of nations: Social, biological, and educational dynamics* (pp. 55–71). New York: Guilford.

Tremblay, R. E. (2000). The development of aggressive behavior during childhood: What have we learned in the past century? *International Journal of Behavioral Development, 24,* 129–141.

Tremblay, R. E. (2001). The development of physical aggression during childhood and the prediction of later dangerousness. In G. F. Pinard & L. Pagani (Eds.), *Clinical assessment of dangerousness: Empirical contributions* (pp. 47–65). NY: Cambridge University Press.

Tremblay, R. E. (in press). Why socialization fails?: The case of chronic physical aggression. In B. B. Lahey, T. E. Moffitt, & A. Caspi (Eds.), *The causes of conduct disorders and serious juvenile delinquency.* New York: Guilford.

Tremblay, R. E., Japel, C., Perusse, D., McDuff, P., Boivin, M., Zoccolillo, M., & Montplaisir, J. (1999). The search for the age of 'onset' of physical aggression: Rousseau and Bandura revisited. *Criminal Behavior and Mental Health, 9,* 8–23.

Underwood, M. K. (2003). *Social aggression in girls.* New York: Guilford.

Underwood, M. K., Galen, B. R., & Paquette, J. A. (2001). Admirations rather than hostilities: Response to Archer, Bjorkqvist, and Crick et al. *Social Development, 10,* 275–280.

Vaillancourt, T., Brendgen, M., Boivin, M., & Tremblay, R. (in press). Longitudinal Confirmatory factor analysis of indirect and physical aggression: Evidence of two factors over time? *Child Development.*

Vaillancourt, T., Cote, S., Farhat, A., LeBlanc, J. C., Boivin, M., & Tremblay, R. (2003). *Trajectories of indirect aggression: Insights from the Canadian National Longitudinal Study of Children and Youth.* Manuscript submitted for publication.

Vaillancourt, T. (in press). Indirect aggression among humans: Social construct or evolutionary adaptation. In R. E. Tremblay, W. H. Hartup, and J. Archer (eds.), *Developmental origins of aggression.* Guilford Press.

Vaillancourt, T., & Hymel, S. (in press). Understanding sociometric status: What does it mean to be popular? *Social Development.*

Vaillancourt, T., Hymel, S., & McDougall, P. (in press). Bullying is power: Implications for school intervention programs. *Journal of Applied School Psychology.*

Vandell, D. L., & Hembree, S. E. (1994). Peer social status and friendship: Independent contributors to children's social and academic adjustment. *Merrill Palmer Quarterly, 40,* 461–477.

Willoughby, J., Kupersmidt, J. B., & Bryant, D. (2001). Overt and covert dimensions of antisocial behavior. *Journal of Abnormal Child Psychology, 29,* 177–187.

Wright, J. C., Giammarino, M., & Parad, H. W. (1986). Social status in small groups: Individual-group similarity and the social "misfit": *Journal of Personality and Social Psychology, 50,* 523–536.

Xie, H., Cairns, R. B., & Cairns, B. D. (2002). The development of social aggression and physical aggression: A narrative analysis of interpersonal conflicts. *Aggressive Behavior, 28,* 341–355.

Xie, H., Swift, D. J., Cairns, B. D., & Cairns, R. B. (2002). Aggressive behaviors in social interaction and developmental adaptation: A narrative analysis of interpersonal conflicts during early adolescence. *Social Development, 11,* 205–224.

6

Adjudicated Females' Participation in Violence from Adolescence to Adulthood
Results from a Longitudinal Study

NADINE LANCTÔT, CATHERINE ÉMOND, AND MARC LE BLANC*

In their recent review of the literature, Le Blanc and Loeber (1998) note that the criminological study of delinquent behavior has focused primarily on between-group differences. As a result, the etiological study of delinquency from an individual perspective has been neglected. This observation is particularly true when examining the evolution of delinquents and violent activities among adolescent females (Pajer, 1998; Wanby, Bergman, & Magnusson, 1999). It is an accepted fact in the literature that females commit less serious offences when compared with male counterparts (Chesney-Lind & Shelden, 1998). This gender difference is observed in official statistics as well as in self-reported surveys. Females are also less likely to continue engaging in delinquent behaviors as they move into

* This research was supported by the Conseil québécois de la recherche sociale, the Fonds pour la formation des chercheurs et l'action concertée du Québec and the Conseil de recherches en sciences humaines du Canada.

NADINE LANCTÔT, CATHERINE ÉMOND AND MARC LE BLANC • School of Criminology, University of Montréal, Montréal, Québec, Canada, H3C 3J7.

late adolescence/early adulthood (Pajer, 1998; Lanctôt & Le Blanc, 2002). However, the gender gap in prevalence and persistence rates is smaller for deviant activities such as drug use (Pajer, 1998; Lanctôt & Le Blanc, 2002).

While the widely cited differences in rates and patterns of offending across gender are informative, these types of aggregate level comparisons do not allow for an examination of the onset and evolution of delinquent and violent behavior of females as they mature into young adulthood. A developmental analysis of delinquent conduct aims to examine the stability and progression of delinquent behavior throughout the life-course. It provides an opportunity to identify distinct pathways, each representing patterns of development that characterize subgroups of individuals (Loeber et al., 1993). The previous treatment of delinquent females as a homogeneous subgroup, which all share a common pathway to involvement in delinquent behavior, has resulted in a lack of theoretical and empirical knowledge in this area.

Only a handful of prospective studies have examined the developmental course of delinquency among females. The common finding throughout this small body of the literature is that the majority of females participate in exploratory delinquency during their adolescence (Ageton, 1983; Dunford & Elliott, 1984; Lanctôt & Le Blanc, 1999). It is unusual, however, for females to persist in serious forms of delinquency. For example, Ageton (1983) reported that over a 5-year period, females' self-reported participation in crimes against the person dropped from 36% to 12%. More recently, Ayers et al. (1999) concluded that females who engage in serious forms of delinquency, such as violence, do so over a shorter period of time than male counterparts. Between the ages of 13 and 15 years, 19% of females as compared to 28% of males in their sample reported having been involved with some extent and with constancy in serious delinquent activities.

Low levels of persistence in delinquent behavior have also been observed among adjudicated samples of female youth. For example, Lanctôt and Le Blanc (1999) reported that 19% of adjudicated females followed a persistent trajectory from mid-adolescence to the end of adolescence. In spite of their high risk to persist in delinquent and violent behavior, relatively few females did so. Maughan, Pickles, Rowe, Costello, and Angold (2000) reported similar findings based on an accelerated cohort design of 9, 11, and 13 year old American youths ($n = 4,500$). Specifically, they found that only 2.3% of females followed a stable high pathway, compared to 11.7% of males. Most of the youths (87.7% of females vs. 68.4% of males) had a stable low pathway. Finally, 10% of females and 19.9% of males demonstrated a declining pattern of involvement in violence.

Another question that arises is whether the level of female involvement in violent activities is similar to their level of involvement in other delinquent or deviant activities. This question is important in fostering the understanding females' violence in a broader context. Studies conducted on the development of delinquency indicate that violence does not come along (Le Blanc & Loeber, 1998). Youths expressing violence are also involved in a myriad of deviant and delinquent conducts. Thus, prevention and intervention strategies need to evaluate a range of risk behaviors simultaneously, and to focus on a subgroup of youths who are more at-risk than to focus on one particular behavior (Thornberry, Huizinga, & Loeber, 1995). It appears that comorbidity of adolescent problem behavior and delinquency is pervasive, and that adolescents who have multiple problems are more likely to have continuing problems (Nottelman & Jensen, 1995). This association between violence and other delinquent/deviant conducts was mostly examined with males' samples; yet, the literature concerned with females' outcomes is quite scarce.

Arguably, there is a lack of knowledge related to the evolution of delinquent and violent behavior among females. In particular, there have been virtually no studies to date that have examined the development of delinquency and violence among females during the transition from adolescence to young adulthood. In effect, Pajer (1998, p. 869) concludes: "Our understanding of the developmental trajectories of antisocial girls and women is so limited,... that as policy makers or clinicians, we do not know how to prevent or treat such outcomes." In light of this shortcoming, it thus seems necessary to improve the current state of knowledge related to the development of delinquent and violent conducts of females. The results of the present study attempt to fill this void.

METHOD

Between 1992 and 1993, 150 adolescent females adjudicated under the Young Offenders Act for a criminal offense (17%; $n = 26$) or processed under the Youth Protection Act for presenting serious problem behavior (83%; $n = 124$) were interviewed. These females were sentenced by the Youth Court of Montreal to probation, to a social follow-up, or to a placement in a rehabilitation center. Between 1995 and 1996, 123 females (82% of the original sample) were interviewed again. A third wave of data collection was conducted in 2000–2001, during which 113 participants (75% of the original sample) were re-interviewed. In total, 97 (65%) females participated in all three waves of data collection. Each time of measurement is respectively designated as mid-adolescence, end of the adolescence, and young adulthood. It should however be acknowledged that a certain age range exists at each occasion of measurement. Mean ages at each testing time were 15.1 (SD = 1.4), 17.5 (SD = 1.4), and 23.0 (SD = 1.5) respectively.

Most of the females (90%; n = 135) were born in Canada; however, a quarter (24%; n = 36) had at least one parent who had immigrated into Canada. The majority of participants (83%; n = 125) had parents who are separated and came from underprivileged families; approximately two-thirds (62%; n = 93) reported that their mother had received welfare at some point in her life.

Participation in deviant and delinquent behavior was measured through a self-report card-sorting task that included 63 delinquent acts. For each behavior, information regarding age of onset, prevalence, and frequency was collected. The psychometric properties of this task are reviewed in the MASPAQ (Le Blanc, 1996). The violence index was created by summing 13 of these self-report items. Four of these items refer to physical violence (gang fighting, fist fighting, striking someone because of being shoved, and striking someone because feeling annoyed). Four items are related to threats and intimidation (threatening others to get something, threatening to force others to do something, threatening to dominate others, and beating someone for no reason). Three items concern the use of weapons or other objects (carrying a weapon, using a weapon while fighting, and throwing objects at people). The last two items represent indirect violence (encouraging others to harm someone they dislike and accusing others of starting a fight). The prevalence and variety of violence are analyzed. Prevalence rates refer to the proportion of the females who participated in violence in the 12 months preceding each interview while variety is operationalized as the number of different types of acts that were committed by females during that period. With respect to differential sample attrition, there were no differences found between females who had been interviewed at all three occasions of measurement versus those who were lost across testing waves, this absence of differences holds for variety (t = 0.522; p > 0.10) and for prevalence (X^2 = 0.009; p > 0.10).

Results are presented in three sections. First, the involvement of females in violence is described for each time of measurement taken separately. Thus, the participation of females in violence is analyzed for 150 females in mid-adolescence, for 123 females at the end of adolescence, and for 113 females at the beginning of adulthood. Secondly, the three times of measurement are considered simultaneously, which allows for an evaluation of the individual development of violent conduct from mid-adolescence to the beginning of adulthood. This developmental analysis considers the 97 females who were interviewed at each period of the study. This identification of different pathways of violence among females is performed in a multivariate data set through k-means cluster analysis. This type of analysis identifies homogeneous subgroups of cases, within a relatively heterogeneous group. Violence is assessed in terms of age of onset and its variety during the 12 months preceding each interview. Analyses of variance (ANOVA) is conducted to determine whether between-groups differences are greater than within-groups differences for each component included in the cluster analysis. Finally, analyses of variance (ANOVA) is also be performed to verify if females of each violent pathway differ in their level of involvement in vandalism, theft, and drug use. This indicates if the development of violence and that of other delinquent conducts follow a similar pathway. These behaviors were included in the self-report card-sorting task. Vandalism and drug use each refer to 5 items and the index of thefts is composed of 13 items.

RESULTS

Participation in Violence during Three Distinct Periods

During the year preceding their adjudication, close to three-quarters (73%; $n = 110$) of females had committed at least one violent act. While this high proportion is not surprising given the nature of the sample, by the end of adolescence, the reported involvement in violent activities had declined substantially. Only 52% ($n = 64$) reported involvement in violence in 12 months preceding the second interview. Finally, at the final testing period when females were entering early adulthood, only 36% of females reported involvement in at least one violent activity in the 12 months preceding the interview. Thus, the prevalence rates of violence decreased considerably from mid-adolescence to young adulthood among adjudicated females. The variety of violent behavior also decreased across the three testing time. Specifically, at mid-adolescence, approximately one third of the females (31%; $n = 47$) reported having committed at least five types of violent behavior. This proportion fell to 8% ($n = 10$) at the end of adolescence and to 4% ($n = 5$) at the beginning of adulthood. Results also indicate that females are participating in a restricted range of violent activities. Despite the fact that there were 13 different types of violent behavior that were assessed originally, on average only 3.3 kind of violent conducts were reported by females at mid-adolescence. This variety is even lower at the second (1.46) and third (0.73) testing wave.

Interestingly, although the majority of females engaged in violence, particularly during mid-adolescence, the variety of means through which violence was expressed was quite restricted. Thus, the prevalence rates and variety of engagement in violent behavior decreased across the three testing times. Next, the developmental trajectories of this sample of adjudicated females will be explored.

WITHIN-INDIVIDUAL VARIABILITY IN VIOLENCE TRAJECTORIES

What shape does the violent pathway take for females during the transition from mid-adolescence to young adulthood? In order to explore this question, the violent trajectories of the 97 females who participated in the study at all three occasions of measurement were analyzed.

In order to identify and distinguish sub-groups of females according to their levels of participation in violence, pathways of violent activity were identified using k-means cluster analysis. Age of onset and variety of violent offending during the 12 months preceding each measurement occasion were included in the analysis. Three sub-groups of females were identified: non-violent (44%; $n = 43$), explorers (42%; $n = 41$), and decliners (14%; $n = 13$). Mean scores relative to females of each pathway are reported in Table 1. The objective that was pursued has been reached, which was optimizing the intra-group homogeneity while maximizing the differences that distinguish the groups. Indeed, analyses of variance show that, for each predictor, the within-group variance is lower than the between-group variance ($p < 0.001$).

The first subgroup identified is composed of 43 (44%) females who engaged in violence for the first time at a later age: 14.7 years old versus 9.2 and 8.4 among explorers and decliners respectively. Females with the non-violent pathway also exhibited a level of violence throughout the course of the study that was significantly lower than the violence among the rest of the sample. Females following this pathway had engaged, on average, in less than one type of violent activity at each time of measurement.

TABLE 1. MEAN SCORES COMPARISON OF VIOLENCE ACROSS THE THREE VIOLENT PATHWAYS

	Non-violent (1) ($n = 43$)	Explorers (2) ($n = 41$)	Decliners (3) ($n = 13$)	F	Differences between groups
Age of onset	14.67 (2.69)	9.20 (2.52)	8.38 (2.47)	57.90***	1 > 2, 3
Variety of violence					
Mid-adolescence	0.63 (0.87)	4.32 (2.13)	9.92 (1.75)	172.68***	1 < 2, 3; 2 < 3
End of adolescence	0.42 (0.85)	1.49 (1.82)	2.23 (1.88)	9.80***	1 < 2, 3
Beginning of adulthood	0.16 (0.43)	1.15 (1.62)	1.38 (2.02)	7.70***	1 < 2, 3

Note: *** $p < 0.001$

The second subgroup of females was named "explorers" (42%; $n = 41$) due to the relatively high variety scores during mid-adolescence ($M = 4.32$), and subsequent low level of engagement in violence by the end of adolescence ($M = 1.49$) and beginning of young adulthood ($M = 1.15$). The final pathway included the smallest number of females ($n = 13$; 14%). These females engaged in a large number of violent activities during mid-adolescence. On average, they reported involvement in approximately 10 different kind of violent behavior. Despite their high levels of engagement in violence, the variety of their violent behaviors also declined over time. By the end of adolescence and the beginning of young adulthood, these females reported, on average, engaging in 2.2 and 1.4 types of violent activities respectively.

Overall, the developmental analysis suggests that violence, as measured in the present study, is not a persistent behavior among adjudicated females of this sample. Although certain females exhibited high levels of violence at points throughout adolescence, there were no identifiable subgroups that remained highly involved in violence, with respect to its variety, in the transition to young adulthood.

VIOLENCE: A SYMPTOM OF A GENERAL DEVIANT SYNDROME?

The question that now arises is whether the levels of females' involvement in violent activities is similar to their levels of involvement in other delinquent or deviant activities. Are the most violent females also the ones that are the most involved in thefts, vandalism, and drug use? Table 2 reports the variety of these conducts during mid-adolescence for each subgroup of females.

TABLE 2. COMPARISON OF THE VARIETY OF THEFTS, VANDALISM, AND DRUG USE ACROSS THE THREE VIOLENT PATHWAYS

	Non-violent (1) ($n = 43$)	Explorers (2) ($n = 41$)	Decliners (3) ($n = 13$)	F	Differences between groups
Variety at mid-adolescence					
Thefts	1.65 (1.99)	3.54 (2.85)	8.00 (3.34)	30.61 ***	1 < 2, 3 ; 2 < 3
Vandalism	0.28 (0.59)	1.15 (1.29)	2.77 (1.42)	28.55 ***	1 < 2, 3 ; 2 < 3
Drug use	2.88 (1.53)	3.48 (1.50)	4.46 (1.05)	6.06 **	1 < 2, 3

Note: *** $p < 0.001$; ** $p < 0.01$

Results indicate that females from the decliner pathway are not only the most violent females; they are also the ones who are the most involved in thefts, vandalism, and drug use. During the 12 months preceding the first interview, these females reported having committed, on average, 8 different types of thefts on a possibility of 13. Among the 5 behaviors related to vandalism in the self-reported survey, they reported almost 3 of them. Their drug use was also quite important since more than 4 types of drugs were consumed among the 5 types of drugs that were listed in the survey. In opposition, females who committed a very low variety of violent acts from adolescence to adulthood were also involved in very few other delinquent and deviant conducts. These results indicate that the involvement in violence is not independent from the involvement in other misconducts. This observation should guide prevention strategies.

DISCUSSION

Results from this longitudinal analysis indicate that although violence tends to be a common behavior among adjudicated females during mid-adolescence, their participation in violence decreases substantially as they progress towards adulthood. The variety of violent behaviors also declines as females progress in age: while 31% of adjudicated females were involved in a high variety of violent conducts (at least five types of violent behavior) during mid-adolescence, this proportion dropped to 4% at the beginning of adulthood. Similar results were observed by Ayers et al. (1999). Moreover, the examination of within-individual variance in violent behaviors indicates that females who do engage in high levels of violence exit out of this behavior pattern quickly, namely prior to entering late adolescence. There were no identifiable trajectories that demonstrated a pattern of high and constant involvement in violence from mid-adolescence until the beginning of adulthood. Rather, results identified only non-violent, exploratory and declining trajectories.

This significant decline of violence throughout females' transition to adulthood could be explained by the social roles that accompanied this transition. The exposition to diverse life events at the beginning of adulthood (entry into the labor market, living with a partner, becoming a parent) could explain the decline in delinquency and violence (Sampson & Laub, 1993). This applies particularly to females. In fact, it might prove difficult for females to be violent towards others while feeling responsible for the well being of their children and the people surrounding them (Broidy & Agnew, 1998). It is also important to recognize that this very low tendency to persist in violence does not necessarily imply that adjudicated females are escaping from maladjustment as they progress toward adulthood.

Females' personal and social difficulties could be expressed with behaviors, namely drug abuse, that cause more prejudice to themselves than to others. Furthermore, these females are more vulnerable than non-violent females to mental health problems and disorders (Pajer, 1998). These avenues need to be examined with attention in further studies.

Finally, results of this study add to the evidence that there is an association between various forms of deviant and delinquent behaviors. In other words, when females are involved in violence, they also tend to be simultaneously involved to a similar degree in theft, vandalism, and drug use. These results lend support for the following clinical and programming recommendations. First, it may be more beneficial to adjust prevention programs to a myriad of deviant and delinquent behaviors simultaneously rather than to focus on one particular behavior (Thornberry et al., 1995). From this perspective, programs aimed at preventing violence among adolescent females should consider violence as a symptom of a more general deviant syndrome. Moreover, programs should be designed to address within-sex heterogeneity. Prevention strategies should focus especially on a subgroup of females who are more at-risk of being involved to a high extent into deviance, delinquency, and violence. The application of a cognitive-behavioral program would be one clinical strategy to consider. This program aims to restructure youths' cognitive thinking. It is designed to help youths improving their social habits, managing their stress, resolving problems with prosocial means, and better regularizing their anger (Le Blanc, Dionne, Proulx, Grégoire, & Trudeau-Le Blanc, 1998). Such a program is actually put into practice in eight units of girls in readaptation centers in Montreal.

It is important to note that these findings must be interpreted in light of this sample's characteristics and the type of violent behaviors that were examined. In essence, any generalization made from findings based on high risk samples must be done with caution due to the selection mechanisms that are at work. In addition, the types of violence measured in this study were restricted mainly to physical forms of aggression directed towards others. Relational aggression, which is a mode of expression largely used by females (Crick & Grotpeter, 1995), was not assessed sufficiently. The lack of gender-sensitiveness of our measure might explain the restricted variety of means through which females expressed violence.

Finally, in order to better prevent violence and its consequences among females, the next step will be to identify the personal and social factors that are associated with a high involvement in violence. Furthermore, the consequences of a high involvement in violence during adolescence on the quality of females' personal and social adaptation to adult life will be examined. Many outcomes will need to be considered, especially the ones related to the internalization of problems.

REFERENCES

Ageton, S. S. (1983). The dynamics of female delinquency, 1976–1980. *Criminology, 21*, 555–584.

Ayers, C. D., Williams, H., Hawkins, J. D., Peterson, P. L., Catalano, R. F., & Abbott., R. D. (1999). Assessing correlates of onset, escalation, and desistance of delinquent behavior. *Journal of Quantitative Criminology, 15*, 277–305.

Broidy, L., & Agnew, R. (1997). Gender and crime : A general strain theory perspective. *Journal of Research in Crime and Delinquency, 34*, 275–306.

Chesney-Lind, M., & Shelden, R. G. (1998). *Girls delinquency and juvenile justice.* Brooks/Cole Publishing Company: Pacific Grove, California.

Crick, N. R., & Grotpeter, J. K. (1995). Relational aggression, gender, and social-psychological adjustment. *Child Development, 66*, 710–722.

Dunford, F. W., & Elliott, D. S. (1984). Identifying career offenders using self-reported data. *Journal of Research in Crime and Delinquency, 21(1)*, 57–86.

Lanctôt, N., & Le Blanc, M. (1999). Les trajectoires marginales chez les adolescentes judicia-risées: Continuité et changement. *Revue internationale de criminologie et de police scientifique, 52(1)*, 31–54.

Lanctôt, N. & Le Blanc, M. (2002). Explaining adolescent females' involvement in deviance. *Crime and Justice: An Annual Review, 29*, 113:202.

Le Blanc, M. (1996). *MASPAQ : Mesures de l'adaptation sociale et personnelle pour les adolescents québécois: Manuel et guide d'utilisation.* (3ʳᵈ éd.). Montréal : Groupe de recherche sur les adolescents en difficulté, École de psychoéducation, Université de Montréal.

Le Blanc, M., & Loeber, R. (1998). Developmental criminology upgraded. *Crime and Justice: An Annual Review, 23*, 115–198.

Le Blanc, M., Dionne, J., Proulx, J., Grégoire, J., & Trudeau-Le Blanc, P. (1998). *Intervenir autrement: Le modèle différentiel et les adolescents en difficulté.* Montréal, Presses de l'Université de Montréal.

Loeber, R., Wung, P., Keenan, K., Giroux, B., Stouthamer-Loeber, M., Van Kammen, W.B., & Maughan, B. (1993). Developmental pathways in disruptive child behavior. *Development and Psychopathology, 5*, 101–133.

Maughan, B., Pickles, A., Rowe, R., Costello E. J., & Angold, A. (2000). Developmental trajectories of aggressive and non-aggressive conduct problems. *Journal of Quantitative Criminology, 16*, 199:221.

Nottelman, E. D., & Jensen, P. S. (1995). Comorbidity of disorders in children and adolescents: Developmental perspectives. In T. H. Ollendick & R. J. Prinz (Eds.), *Advances in Clinical Child Psychology, 17*, 109–155.

Sampson, R. J., & Laub, J. H. (1993). *Crime in the making: Pathways and turning points trough life.* Cambridge: Harvard University Press.

Thornberry, T. P., Huizinga, D., & Loeber, R. (1995). The prevention of serious delinquency and violence: Implications from the Program of Research on the Causes and Correlates of Delinquency. In J. C. Howell, B. Krisberg, D. J. Hawkins, & J. J. Wilson (Eds.), *Serious, violent, & chronic juvenile offenders (pp 213–237).* Thousand Oaks: Sage.

Pajer, K. A. (1998). What happens to bad girls? A review of adult outcomes of antisocial adolescent girls. *American Journal of Psychiatry, 155*, 862–870.

Wangby, M., Bergman, L. R., & Magnusson, D. (1999). Development of adjustment problems in girls: What syndromes emerge? *Child development, 70*, 678–699.

7

Race, Gender, and Aggression

The Impact of Sociocultural Factors on Girls

MARGARET A. JACKSON

In the street or in school, it's the same. I don't feel I belong. But I learned that if somebody beats on me, I'd better beat back or I'll keep getting hurt. Actually, now I get respect because of it.

Lena, young immigrant girl, age 14

Lena's words capture the dilemma experienced by many young marginalized girls today, but which seem especially true for young immigrant and refugee girls (Chesney-Lind, 2001; Mayeda, Chesney-Lind, & Koo, 2001). To fit in, to survive, they may turn to aggression; otherwise they may find themselves the target for aggression. Numerous authors in this text focus upon individual risk factors to explain and/or predict why some girls are more prone to aggressive and violent behavior than others. In the present chapter, the examination shifts to consider the social context within which the particular factors of race and gender can prove to be "risky" for girls.

Evidence that the social location of immigrant and refugee girls constitutes a form of risk in and of itself comes from a 1993 Working Group Report in which the members indicate that such girls "experience higher rates of violence due to the impact of racism and sexism in their communities and the host society and due to dislocation as the result of immigration" (Barron, 2001, p. 1). As Jiwani (1998) comments, the girls are "caught

MARGARET A. JACKSON • School of Criminology, Simon Fraser University, Burnaby, British Columbia, Canada, V5A 1S6 between two cultures where their own is devalued and inferiorized, and where cultural scripts in both worlds encode patriarchal values" (p. 3). As well it appears that refugee girls are actually in a more vulnerable position than refugee boys in this regard (Barron, 2001).

In some cultural contexts girls are less valued than boys and, as a result, are at higher risk for neglect and abuse. Their participation in educational endeavors, for example, is often prematurely curtailed and they are subject to sexual abuse, assault, and exploitation in greater number than are boys (Cameron, 2001). For the above reasons, as well as the fact that girls are an understudied population for this topic area more generally, the focus for this chapter will be upon immigrant and refugee girls.

It is the intent of this chapter to take a closer consideration of the sociocultural factors which may contribute to and have an impact on, the immigrant and refugee girls' vulnerability to both being aggressed against and acting aggressive themselves. Framing the analysis throughout, the voices of the young women themselves serve as the data. In the attempt to make meaning of their experiences, the theoretical lens employed is feminist and rights-based. The rights-based perspective is appropriate as it is evident that these factors of race and gender "place the immigrant and refugee girl-child at greater risk for all forms of discrimination and human rights violations" (Cameron, 2001, p. 3). In essence, examining how these sociocultural factors uniquely intersect (Jiwani, Janovicek, & Cameron, 2002) for the girls provides an understanding which should be contrasted with a similar focus placed on the impact of individual factors, such as mental health status, on this vulnerability.

The concept of interlocking systems of domination forms the theoretical basis for the former analysis (Razack, 1998). It is critical, as Razack argues, to consider in a historical manner the meaning of race, economic status, class, disability, sexuality, and gender as they converge to socially construct immigrant and refugee girls within hierarchical social structures (Barron, 2001). In this chapter, the focus is limited primarily to the examination of the impact of race and gender, or more accurately, the processes of racialization and gendering upon the aggressive outcomes for the girls. The study of processes rather than static factors allows for a deeper appreciation of how these categorizations are constructed through continuous interactions in society, continuous constructions of "other" and "self" in hierarchical ways (Chan & Mirchandani, 2002). There are parallels to this kind of analysis with Moretti's (2001) study of self-other representations in her analysis of relational and overt aggression in adolescent girls and boys.

STUDY I: THE VOICES OF IMMIGRANT
AND REFUGEE GIRLS

Three interrelated Feminist Research, Education, Development, and Action Centre (FREDA) Centre studies are discussed.[1] The present author was director of the Centre when the studies were conducted. The first study involved 59 immigrant and refugee girls of color in 14 individual interviews and 6 focus groups. They or their parents were born in other countries. Among the 18 countries of origin were China, Ethiopia, Pakistan, and Zaire.[2] The age requirement for participation was that the girls be between 14 and 19 years of age. The questionnaire was developed with input and feedback from a group of young immigrant and refugee girls. As well, young women of color led the interviews and focus groups. This first study focuses primarily on the processes that can intersect to increase the girls' vulnerability to marginalization and aggression.

The girls were asked to talk about their experiences in school and with family and friends. It is a "lived realities" approach which can then be used for comparison with the intended outcomes of relevant policies and programs developed to assist the girls. One question, for example, after the girls were requested to define "safety" and "respect," inquired how they felt about their treatment in the school environment: safe, respected? Their responses could then be compared with current attempts to secure that safety and respect by way of such initiatives as anti-bullying and multicultural programs.

Turning to the findings, the most prominent issue to emerge from the interviews and focus groups was what the girls described as a struggle for power among young people from different cultural groups. Those struggles were often described as violent, as seen in bullying behaviors. Many girls pointed to racism as a key cause underlying violence in the schools and they recognized intercultural tensions as a feature of school life (Jiwani et al., 2002).

A quote from an interview with a self-described Persian girl sets out the intercultural divisions that seem to underlie the tensions:

---

[1] FREDA is one of five research centres across Canada originally funded by Health Canada and SSHRC (Social Sciences and the Humanities Research Council) to undertake research in the area of violence against women and children.

[2] The first report is entitled, "Erased Realities: The Violence of Racism in the Lives of Immigrant and Refugee Girls of Colour" and was authored by Yasmin Jiwani, Nancy Janovicek, and Angela Cameron. It was funded by Status of Women.

> You know in high school people are like that. They talk behind each other's
> backs. I don't know why. They hate them because of their culture, where they're
> from. Because people in this school hang out with each other... They just like
> hanging out with their own country people. (Jiwani et al., 2002 p. 67)

Many of the girls talked about the difficulty of fitting into the dominant
culture. It is true that girls who are seen as being different because of race,
gender, sexual orientation, disability, and/or class generally are at greater
risk of being taunted and targeted for violent acts because our society
tends not to value those who are different (Jiwani et al., 2002). This can be
observed not just in the school environment but in the wider community
as well.

Among the most vulnerable appear to be those girls who have recently arrived in Canada. In schools, recent immigrants are called FOBs,
an acronym for "fresh off the boat." One interviewed girl from Persia defined it this way: "FOB is like fresh off the boat. It means that you're really
geeky and you don't know how to speak and stuff. You dress stupidly or
whatever, right?" (Jiwani et al., 2002, p. 68)

Assimilation is one answer for the girls but can entail a loss of
identity with their own culture or negotiating a balance between the
two, often competing, traditions. One interviewed girl described it this
way, "sometimes I feel like I have to lose my 'true' identify to fit in"
(Jiwani et al., 2002, p. 68). The process of identity formation then can
clearly be problematic for these girls. Their sense of belonging is influenced by their particular location in a culture, on the one hand, and
the disjuncture of that location from the dominant culture's norms, on
the other. This disjunctive affect about self clearly has an impact on the
girls' feeling of status and worth, a finding consistent with those of Artz
(1998), Crick and Dodge (1996), Crick and Werner (1998), and Moretti
(2001).

From the interviews, it became evident as well that schools are often
seen as sites of external control rather than serving as places of support or
safety. Schools are where the tensions become crystallized, and where many
girls expressed frustrations with what they experienced as discrimination
against immigrant and refugee girls. A South Asian girl commented that,
"from what I've seen, the kids fear it (racist acts in school) so they won't go
and tell people about it. They'll just keep it inside. And I think that sooner
or later, it's just going to make them explode. So if I could give advice,
I'd tell them, number one, go to a person who you know you can trust. I
wouldn't say first to go to somebody at school" (Jiwani et al., 2002, p. 71).
As Corrado, Odgers, and Cohen (2000) found in their study of incarcerated
girls in Canada, "authorities" making decisions about troubled girls, in the

name of protecting them, can actually often remove them from their social context of support and incarcerate them.

In addition to general challenges at school, the girls also identified problems with language as an obvious reason for feeling marginalized in schools. Often these young women are streamed into alternative classes because they have not yet developed efficient language skills. A Thai girl, who lives in a small British Columbia Interior town, explained that for the first two weeks of school she did not understand a word that was said in class. When one of her parents explained this to the teacher, she was subsequently placed in remedial classes because English as a Second Language (ESL) classes were not available (Janovicek, 2001).

As well, the girls can be taunted for their accents and for the clothes they wear. Their own parents, who encourage them to fit in, often do not have the economic resources to purchase high fashionr clothes that are almost mandatory in many popular school groups (Janovicek, 2001).

Having examined how the processes of racialization and gendering can impact on the girls' vulnerability to marginalization and aggression, we now take a look at the "flip side", that is, how those same processes can come together to increase their vulnerability to commit acts of aggression themselves.

STUDY II: IMMIGRANT AND REFUGEE GIRLS ON PROBATION

The second supplemental FREDA study (Barron, 2001) interviewed eight girls who were either on probation or had been on probation. Half of the respondents had been charged with assault (Barron, 2001). The basic questionnaire employed in the first study was also used for the second (with some modifications because these girls were not as likely to be in school at the time of the interview and because the focus was more upon their criminal justice experiences). In the questioning, the girls were asked about specific areas dealing with "the kinds of violence the girls were knowledgeable about, including questions about racism, health issues, and survival strategies" (Barron, 2001, p. 13). For example, with regard to the last issue of survival strategies, the girls were asked what they learned to do to cope.

Barron (2001) notes that first "the girls only appeared to recognize racism as a factor in violence when asked if they would define racism as being violent" (p. 24). One girl said yes, explaining that "Even though the person isn't physically [hurt], it hurts them emotionally inside, you know, and I think that hurts more cause when someone hits you, it could be over, but when someone says something about your race, you could be thinking about that for the rest of your life, and you'll have doubts about that kind of race" (p. 24).

Unlike respondents in the first study, few girls included race as a factor in triggering aggressive encounters. One example can be seen in the response made by a girl against another visible minority girl: "When you fight, it's nothing about race, it's all about popularity . . . You don't just hate someone because of what they are, but how they treat you" (p. 23).

The same girl indicated she had been called racist names when she was in grade 7, and it offended her at the time, but now she says she is proud to be referred to as "China-woman." This kind of racist naming gets explained away by another girl who offers the rationale that the person does not intend to be racist, they are just "mean" spirited individuals. They also expressed the belief that there was more conflict between different visible minority communities than between people of color and white people (Barron, 2001). Thus the process of "conventional" racialization by the dominant culture becomes obscured.

The case of another girl, Amy (not her real name), is relevant to the discussion on how a girl's experience of violence against herself can lead to her own involvement with violence against others. Amy was charged with assault and admitted to the charge saying, "my mom hit me, so that's when they took me away. When I went into care, I didn't know anything right, so I assaulted my foster mom and that's how it all started" (Barron, 2001, p. 17). The situation is parallel to a case reported in Chesney-Lind (2001). And again, quoting Barron:

> She further explains that her mother, who cannot speak English was not given any support after she and her father immigrated to Canada from Hong Kong and then her father left the family without financial resources. It is ironic and disturbing that Amy's charges of assault and uttering threats stemmed from a process of her being placed into care for her own 'safety' from her own mother. (p. 25)

Amy's experiences exemplify how a particular social location can have a negative impact on how an individual is perceived and processed as a risk. Here the concept of risk can work to the disadvantage of these girls. It is worthy and relevant to note the emphasis on the determination of risk for decisionmaking about girls on probation, e.g., that is evidenced in the British Columbia Youth Community Risk/Assessment instrument. One risk factor of concern in that instrument, for example, is the fact that "the youth is facing difficulties or conflicts relating to cultural, ethnic, or religious adjustment, including conflicts or adjustments with peers or family" (Barron, 2001, p. 18). But the question has to be asked, whose risk has priority in decisionmaking here, the risk of the girl to the community or the risk *to* the girl in the community? These are policy and rights questions.

There appears to be the assumption that the problems facing the immigrant and refugee youth who has come to the attention of the justice system arise from difficulties in her or her family's adjustment to the dominant white society. The difficulties of adjustment are articulated as difficulties of not integrating sufficiently, or not releasing cultural traditions sufficiently to fit in. This was confirmed as problematic in a small probation file review on the girls interviewed. In one file, it is indicated that "family members barely speak English and it's been difficult to contact anyone at home despite numerous phone calls and random home visits" (Barron, 2001, p. 18). This was taken to provide evidence of poor parental supervision.

In another file reviewed by Barron, the mother's situation was used to support a similar allegation of poor family supervision. It was an arrangement in which the mother of the girl on probation was the sole caregiver and had to work at three jobs to support herself and her daughter. In this case, the so-called family was required to undergo counseling to improve parenting and conflict resolution skills. Thus the same criminal justice program is used to monitor both the girl's and the immigrant mother's behavior.

The above case profiles yet another systemic factor that has an impact on the increasing risk to the immigrant and refugee girl, that is, poverty (for more detailed discussion of this factor's influence, see also Reitsma-Street's chapter in the present text). It is already evident that there are links between poverty and discrimination against women and children (UN Working Group on Girls, 1995; Barron, 2001). These connections are proven here in Canada for immigrant and refugee women and their offspring. With their lesser economic status and restricted labor force involvement, they are vulnerable to being assessed as second class citizens (Cameron, 2001). One example to illustrate this situation is the one whereby the professional credentials of many immigrant and refugee women are not recognized in Canada; another is the disadvantaged and still unresolved situation of domestic workers at risk (National Association of Women and the Law, 1999; Parrenas, 2001).

Barron (2001) concludes that it is the risk assessment process in the justice system that contributes to the immigrant and refugee girls' vulnerability to getting caught up in that very system. In essence, the emphasis on the individual girls' problems of adaptation to the dominant society denies the systemic prevalence of violence in their lives. As we have seen, it is the system, in this case the justice system, that may set these young women of color up for failure, through the system's own technologies of assessment.

And it is the intersection of processes tied to race, gender, and poverty, rather than individual deficiency factors, that figures most prominently in the equation.

Clearly the results from this small pilot study[3] suggest the need for a fuller, more systematic examination of justice system decision making for this population to be undertaken.

STUDY III: THE VOICES OF SERVICE PROVIDERS WORKING WITH THE GIRLS

The third FREDA study (Janovicek, 2001) examined the perceptions of service providers who work closely with girls and provides confirming information for the other two projects' findings.[4] Five roundtables were conducted with 38 service providers, 10 of whom work with street-involved girls, 10 with lesbians, bisexual, and transgendered girls, 8 with Aboriginal girls, and 6 with girls with disabilities. In addition, individual interviews were conducted with four service providers with immigrant and refugee girls. The goals of the roundtables were to gain an understanding of the girls' lives and to discuss ways to support girls. The participants were asked to comment on the factors influencing girls' identity formation, their vulnerability to violence, the barriers the girls face, and how they understand and respond to systemic disadvantage. Finally, the service providers also discussed the policies' impact on girls' lives and made recommendations for reform (Janovicek, 2001).

Those interviewed point out that a lack of services for these marginalized girls makes them more vulnerable to violence. Girls who do not meet the dominant society's expectations will not be seen as fitting in. The participants argued that existing services are more likely to be based upon models of social control and punishment than assistance and support. These responses appear to be derived from more general societal perceptions that the youths are out of control and need to be reformed. Improving services therefore would require a shift in the perception of both service providers *and* the community about young people from the margins (Janovicek, 2001).

---

[3] The second report is entitled, "The Invisibility of Racism: Factors that Render Immigrant and Refugee Girls Vulnerable to Violence, and was authored by Christie Barron. It was funded by SSHRC, Grant No. 829-1999-1002.

[4] The final report of that project is entitled, "Reducing Crime and Victimization: A Service Providers' Report," and was authored by Nancy Janovicek. The study was funded by the National Crime Prevention Centre, Community Mobilization Program, Ministry of Justice, Canada.

One quote from a service provider nicely capsulates the general sense of the respondents with regard to the role the system plays in creating the disadvantaged state for these marginalized girls:

> I think it's set up though to alienate some children in the interest of others, the whole system . . . institutions, penal institutions . . . . They're creating it for those people who they've set up to put there. And most of them don't expect their golden children to be there and they end up there. This is where we have the therapists and all the psychologists and the psychiatrists justifying why this person's behavior would be like this. You never hear such justification for the poor kid or the racialized kids who get institutionalized. (Interview with Service Provider working with Immigrant and Refugee Girls, Janovicek, 2001, p. 5)

Peled, Jaffe, and Edleson (1995) make the point that the clinicians making such assessments are often white, male, and from a higher socio-economic class than those they see as clients or patients.

The service-providers also felt that conflicting cultural values between the family and the dominant society are a major problem for the youths (Janovicek, 2001). First there may be disciplinary measures taken in the immigrant or refugee home that conflict with Canadian norms. Certain types of spanking are examples of that kind of measure which is legally sanctioned in Canada, but which is often practiced in other countries. Sexual mores represent another common area of conflict. Though sexuality can be a hidden issue in many immigrant and refugee communities, in the Canadian culture, women of color are often sexualized in the media and other means of communication. Therefore mixed messages are externally delivered to the girls but silence at home on the topic does not allow them to understand the messages. Other issues such as HIV/AIDS, homosexuality, and acceptable sexual practice can be similarly hidden (Janovicek, 2001). As a result, although most of the girls interviewed in the first two studies indicated they were proud of their heritage and family, the family itself does not evolve as the site for support or clarification on the sensitive issues which make the girls even more vulnerable to negative external influence.

The service providers interviewed also identified schools as a primary site of violence for the girls. According to them, "intercultural tensions among young people are seldom understood to be a manifestation of racist and patriarchal relations" (Janovicek, 2001, p. 10). Rather, it is argued in the report, the media and teachers tend to emphasize bullying as the problem. Again, individual children are blamed with little attention paid to the sociocultural dimension. It is obvious though that the process of racialization in the school system is demonstrated in the negative experiences identified (Canadian Council on Social Development, 2000). And these experiences can trigger a downward spiral in which girls drop out of school, become alienated from their family, hit the street, and become targeted for prostitution and aggression.

It is true that power plays can be involved in the tensions resulting in bullying. Defending the pecking order protects a particular group's social location, and, power relations are also played out within cultural groups on the street as well as in school. As one service provider analyzed:

> I think there is an expectation that if you don't exert your power over somebody, then you are on the bottom of the pecking order... It's no different on the street but the level of competition then becomes physical because the only thing that you have left are your fist or your words... I think that we've created a population of young women who just believe that they need to victimize someone else to get their own power back because what they've been taught is you're either a victim or a victimizer. (Janovicek, 2001, p. 4)

This kind of thinking is consistent with what Artz (in the present book) found with her interviews with girls in custody (for example, "violence is wrong, and I only hit people I *have* to"). Thus, aggression which occurs within a peer group sorts out who possesses the control in the group—and this can happen within gender groups as well (Janovicek, 2001). According to the service providers, the girls are the most vulnerable. They agreed that, through the use of violence and sexual domination, boys maintain control over groups of girls on the street (Janovicek, 2001).

One service provider explained how this translates into a survival strategy: "In the squats, it's just a given. I've heard young women say, 'Just choose now who you're going to have sex with because you're going to have sex with somebody to stay here because that's the way it's run.' The guys are making that really clear. That's just the trade-off and that's the power in the squats" (p. 16). But teachers and the media tend not to acknowledge that fights and conflicts also often have a racialized edge. When young people of color do defend themselves against racist slurs and/or bullying, teachers tend to blame them for provoking fights and being the bullies (Janovicek, 2001).

The interviewees also commented that students, as we have seen to be true in the interviews with the girls themselves, often do not seem to find racism a problem. They indicated that they find students who were born here seem to find an affinity with the dominant culture and see immigrant and refugee kids as "other" (Janovicek, 2001). The latter perception is consistent with what Barron (2001) found in her study, when interviewing immigrant and refugee girls on probation, in the referencing of recent immigrants as FOBs.

And, as was true with the findings from the other two studies, the service providers also identified language difficulties as generally contributing to the girls' challenges in school and their feelings of alienation in particular (Janovicek, 2001). Often the girls' participation in English as a second language (ESL) classes results in them feeling further marginal- ization as second class citizens. But the most challenging issue for the girls though, according to Janovicek (2001), remains the one of different sets of cultural values that frequently conflict with one other. Girls in abusive dating relationships, for example, may continue in the relationship just to defy their parents' cultural values. Because of this, they are particularly vulnerable since, as stated previously, they often do not feel they can turn to their parents for help and understanding (possibly affecting feelings of attachment, see Moretti chapter, this book). Intersecting with the other difficulties with language, gender, and poverty, it appears then that the tensions between cultural values that affect expectations of one's behavior in society can create serious dilemmas for the girls.

DISCUSSION AND CONCLUSIONS

In reviewing the findings from the three studies, through the theoret- ical lens initially set out, several common themes emerge:

First, the same systemic processes of discrimination can disadvantage the girls and make them more vulnerable both to becoming targets of aggression and for becoming aggressive themselves.

Second, it is clear that the racialization process for the immigrant and refugee girls can work both within the dominant culture and within the racialized culture itself. That is, the girls may come to internalize the dom- inant culture's racialized view of themselves as being inferior (Mayeda, Chesney-Lind, & Koo, 2000). As well, the girls provide evidence of feel- ing discriminated against, especially in the school setting, but they may not connect that same process with their own peer experiences in conflict situations. They recognize hierarchies amongst different "minority" cul- tural groups, but construct them as power hierarchies, not necessarily as explicitly racial ones.

Third, tensions from conflicting cultural expectations make the girls more vulnerable. Thus, many of the girls interviewed expressed mistrust of school authorities to assist in support and counseling, and did not nec- essarily see their families as locations for clarification on troubling issues about sexuality and bullying.

Fourth, vulnerabilities arising from the girls' social location can result in their being considered as "risky" from the dominant society's perspec- tive, as was the case for the girls on probation.

Finally, when trying to come up with solutions, all the above findings can be further analyzed through a rights-based lens, whether it is through application of Section 15 equality provisions of the Canadian *Charter* or the U.S. *Bill of Rights*, or, through such instruments as the provisions of the *UN Convention on the Rights of the Child* (see Woolard and Connolly et al.'s chapters in this book for further consideration of the role of law on these matters). It is evident that because of discrimination, the girls' rights to well-being and safety are jeopardized, and should be available to legal remedies—although broad stroke legal solutions are probably not the most effective for dealing with school and street level changes in attitudes and action.

SELECT RECOMMENDATIONS FROM THE STUDIES

THE INTERVIEWED GIRLS

The girls who were interviewed identified different solutions to these tensions in schools. Among them, they proposed a program that would bring different groups together for a bonding type of experience. They could then work their problems out together, and come up with solutions together (Jiwani et al., 2002). From Barron's (2001) study, one girl indicated that she felt "the best way to prevent violence was to have 'more group activity, 'cause I think the more group activity they have the more different races will come to it, not just like one kind of race. That could help like get along more and get to know each other 'cause like I think the reason why racist people don't like other races is because they don't know them very well" (p. 29). Thus the girls obviously felt programming that would facilitate the bringing together of diverse groups would assist in resolving these tensions.

BARRON/SSHRC CHILD STUDY

From her study on girls on probation, Barron (2001) argues that there are definite problems with ESL classes in the school setting because the girls taking them are labeled as inferior and are made fun of, which discourages them from taking the classes. Her recommendation therefore is similar to what others have also proposed: change the program's description from remedial English programs for those with language limitations to calling them additional bilingual classes for those who already have competence in one language.

Shariff (2002) also examined anti-violence programs and found that few appear to have an impact on reducing violence in the schools. The few that are effective usually contain a grass-roots component, as they involve representatives from the community. These programs are not standardized to fit all and do not rely on the usual approaches to antibullying, anger management, conflict resolution and behavior modification. Indeed, this approach seems to have been introduced as a topic largely irrelevant to the everyday lives of these children, in particular the young immigrant and refugee girls who constitute our focus. Teaching children about rights in school has also been shown to be effective in reducing the number of bullies and racists (results from a Nova Scotia study, as reported in *The National Post*, 2001, June 30, p. A4).

In addition, it was recommended that teachers and counselors from the same cultural communities should be hired so that they can act as role models for both immigrant and Canadian born students.

Finally, there is the recommendation that peer mentor programs for recent immigrant students be developed.

SERVICE PROVIDERS' STUDY

The service providers suggested some points of intervention: first, that curricular development in schools needs to move away from the multicultural emphasis on difference. It has been argued that multiculturalism policies are in fact dangerous because they give the illusion that something is being done to harmonize inter-cultural relations, while in fact not addressing the inequalities that emanate from the lack of respect for diversity. The service-providers also felt that the provincial government needs to take a more proactive stance in promoting equity for girls from marginalized communities. *Zero-tolerance* and bullying policies are often insufficient because they mask the power relations behind school violence. Furthermore school policies tend to be blind to gender issues, and thus perpetuate patriarchal relations in the school system itself.

Traditional services often employ a "quick fix" approach to the problems. Proponents of this approach expect that the girls will demonstrate positive changes in a few weeks. One service provider argued that this is an unrealistic expectation because years of abuse and marginalization cannot be cured in a few weeks. Thus, as they are presently established, intervention programs can set girls up for failure. This makes them more vulnerable to violence since they believe that they have failed or have been found lacking once again. It was also recommended that teachers should be more active in monitoring and addressing racism in the schools. They need anti-racist training themselves so that they can also monitor their own behavior.

In conclusion, effective programming for girls needs to consider all of the intersecting factors discussed above. We are in agreement with the conclusions of Chesney-Lind (2001) in this regard: "Finally, programs should invariably work to empower girls and advocate for change that will benefit them. This entails not only building on girls' innate strengths, skills and creativity to develop their voices and their abilities to assert themselves, but also identifying and challenging barriers (such as race, gender, and poverty) that girls, particularly marginalized girls, face in our society" (parentheses added, p. 6).

REFERENCES

Artz, S. (1998). Where have all the school girls gone? Violent girls in the school yard. *Child & Youth Care Forum, 27*, 77–109.

Barron, C. (2001). The invisibility of racialization: Factors that render immigrant and refugee girls vulnerable to violence. Unpublished manuscript. Vancouver: Feminist Research, Education, Development, and Action (FREDA) Centre for Research on Violence against Women and Children.

Cameron, A. (2001). From rhetoric to reality: Canada's obligations to the immigrant and refugee girl child under international law. Unpublished manuscript. Vancouver: FREDA Centre for Research on Violence Against Women and Children.

Canadian Charter of Rights and Freedoms (1982). Available at: *www.pch.gc.ca/ddp-hrd/canada/guide/index_e.shtml*.

Chan, W., & Mirchandani, K. (2002). *Crimes of colour.* Peterborough, Ontario: Broadview Press.

Chesney-Lind, M. (2001). What about the girls? Delinquency programming as if gender mattered. *Corrections Today, 63,* 38–44.

Convention on the Rights of the Child. 20 November 1989, 1989 UNTS 1992/3.

Crick, N., & Dodge, K. (1996). Social Information-processing mechanisms in reactive and proactive aggression. *Child Development, 96,* 993–1002.

Crick, N., & Werner, N. (1998). Response decision processes in relational and overt aggression. *Child Development, 69,* 1630–1639.

Corrado, R., Odgers, C., & Cohen, I. (2000). The Incarceration of female young offenders: Protection for Whom? *Canadian Journal of Criminology, 42,* 189–207.

Immigrant Youth in Canada (2000). Canadian Council on Social Development. Ottawa.

Janovicek, N. (2001). Reducing crime and victimization: A service providers' report. Vancouver: FREDA Centre for Research on Violence Against Women and Children.

Jiwani, Y. (1998). The Girl Child: Having to 'Fit'. Vancouver: FREDA Centre for Research on Violence Against Women and Children.

Jiwani, Y., Janovicek, N., & Cameron, A. (2002). Erased realities: The violence of racism in the lives of immigrant and refugee girls of colour. In H. Berman & Y. Jiwani (Eds.), *In the best interests of the girl child* (pp. 45–88).The Alliance of Five Research Centres on Violence, Status of Women Canada, Ottawa.

Mayeda, D., Chesney-Lind, M., & Koo, J. (2001). Talking story with Hawaii's youth: Confronting violent and sexualized perceptions of ethnicity and gender. *Youth & Society, 33,* 99–128.

Moretti, M., & Odgers, C. (2002). Aggressive and violent girls: Prevalence, profiles and contributing factors. In R. R. Corrado, R. Roesch, S. D. Hart,. & J. Gierowski (Eds.), *Multiproblem violent youth.* Amsterdam: IOS Press.

Moretti, M., Holland, R., & McKay, S. (2001). Self-other representations and relational and overt aggression in adolescent girls and boys. *Behavioral Sciences and the Law, 19*, 109–126.

National Association of Women and the Law (1999 March). Gender analysis of immigration and refugee protection legislation and policy (Submission to Citizenship and Immigrations Canada).

Parrenas, R. (2001). *Servants of globalization: Women, migration, and domestic work.* Stanford: Stanford University Press.

Peled, E., Jaffe, P., & Edleson, J. (1995). *Ending the cycle of violence: Community responses to children of battered women.* Thousand Oaks, CA: Sage.

Razack, S. (1998). *Looking white people in the eye: Gender, race, and culture in the courtroom and classrooms.* Toronto: Oxford University Press.

Shariff, S. (2002). Rhetoric or reality? An analysis of the impact of school anti-violence initiatives on racialized immigrant and refugee girls. Unpublished manuscript. Vancouver: FREDA Centre for Research on Violence Against Women and Children.

Smyth, J. (2001, June 30). Teaching children about rights leads to fewer bullies, racists. *The National Post,* Saturday, p. A4.

United Nations High Commissioner for Refugees (UNHCR) policy on refugee children. UNHCR EXCOM Subcommittee of the Whole on International Protection, 54th Sess., 23rd Meeting UNHCR Doc. EC/SCP/82 (1993).

Working Group on Girls (Non Governmental Organizations (NGO) Committee on UNICEF) (1995). Clearing a path for girls: Summary of NGO's report from the field on progress since the Fourth World Conference on Women, Beijing, China, 1995. Available at: *www.girlsrights.org.*

Youth Community Risk/Needs Assessment Rating Guidelines (1999). British Columbia Ministry for Children and Families. Victoria: Provincial Government of British Columbia.

8

Revisiting the Moral Domain

*Using Social Interdependence Theory to Understand
Adolescent Girls' Perspectives on the Use of Violence*

SIBYLLE ARTZ

In my ongoing research on understanding adolescent girls' use of violence,
I have long been haunted by a remark made to me by a 14-year-old girl
who was trying hard to help me to see the rationale for her use of violence.
As she pointed out, "Violence is wrong, and I only hit people I *have* to." She
was not alone in making this claim. All the girls I have spoken with over
the years have told me one by one, "I never hit anyone unless I have to,"
and "I only hit people who deserve it." For them, the use of violence was
not desirable, but none-the-less required. In other words, for them, there
appeared to be a moral imperative for their actions.

The girls' words, their narrative of self and other, particularly their use
of "I" statements, seemed to underline the notion expressed by a number
of researchers who study moral action that such behavior is situated in
identity and experience, and given that we are all self-interpreting beings,
the direction and meaning of personal action provide clues to explanations
for behavior. As Gilligan (1988), one of the first researchers to be concerned
with a positive grasp of girls' and women's morality, notes "The close ties
I have observed between self-description and moral judgment illuminates
the significance of how ... different images of self give rise to different vi-
sions of moral agency" (p. 7). Porter (1991), in her book, *Women and moral
identity*, also suggests that, "As self-interpretive beings we attach different

SIBYLLE ARTZ • School of Child and Youth Care, University of Victoria, Victoria, British
Columbia, Canada, V8W 2Y2.

meanings to experiences. Moral action is influenced by a host of motivations that affect our self-understanding, our interpretation of situations and the ultimate outcome of moral judgments" (p. 148).

Gilligan and Porter, however, differ in how they tie self-interpretation to moral action. Gilligan (1988), much like her mentor Kohlberg (1981), ties that self-description to a stage theory of moral development. For Kohlberg, moral development is grounded in universal principles and proceeds in an invariant and systematic way through three stages, each with two levels: the first stage is pre-conventional morality grounded in punishment and obedience, then instrumental relativism. Next comes conventional morality grounded in interpersonal concordance and then law and order. The final stage, post-conventional morality, is grounded in social contract legalism and then a principled conscience guided by ethics of impartial universal justice. In Kohlberg's system, girls often lag behind boys in their moral development because they largely fail to invoke an impartial application of rights-based rules and universal justice and appear to stay focused on interpersonal concordance—that is concerned with pleasing or helping others, being "nice" and "good" and not with universal justice.

Gilligan (1988) takes exception to Kohlberg (1981) in that she disputes the moral inferiority of girls and proposes instead that girls' morality is grounded not in the justice orientation that Kohlberg claims for all human beings, but in a care orientation that makes primary the preservation of relationships. According to Gilligan, Kohlberg's system describes primarily male moral development and is inadequate for females. She suggests that the developmental course of morality for females is premised initially on being responsible solely for the needs of self, then, as girls mature, becomes focused on a responsibility for meeting the needs of others *before* self, and finally when moral maturity is achieved, is anchored to a balanced approach that promotes taking responsibility for meeting the needs of both self and others. Gilligan thus claims different underlying cognitive structures for males and females. But Porter (1991) disagrees with both Gilligan and Kohlberg. She contends that in construing moral decisions as the outcomes of underlying developmentally driven cognitive structures, stage theory based systems fall short by not taking seriously the importance of self description and instead abstract self from world and fail to take into account both the agency of persons as self-interpreting beings and the personal context of moral dilemma.[1]

Stage theory aside, there is strong agreement that interpretation of self and world is key to moral action. Katz (1988), in examining the use of violence suggested that the key to behavior that is otherwise not espoused

---

[1] For an in-depth discussion of limitations of conceptualizing moral decision making as the product of individual moral development see Porter (1991).

but none-the-less practiced, can be found in an analysis of the conditions and interpretations that are the context for such behavior. Moretti, Holland, and MacKay (2001) have also offered evidence of the importance of self-representation or self-interpretation to indirect and direct use of aggression in girls. Thus, if one is to understand moral judgment, one must first of all understand the interpretive, contextual basis of that judgment. Analyzing first for moral developmental stage may foreclose, rather than assist such an inquiry.

In my earlier research I had already looked for evidence that pointed to moral developmental stages either as described by Kohlberg (1981) or by Gilligan (1983, 1988) and given that I was studying adolescent girls, listened for the "Different Voice," the voice of care and responsibility for relationship, the voice described by Gilligan as uniquely female. Having done that over time, I had concluded that in the narratives provided by my female research participants there was little evidence of that different voice (Artz, 1998). Instead, given the emphasis on having to use violence against even one's friends and acquaintances if conditions demanded it, I found some evidence of the self-centered and self-serving moral reasoning characteristic of Kohlberg's pre-conventional moral stage (Colby & Kohlberg, 1987). This finding was consistent with the position taken by numerous other researchers that adolescent and adult females and males who offend against others consistently demonstrate a pre-conventional approach to moral reasoning and are therefore delayed at this stage since the expectation is that they should be moving out of this stage around the age of 10 and have left this stage behind by age 13 to 14 (Arbuthnot, 1984; Blasi, 1980; Taylor & Walker, 1997; Trevethan & Walker, 1989).

I had, however, also concluded that while statements claiming that victims "had" to be beaten, that is, were responsible for their own victimization because they acted in ways that demanded the exercise of violence against them, may well be indicative of a self-serving orientation towards questions of right and wrong, other explanations were also both possible and perhaps more powerful. Porter (1991) and Katz (1988) both allow for an examination of the social conditions that give rise to justifying violent aggressive and violent action as the basis for a more fully rounded understanding of moral action, but neither Porter or Katz have developed a framework for examining these conditions beyond a strong affirmation of the inseparability of self, context, and behavior. Others, for example, Taylor and Walker (1997), note the links elsewhere in the moral development research between coercive parenting, low levels of attachment, and delayed moral development and emphasize the importance of working towards improving moral development as Gibbs, Arnold, Ahlborn, and Chessman (1984) and Arbuthnot and Gordon (1988) have done through improving the "moral climate." But Taylor and Walker characterize moral climate in terms of Kohlberg's stage theory and provide no additional information about the social conditions that perpetuate a delayed climate and with it a delayed individual other than that morally delayed climates are populated and dominated by morally delayed people.

I continued to research the personal narratives of girls who use violence, but had not pursued either the development or the discovery of a framework that further explained moral climate until Magnuson (1999, 2002) prompted me to take up this question again. Magnuson's application of Johnson and Johnson's (1989, 1998) research on the goal structures of social interdependence theory offers what had thus far been missing for me, a promising framework for examining the conditions that promote moral experience.

As Magnuson (2002) points out, it is the "characteristics of social structure and not individual traits,"(p. 5) that in Johnson and Johnson's (1998) terms, structure a "hidden curriculum that permeates the social and cognitive and with it moral development of children, adolescents, and adults... [and has] a set of values inherently built in" (p. 3) are central to understanding individual action. These conditions provide us with clues as to how people may be interpreting self and world and how they may be morally positioned with regard to their actions.

THE CONDITIONS OF MORAL EXPERIENCE

The three conditions of moral experience identified by Johnson and Johnson (1989, 1998), assume different but equally compelling social values and give rise to very different forms of self-representation and with that, different grounds for moral action Magnuson (1999, 2002).

COMPETITION

In social conditions premised on competition, people engage in a zero sum game that pits them against all others in a battle for extrinsically motivated gains and rewards. The right thing to do, then becomes whatever it takes to win, to dominate, to get or keep for oneself what is desired. Under these conditions, the winner takes all and must forever defend her or his position.

INDIVIDUALISM

In social conditions premised on individualism, people focus on their personal needs and must negotiate meeting these needs with others also engaged in the same undertaking. The right thing to do emerges out of an observation of the rules of fair play that dictate that each individual has the right to equal access. Under these conditions, winning is premised on successfully persuading others that one's needs are more undeniable than theirs and that one ultimately has the greater right to the ends that others are also pursuing.

COOPERATION

In social conditions premised on cooperation, people are committed, even dedicated to, a common community of practice or cause, a shared purpose and a set of agreed upon standards that they both aspire to and uphold. The right thing to do is to work for the common cause and to achieve excellence in terms of that cause. Under these conditions, winning is premised on successfully cooperating such that the group meets the agreed upon end, the common goal. Even where personal action is concerned, such action is always examined in the light of the commonly agreed upon standards and goal.

These three conditions became the framework against which I re-read previously analyzed data and re-examined earlier questions about adolescent girls' perspectives on their use of violence. In so doing, I am not suggesting that this framework be applied exclusively to girls. In fact, given the research on the developmental challenges faced by males (c.f., Garbarino, 1999; Pollack, 1998) this framework may well hold a great deal of promise for boys. I confine myself here, as a first step, to an analysis of data on girls and suggest that, in future, a similar analysis of data on boys be included along with an analysis of gender differences.

REVISITING PREVIOUS RESEARCH

SOURCES OF THE ANALYSIS

In examining previously analyzed data, I re-opened the transcribed interviews that focused on my earlier informants' ways of understanding themselves, their life worlds, and the ways in which they made sense of their own and others' behavior particularly with respect to the use of aggression and violence. These were the six key informants who participated in a fourteen-month long study of violent school girls (Artz, 1996, 1998), to which I added interview data from seven adolescent key informants involved in research on violence prevention conducted over a 5-year period in a school district on Vancouver Island (Artz, 2000), seven female young offenders residing in a Vancouver Island custody center (Artz, Blais, & Nicholson, 2000), and four adolescent females interviewed while making a documentary on girls who use violence (Artz, 2002). Given Magnuson's (1999, 2002) findings about a social interdependence anchored in competition, I looked especially for evidence of competition, and it was everywhere to be found.

Evidence of Competition

Evidence of competition abounded in the transcripts. As one girl explained, "When you're a teenager you're in kind of a conflict position where you have to keep your own position and not let people put you down" (Artz, 1998, p. 192). In order to make sense of the varieties of competition experiences discussed by the research participants I have organized these into categories focusing on self-description, description of family, peer relations, and the social conditions in the research participants' schools and custody centers.

Self-Descriptions Premised on Competition

I took self-descriptions in which girls ranked, compared, or somehow measured themselves against others as evidence of competition and found that every girl I talked to had in fact spoken about herself in this way. Schoolgirls who used violence described themselves as "usually the tougher person who'd be like the tougher one that people would have to back down against." They also spoke of labeling themselves as being one of "the scummy people," or of being labeled as "stupid" by teachers, or as "bitches," "sluts," "ho's" by family members and their peers, and talked about being "losers" and being "ugly" and feeling like "an outcasted little person" (Artz, 1998). Incarcerated girls also described themselves as being called "bitches" and "sluts" and so forth, as being termed "ugly" and "dirty," and as being seen as and seeing girls in general as meaner and more vicious than boys (Artz et al., 2000). The labels that they dealt with were always comparative, that is, formulated as greater or lesser than others, and often negative, even demeaning. One girl recently told me, "I'm a girl that can defend herself and stand up for herself. I'm named a bully." Another said, "I won't back down, I'm not like that. I can't really do that just because of my reputation of who I am. If I do, rumors will fly around [and they'll say], oh my god, this chick won, she backed down."

One extreme example of experiencing herself as competitive came from a young woman who had spent a number of years moving in and out of custody often for violent offenses:

> I used to see how long sessions [in jail] I could get. I wanted to see if I could go
> up for arson or attempted murder. I have so many charges on my record. I have
> an accessory to murder. I have an arson, a causing accidental death. It was an
> accident, but it was still a death. I have all this crap on my record and it's like
> the way I was. (Artz et al., 2000, p. 15)

In describing themselves, these girls often referred to family, and when discussing family and peer relations they talked about feeling pitted against those closest to them.

FAMILIES AS BATTLEGROUNDS FOR DOMINANCE AND CONTROL

All the participants in my various studies, despite speaking about loving their family members, described their families as networks based on battles for control and dominance where fathers fought with mothers, some mothers fought back almost on a daily basis, parents fought with children, and siblings fought with each other. The girls talked about fathers who used intimidation and violence against their mothers, and who also in some cases entered into sibling rivalries with them over attention from their mothers. As one girls stated about her stepfather, he "is not like a father unless he has to be." Instead, he "acts like a brother" to her, listens to her music, talks the way she and her friends do using expressions like "dude" and relates to everything she does in the same way that she and her friends do. This led to a kind of rivalry that she described as "constantly fighting like brother and sister" and created some problems for Sally because as she put it, "I do need him to act like a parent."

Following in this vein, the girls described their mothers as either entering into the fray and competing for dominance with fathers or taking diffident and defensive roles that left their daughters feeling defenseless in the face of the fathers' aggression (Artz, 1998, Artz et al., 2000). They also talked about alliances with their siblings against their parents, especially fathers, but they also talked about intense rivalry among siblings, "My sister used to kick my ass every day and I'd be up there and I'd go, "Want to fight?" And then I'd run away. I've been doing that since I could talk (Artz et al., p. 19).

Much of what the girls talked about is expressed in the example that follows:

> All our fights start over stupid things, just little stupid things, and they always
> seem to happen on vacation or something like that. 'Cause Christmas time
> we'd always get in a fight, and the family would split up. My dad would go
> somewhere for a couple of days before Christmas, then come back. My sister

and I got in a big huge fight [over who could wear a particular pair of shoes] on Valentine's Day, and I ran away...(Artz, 1998, p. 87)

As one girl summarized her family experience, "I guess my family has a lot of hate for each other, like everybody and stuff. Like I hated my mother and felt hated by her...taken for granted by her..." (Artz et al., 2000, p. 20). Another girl talked about her ongoing verbal and sometimes physical battle with her father, a battle in which she sided with her mother and fought on an almost daily basis against his dominance of the household and the expectation that she should clean up after him. As she stated,

I think he should do more around the house. And he's such a slob. I mean half the stuff around this house is from him. I mean all this shit right here, all those papers there are his...he's just a slob and he walks into the house with his big work boots on and tracks dirt everywhere and it pisses me off...and when I say, "Take your damn boots off your feet for the last time!" he goes, "I'm doing business, so get out of here." (Artz, 1998, p. 116)

The competitive dynamics that the girls described as characterizing their home lives did not stop once they left the family sphere of influence; very similar interactions and values were described as persisting in their relationships with peers, even those they called their friends.

Peer Relationships and Friendships Premised on Rivalry, Competition, and Dominance

All the participants in my studies talked about being in constant competition with peers and friends. One girl talked about having a relationship with her best friend that was the kind of friendship where "she wanted to see me get pushed around, and I would love to see her pushed around too" (Artz, 1996, p. 100). Other girls described their experiences with friends and peers as follows:

Other girls...I don't like other girls my age...everything is...they're competition. [and] They see you as competition. You can never walk down the street and look at a girl and smile because that girl is glaring at you. She's sizing you up...The majority of girls are just bitches. And you try and fit in with them and all that stuff and suddenly, I don't know, they're just competition...competition for guys, anything, the best clothes, the prettiest, everything is a competition, *everything* is a competition. (recently transcribed interview)

When asked about how they thought and felt about the way in which they perceived other girls, one girl explained that,

Personally, like I can't say that I like everybody, right? So I have my share of girls that I totally hate...My share of girls that I victimize....I victimize a girl because she pissed me off, or she did something...that I want to get her back for... Like she looks at me the wrong way... [or like the girl I assaulted] she told a lie about my boyfriend... (Artz et al., 2000, p. 30).

As a schoolgirl who participated in my research explained, she felt caught up in what she called the "pretty power" hierarchy where,

Girls fight over who's prettier than who, about popularity, about guys. Why fight over boys—I think we're all in a constant competition with each other because a lot of us have the same taste. All of us like one person—say one guy is good looking, we're all in a fight over who's getting who. Why is that so important? Some of it has to tie in with the popularity thing, whether or not you have a boyfriend, and people are like "Oh my boyfriend and oh blah, blah blah." (Artz, 2000, p. 48)

All the girls interviewed concurred that, "Guys is always a big one. Like boyfriends and stuff," (recently transcribed interview) when discussing the focus of their competition with each other. In describing how one got to the top of the "pretty power hierarchy," (Artz, 2000, p. 47) one girl explained:

First of all, [to be a leader] it depends on how long you've been here [a custody center, a school, a neighborhood]. Second it's how big you are and who you hang out with and how you act and how you treat people. Leaders are the ones who are the prettiest or who are accepted by the boys and maybe a little bit like me. I'm a victimizer... victimizers are basically on top. (Artz et al., 2000, p. 25)

The girls' competitive and hierarchical experiences of their peers and friends reached also to the way in which they described the social conditions in their schools and the custody center.

THE GIRLS' EXPERIENCES OF THE SOCIAL CONDITIONS IN THEIR SCHOOLS AND CUSTODY CENTER

For the girls involved in my research, their schools and custody center were places where they believed that they continuously had to compete for positions of dominance. As one female custody centre resident explained,

We're all tight in here, boys and girls, but you can't say it's going to be right with all the girls... One's going to be prettier and one's going to be uglier [and if you're uglier] you're going to get victimized... Like "Oh you slut, I'm going to kill you. I'm going to stab you. I'm going to shake you in here. Like I'm going to vent[2] you. All of ten girls against you two, or you three. It's going to be all of us against you guys and stuff. Nobody likes you. If you rat us out, we're going to beat the shit out of you. And if you leave here, and we see you, you're going

---

[2] "Venting" is threatening a girl with verbal physical and sexual victimization through the air vents between cells.

to be in an alley and we'll pimp you" ... They say harsh stuff like that ... It's like you have to watch out no matter what, and no matter where you are or anything. You have to watch out. (Artz et al., 2000, p. 27).

Girls in custody reported being verbally, physically, and sexually victimized by boys and girls, with those lower on the hierarchy [read less physically appealing and strong] experiencing more victimization, but with no girls escaping the sexual harassment meted out especially by the boys but also by other girls on a daily basis (Artz et al., 2000).

Schoolgirls who participated in my research talked about how difficult the social conditions in their schools were because in their social worlds fights happened every day and people were "mean" and their reputations were constantly on the line, where they felt they were "living on the edge" and where others organized beatings against them or challenged their reputations, where they routinely experience sexual harassment and sexual objectification, they engaged in battles with teachers and administrators and had little hope of feeling safe (Artz, 1998). As one girl who had dropped out of school because she was afraid of getting beaten up again said, "I don't like the world right now, I think it's a piece of shit" (Artz, 1998, p. 97).

The girls in my studies described a world in which they needed to constantly struggle and compete for social survival, where even if they had a reputation for dominance and regularly intimidated others, they felt that they had to watch their backs and constantly defend their reputations and social positions. For these girls, violence was indeed wrong but always a necessity. Their survival depended on it at home, at school, and in custody.

IMPLICATIONS FOR UNDERSTANDING GIRLS' USE OF VIOLENCE

If competitive social conditions and with these a grasp of self, other, and world that suggests an ongoing struggle for personal and social survival do indeed contribute to girls' use of violence as my re-examination of my research data suggests, then much may be gained from investigating the social structures that are the life worlds of violent girls for the "hidden curriculum," identified by Johnson and Johnson (1998). This curriculum shapes the existential understanding of those who live within it, permeates their interpretive capacities, and may well be fundamental to explaining their behaviors. If the hidden curriculum is central to our understanding girls' use of violence, then we are required to treat their behaviors as symptomatic of their social structure. If competition is a driving force, we can then very likely expect a means-end, win-lose survivalist morality based on extrinsic rewards. We can then also work towards shifting the curriculum away from these principles and assumptions toward a more cooperative and collaborative mode. As Kelly (2003) points out,

> The vast body of developmental research has revealed that at birth, children do not have mind-sets that predispose them toward delinquency, drug use, or any other form of deviant behavior. To the contrary, these studies have pointed unanimously to an inborn state of healthy mental functioning in children, which includes a natural interest to learn, an intrinsic ability to act in mature, common sense, non-deviant ways and a natural desire to use and expand their abilities in legitimate and pro-social directions. (p. 58)

Kelly argues emphatically for caring, supportive, non-judgmental, non-punitive relationships between troubled children and youth and adults as the basis for behavioral change. He argues just as emphatically against treating young people who use problematic behavior as a way of dealing with the world as damaged, defective, and somehow "*missing* some essential factor (e.g., social skills, assertiveness, functional cognitions, self-esteem, impulse control, etc.) which if supplied from *outside–in*, would prevent or control their dysfunctional tendencies" (p. 2). Kelly notes the importance of creating opportunities for healthy psychological functioning through inclusion, relationship building, and community partnership, in other words, through collaboration and communication—not competition based external reward systems, the very systems that are so often that basis for intervention in the youth custody centers to which adjudicated violent girls are sentenced (Artz et al., 2000).

Certainly more research needs to be done on the moral conditions discussed here and their relationship to stage theories of moral development. Magnuson (1999, 2002) has already contributed to such research and, like Porter (1991), has suggested that our current stage theories of moral development fall short because they assume only an individualistic basis for moral decision-making and because they ultimately abstract the individual from her or his context. Neither Kohlberg (1981) nor Gilligan (1983) offer a system for understanding morality that allows for a clear understanding of the self-in-context that is the agreed upon basis for the emergence of moral voice. Further, in offering us only a "male" and a "female" voice, these two systems do not allow for the many within group differences among males and females, or for the possibility of shared contexts that because of the "inseparability of the self and the context," (Porter, 1991, p. 170) inform sexual identity, gender, moral identity, and moral action along with a host of other symbolic interactions between people and groups.

We come again to the importance of examining the social conditions of our actions. Our "take home" message can be that while we further explore these questions through research, we can also shift our understanding of girls who use violence. If we move away from deficit based models that construct girls who use violence as morally delayed and perhaps not even "properly female" given the absence in their discourse of the voice of care, we can move towards models that take into account girls' lived experiences, their meaning making processes grounded in the hidden curriculum that informs their self-other representations, and help them to use their interpretive capacities as a basis for change.

REFERENCES

Arbuthnot, J. (1984). Moral reasoning development programs in prison: Cognitive developmental and critical reasoning approaches. *Journal of Moral Education*, 13, 112–123.

Arbuthnot, J., & Gordon, D. (1986). Behavioral and cognitive effects of a moral reasoning development intervention for high-risk behavior disordered adolescents. *Journal of Consulting and Clinical Psychology*, 54, 208–216.

Artz, S. (1996). The life worlds and practices of violent school girls. (Doctoral dissertation, Victoria, BC: University of Victoria, 1996).

Artz, S. (1998). *Sex, power, and the violent school girl*. Toronto, ON: Trifolium.

Artz, S. (2000). 'Considering adolescent girls' use of violence: A researcher's reflections on her inquiry.' *The B.C. Counsellor*, 22, 45–54.

Artz, S. (2002). Vancouver conference on aggression and violence in girls. Educational video, Victoria, BC, Ottawa, ON: Justice Canada, Youth Justice Policy.

Artz, S., Blais, M., & Nicholson, D. (2000). *Developing girls' custody units*. Unpublished report to Justice Canada.

Blasi, A. (1980). Bridging moral cognition and moral action: A critical review of the literature. *Psychological Bulletin*, 88, 1–5.

Colby , A., & Kohlberg, L. (1987). *The measurement of moral development, volume I: Theoretical foundations and research validation*. Cambridge: Cambridge University Press.

Gibbs, J., Arnold, K., Ahlborn, H., & Chessman, F. (1984). Facilitation of sociomoral reasoning in delinquents. *Journal of Clinical and Consulting Psychology*, 52, 37–45.

Garbarino, J. (1999). *Lost boys: Why our sons turn violent and how we can save them*. New York: Free Press.

Gilligan, C. (1983). *In a different voice: Psychological theory and women's development*. Cambridge, MA: Harvard University Press.

Gilligan, C. (1988). Remapping the moral domain: New images of self in relationship. In C. Gilligan, J.V. Ward, & McLean Taylor (Eds.), *Mapping the moral domain*. Cambridge, MA: Harvard University Press.

Johnson, D.W., & Johnson, R.T. (1989). *Cooperation and competition: Theory and research*. Edina, MN: Interaction Book.

Johnson, D.W., & Johnson, R.T. (1998). Cooperative learning, values and culturally plural classrooms. In M. Leicester, C. Modgill, & S. Modgill (Eds.), *Values, the classroom and cultural diversity*. London: Cassell, PLC.

Katz, J. (1988). *Seductions of crime: Moral and sensual attractions of doing evil*. NY: Basic.

Kelly, T. (2003). Health realization: A principle-based psychology of positive youth development. *Child and Youth Care Forum*, 32, 47–72.

Kohlberg, L. (1981a). *The meaning and measurement of moral development*. Worcester, MS: Clark University Press.

Leschied, A., Cummings, A., Van Brunschot, M., Cunningham, A., & Saunders, A. (2000). *Female adolescent aggression: A review of the literature and the correlates of aggression* (User Report No. 2000–04). Ottawa, ON: Solicitor General Canada.

Magnuson, D. (1999). *Social interdependence: The goal structure of moral experience.* (Doctoral dissertation, Minneapolis, University of Minnesota, 1999).

Magnuson, D. (2002). Qualities of moral experience under cooperative, competitive and individualistic conditions. Unpublished manuscript, Cedar Falls, Iowa, School of Health, Physical Education and Leisure Services, University of Northern Iowa.

Moretti, M., Holland, R., & McKay, S. (2001). Self-other representations and relational and overt aggression in adolescent girls and boys. *Behavioral Science and the Law, 19,* 109–126.

Peplar, D., & Craig, W. (1999). *Aggressive girls: Developmental disorders and outcomes.* Downsview, ON: LaMarsh Centre for Violence and Conflict Resolution, York University.

Pepler, D., & Sedighdeilami, F. (1998). *Aggressive girls in Canada.* Ottawa, ON: Human Resources Development Canada.

Pollack, W. (1998). *Real boys: Rescuing our sons from the myths of boyhood.* New York: Henry Holt.

Porter, E. (1991). *Women and moral identity.* North Sydney, NSW: Allen & Unwin.

Taylor, J., & Walker, L. (1997). Moral climate and the development of moral reasoning: the effects of dyadic discussions between young offenders. *Journal of Moral Education, 26,* 21–43.

Trevethan, S., & Walker, L. (1989). Hypothetical versus real-life moral reasoning among psychopathic and delinquent youth. *Development and Psychopathology, 1,* 91–103.

Whithecomb, J. (1997). Causes of violence in children. *Journal of Mental Health, 6,* 433–442.

9

Connecting Policies, Girls, and Violence

MARGE REITSMA-STREET*

Hungry and alone, Kimberly Rogers died in August 2000. She was serving a six month sentence of house arrest in Sudbury, Ontario for the crime of collecting student loans while on welfare (MacKinnon & Lacey, 2001). Although Kimberly had been the first person to appeal successfully the automatic suspension of welfare upon conviction for welfare fraud, she could not support her unborn baby and herself on the meager benefits. Had she gone to college several years ago she would not have been convicted for completing college successfully while collecting both student loans and welfare. It had been legal to do so before. But in 1997 new welfare laws and policies made this option illegal.

Violence of girls is not the primary focus of this chapter in the way it is in most chapters of this book. Rather there is an examination of the trend towards restrictive welfare and punitive justice policies that increases the vulnerability of girls to violence especially if living in low income communities. The restrictions limit the capacity of girls to develop and live as citizens. Concern about the trend is illustrated in a dramatic event that took place in a city thousands of miles away from where Kimberly died.

* This chapter is dedicated to Dr. Jennifer Keck of Sudbury Ontario who until her untimely death was an active member of the Committee to Remember Kimberly Rogers. Thanks to Heather J. Michael for assistance in preparing this chapter, and helpful comments of editors.

MARGE REITSMA-STREET • Studies in Policy and Practice in Health and Social Services, Faculty of Human and Social Development, University of Victoria, Victoria, British Columbia, Canada, V8W 2Y2.

Several girls and young women in Victoria, British Columbia, had been inspired by the efforts of Kimberly Rogers to better herself through schooling and to struggle against the injustice of new welfare laws. They named themselves the Victoria Anti-Poverty Coalition Kimberly Rogers Womyn's Brigade. On April 26, 2002 they occupied a politician's constituency office, told staff to leave, locked the doors, and gave a statement to the press protesting the restrictive new welfare policies in British Columbia. On the windows they pasted signs stating "No jobs, no welfare, no housing" and "Death sentences for the poor." The politicians, media, and police argued the protestors were "aggressive," having intimidated and "rough housed" staff (Curtis, 2002). Those charged with assault and obstruction disputed these reports of violence as did eyewitnesses (Kelly, 2002). Police dressed in full riot gear responded to the protesters' actions by using a battering ram to forcibly remove the women from the office and by pepper spraying three girls who sat on the street in front of the police wagons. The protestors agreed to plead guilty to mischief and were given conditional discharges while a charge against the police for excessive use of force was dropped.

One could argue Kimberly Rogers and members of the Kimberly Rogers Womyn's Brigade committed acts of violence, damaging the welfare of others and themselves. One could also state those acting on the authority of municipal, provincial and federal laws acted violently: indirectly by passing laws that limited the capacity of women on low incomes to feed and better themselves, and directly by pepper spraying young women protesting welfare cuts. This chapter, however, disrupts the usual focus on aggressive and threatening acts of individuals, whether girls or police. Instead the focus is on key recent societal policies that threaten the welfare of young women and expose their vulnerability to violence. Although restrictive welfare and punitive judicial policies negatively affect boys as well as girls (e.g., Platt, 2001), I will not compare the impact of policies on girls versus boys nor examine who is more unjustly treated. A focus on gender differences or discrimination diminishes the opportunity to clarify the submerged and missing experiences of girls. Furthermore, concentrating on girls and comparing changes in policies over time rather than by gender, can have fruitful implications for research and policy changes benefiting both girls and boys.

POLICING THROUGH POLICIES

The concept of "policing girls" (Reitsma-Street, 1998) frames the examination of changes in Canadian and American welfare and youth justice laws. Policing processes regulate and enforce particular attitudes and behaviors. They include informal activities that reinforce behaviors through shame or praise, and formal institutional processes produced through policies and laws. Policing processes are engaged in by everyone. The more influential ones are created by persons taking positions of power in households and communities: the policies and practices they legislate can be enforced by giving or withholding resources, and by authorizing the use of force. The concept of policing points to the myriad of processes or "techniques" (Donzelot, 1979: 8) used by persons to convince and pressure girls to incorporate particular feminine attitudes, behaviors, and identities that "keep them in their place" (Carlen, 1995: 215). Researchers of American, European, and Canadian girls conclude girls are not just socialized, but policed to grow up good and pressured to take care of others before themselves. Taking care of others includes the responsibility to keep society wholesome and pure and to defend one's reputation and pick productive partners (Artz, 1998; Cain, 1989; Reitsma-Street, 1998; Schlossman & Wallach, 1978).

Historically policing processes included policies and practices that limited girls access to education and adequate paid work, pushed them into performing a disproportionate amount of relational and provisioning work for those they love, while making invisible the attendant costs of economic dependency, the burden of unpaid heavy work, and the devalued status of less productive citizens (Brown & Gilligan, 1992; Kostash, 1987; Sharpe, 1994; Smart, 1976). Informal and formal policies have changed over time. There is even cautious optimism that policing girls to fulfill narrow expectations about beauty, femininity, and dependency have eased with increased access to education, respect for diversity, and public denunciation of relationship violence (Bhavnani, Kent, & Twine, 1998; Rosenberg & Garofalo, 1998).

New purposes and variations of policing processes, however, have emerged. Girls and women are now pressed to become responsible for the double future of homemaker and laborer (Kearney, 1998; Walkerdine, Lucey, & Melody, 2001) and the triple obligations of domestic, employment, and volunteer community work (Hancock, 2002; Neysmith & Reitsma-Street 2000). In anti-poverty and anti-violence programs it is girls who are expected to shoulder the extra responsibilities for ensuring peaceful relationships, consensus building, and developing social capital as well as human and financial capital (e.g., Rankin, 2002). When pressures to fulfill multiple obligations increase at the same time policies restrict opportunities, girls find themselves working harder to defend their limited options, sometimes using illegal and violent activities to do so. Those who do not or cannot succeed, encounter serious penalties: unsafe working conditions and inadequate housing; anxiety, anger, and depression; denial of social and housing benefits; and more criminal records and custody sentences if convicted of violating either justice or social policies (Chesney-Lind, 1999; Platt, 2001). Kimberly's sentence for welfare fraud exemplifies the new harshness: a sentence of 6 months house arrest, 18 months probation, and repayment of student loans and welfare overpayment. The following sections explore the trend towards increased use of restrictive social policies and punitive youth justice laws to police girls.

RESTRICTIVE SOCIAL POLICIES

Criminologist Pat Carlen argues there are "malign institutional" policies and practices that deliberately favor some persons at the expense of others or that purposively restrict opportunities of people (1995, pp. 213–214). In the recent past, correctional policies restricted education for girls to training programs for low wage service jobs; liberal arts education or apprenticeships for well-paid trades were the exception, not the norm (Ackland, 1982; Brenzel, 1983; Chesney-Lind & Sheldon, 1998). Practices instructed correctional workers to attend more carefully to anger management, normative heterosexual behavior, and vaginal maladies of girls than their need for financial management skills or assertive healthy sexual expression (e.g., Geller, 1987). Most restrictive are the malign policies that tore generations of black and native children from their communities, selling them into slavery or locking them in residential schools for most of the year where their language, culture, and family ties were systematically destroyed (Fournier & Crey, 1997). More invisible than malign policies are "antisocial" policies. In his book *Anti-Social Policy*, Squires (1990) examines policies and practices that are "frequently disciplinary in practice and profoundly 'anti-social' in their consequences" (1990, p. 2). Policies are antisocial when they exclude girls from education and train girls for insecure, poorly paid jobs with few medical and pension benefits while disregarding the relationship, household, and community obligations that girls and young women are expected to, and often want to fulfill (Hancock, 2002; Rose, 1993).

From the 1960s until the 1990s, there had been a perceptible *decrease* in both malign and antisocial types of policies, improving opportunities of girls and women in Western European and North American countries (e.g., Evans & Wekerle, 1997; Headey, Goodin, Muffels, & Dirven, 1997). More female citizens became eligible for modest social assistance and social housing. Access to higher education and health care increased significantly, although millions remain excluded in the United States as it has no universally medical insurance policy. Minimum wages and employment standards improved. There were minimal gains, however, in public support for quality child, home, or elder care, except in non- English speaking states such as Quebec, France, Denmark, and Holland (Knijn & Kremer, 1997). Often excluded from access to the benefits of these policies are those girls classified as refugees, immigrants, and illegals who provide cheap labor in service industries and homes of wealthier citizens (McWatt & Neysmith, 1998; see also Jackson's chapter in this book).

By the turn of the 21st century Canadian citizens continue to have access to publically governed and funded primary education as well as hospital and doctor services despite strong pressures to shrink these public services in favor of more private ones. There were even modest improvements in 2002 to a national monthly children's benefit program geared to low income families in the paid labor market. But there remains minimal support for public quality childcare, a policy that deeply affects children and the girls and young women who are their primary caretakers (Ferguson, 1998; Knijn & Kremer, 1997). Moreover, other progressive trends are being systematically reversed in the 1990s. New types of "antisocial" and "malign" policies make more girls vulnerable to violence and restricted opportunities, especially those from poor neighborhoods. For instance, the public guarantee and obligation to provide for persons in need in Canada, that had been legislated 30 years ago in the federal *Canada Assistance Plan*, was abolished in 1996. Enforceable national standards for citizens in need have diminished; no longer are there laws for instance prohibiting forced employment of needy persons. By the mid 1990s there were deep federal and provincial cuts to all social, housing, education, and health services. More cuts followed in British Columbia when a new government took office in 2002 (Rice & Prince, 2000; Friends of Women and Children Report Cards, 2002). Throughout Canada, there are now more food banks and food cupboards than McDonald fast food outlets. Homelessness, hunger, and fear of violence are growing in this rich country (Layton, 2000).

The reversed trend is clearest in the new welfare laws and policies. It was the *Ontario Works Act* of 1997 that cut eligibility to welfare and increased sanctions in Canada's most populous province for poor young women like Kimberly Rogers who wanted a college degree and a better job. The Kimberley Rogers Womyn's Brigade were protesting the new British Columbia *Employment and Assistance Acts*, approved in 2002, that affects 6.5% of the province's population as well as their neighbors, friends, and local businesses (National Council of Welfare, 2002). The two year maximum of benefits in British Columbia for single persons not able to prove serious disabilities is harsher than any other welfare policy in Canada and Europe. Previously, benefits had been far from adequate especially for single young persons (Goldberg & Long, 2001). In 2002 benefits were cut up to 40%. Virtually all job earnings and support payments are taxed at 100%.

Girls under and over 18 years of age are totally ineligible for any welfare assistance until they prove—with written documents—they have lived independently and productively for two years, except if fleeing an abusive household or seriously disabled. Youths (and adults) are ineligible for benefits if they want to finish high school, take an apprenticeship course, or pursue post-secondary education unless they offer proof of serious disabilities. If eligible, girls may take short term job training programs in tourism or hospitality services offered by for profit companies; ironically, these programs are paid for by public funds (Reitsma-Street, 2002).

In the United States "welfare as we knew it ended" in 1996 with the *Personal Responsibility and Work Opportunity Reconciliation Act* (Whitaker & Time, 2001, p. 77). Federal and state programs for poor families and communities, called Aid to Families with Dependent Children, that had always been less generous and publicly supported than similar programs in Europe and Canada, were abolished along with any guaranteed support for families in need. The new Temporary Assistance for Needy Families programs drastically restrict eligibility and welfare payments for families. Assistance ends in five years, often sooner. Expectations to work for welfare and involuntary volunteering have increased along with more penalties for late, incomplete reporting and fraud.

These examples of new restrictive social policies in Canada and the United States, police girls and young women, especially if poor, to stay in relationships and school, regardless of violence or quality of life. Girls are pushed to accept any paid job, even if inadequate remuneration, illegal, or unsafe (Mosher, 2000). Rose (1993) and Mink (1998) argue that historically American welfare policies prepared girls to see few options besides marriage, domestic duties, parenting and volunteering. The current welfare laws push girls into low wage service or piece-work with minimal rights to publicly funded services. If girls have to live on limited income with inadequate resources to provide for necessities, they are particularly vulnerable to the policing and violence of family members, neighbors, and professionals who judge their suitability, eligibility, and performance as a condition of receiving a few health, education, housing, and social benefits.

What will be the impact of these restrictive policies on girls? Ehrenreich and Piven (2002) ask what happens to girls, women, mothers, and children when people are freed from welfare dependency to go into the job market but there are no jobs, no childcare, and no welfare. The poverty rate for Canadian youth under the age of 18 was remarkably high in the 1980s rising to 21% in 1995 (National Council of Welfare, 2001, p. 5). The urban poverty rate in 1995 was highest for female youth age 15 to 24 at 32.9% (Lee, 2000, p. 28). One in three youths were poor in the large American cities by the late 1980s, and over 40% for African-American and Latino households (Greene,

1993; Schnaffner, Shick, & Stein, 1997, p. 192). These high poverty rates existed *before* the recent cuts and restrictive policy changes just described. It is expected female youth poverty rates will increase in Canada and the U.S. as the consequences of more restrictive welfare, educational, work, and other social policies ripple outward. In studies of those leaving or pushed off welfare by the new laws, researchers found very few youths or families were better off than before, while close to 90% experienced more unmet medical needs, hunger, utilities cut off, and no addresses (e.g., Bezanson & McMurray, 2000; Hancock, 2002; Patriquin, 2001; Lindhorst, Mancoske, & Kemp, 2000). Unless costs of living decrease dramatically and access to good jobs increases, it is expected the trend towards restrictive policies will prompt more girls and young women from poor communities to earn money and status through any job they can find whether in service industries, the new call centers and sweat shops, sex trade work, selling of drugs, or petty theft. Girls will be exposed to more risks of violence due to unsafe working conditions, poorly restricted labor relations, and sharp competition.

PUNITIVE YOUTH JUSTICE POLICIES

Girls and young women in the 19th century were tried as adults and subjected to adult sentences whether convicted of murder or shoplifting. The punitive nature of adult criminal laws and policies was substantially modified in the 20th century by the rehabilitative purposes and processes of special youth laws, youth courts, youth sentences, and youth workers. As we move into the 21st century, the return to punitive policies for youth is striking despite their high financial costs, their questionable impact on reducing fear or recidivism, and serious debates about the accuracy and causes of actual levels of crime (e.g., Chernoff & Simon, 2000; Doob & Sprott, 1998; Hallet & Hazel, 1998; Platt, 2001; Steffensmeier & Allan, 1996; Winterdyk, 2000).

The rates and numbers of Canadian and American youths convicted and sentenced to custody have increased significantly in the last 20 years. Platt (2001, p. 147) concludes "juvenile offenders are now regarded as adult criminals in-the-making" while both Platt (2001) and Childs (1997) find more American black youths end up in prison than in college. In Canada, the shorter, determinate custody sentences introduced in the 1984 *Young Offenders Law* were an improvement over the longer, indeterminate ones authorized in the previous *Juvenile Delinquents Act* (Doob, 1992). But as the *Young Offenders Act* was amended over the years, the maximum sentence increased from two to three, then to five, and finally up to ten years for serious offenses (Fetherston, 2000). Public organizations were quoting a Canadian statistical report in the mid-1990s that concluded Canada incarcerates youths at twice the rate of the U.S. per 1,000 youth population; both countries have much higher custodial rates than European ones (House of Commons, 1997, p. 3; National Council of Welfare, 2000, p. 63). The rates and lengths of open and secure custody sentences of girls convicted in Canada have steadily increased over the years from 18% in 1992 to 27% by 2000 (Canadian Centre for Justice Statistics, 1990–2000).

Besides the obvious increase in longer sentences and custody rates for convicted girls, there is a subtler approach in how Canadian and American youth justice laws police girls. In Canada, status offenses had been abolished in the 1984 *Young Offenders Act* but status-like offenses have reemerged, named administrative offenses. These are breaches of restrictions imposed by youth justice officials (Reitsma-Street, 1993) and include offenses such as: escape from custody; failure to appear in court; breaches of curfew, treatment, community service obligations, and other conditions of a probation order. Many of the administrative offenses fall under the broad Section 26 provision which was legislated as a 1986 amendment for youth who "willfully fails or refuses to comply with an order." Of total charges against girls, 6.1% were for administrative offenses in 1986, increasing to 20.9% in 1988 and rising steadily through the 1990s. By 2000, 33.8% or one in three of all principal charges against Canadian female cases were for administrative offenses (Reitsma-Street, 1999; Canadian Centre for Justice Statistics, 1999–2000). Administrative offenses may appear minor, but they are not minor in consequences. They push girls further into the youth justice system, turning a girl into a multiple offender or recidivist. More Canadian girls are sentenced to custody on administrative charges than for either minor or major violent crimes (Conway, 1992; Reitsma-Street, 1999). In one study, breaches of court orders comprised 45% of the girls' current charges and 69% of previous ones (Corrado, Odgers, & Cohen, 2000).

Following passage of the American *Juvenile Justice and Delinquency Prevention Act* in 1974, female status offenders were also deinstitutionalized in the U.S. State diversion programs started up, funded in part by federal dollars. But the definition of status offense has been narrowed over time so that running away from a court-ordered foster home can transform a girl from a status offender into a delinquent. Although the JJDP Act was reauthorized in 1992 with federal funds committed to gender-specific services for prevention of delinquency, MacDonald and Chesney-Lind (2001) report there remain campaigns to amend and overhaul the law, remove the provisions aimed at gender equality, criminalize status offences, and get tough on serious crimes.

There have been sustained efforts to change youth justice laws as a way to get tough on serious crime in many countries with exceptions such as France and Scotland (Hallett & Hazel, 1998; Hackler, 2000). There are also movements to promote alternatives to court proceedings and custodial sentences (House of Commons, 1997). In Canada the new *Youth Criminal Justice Act* (or *YCJA*) became law in April 1, 2003 and embodied both the punitive direction and search for alternatives. Its development and provisions are reviewed by Connelly in this book. In brief, the new name turns attention away from the young offender and instructs people to focus on the criminal behaviors in a situation and a just response. The principles and preamble of the new *YCJA* include prevention of crime, rehabilitation of youth, and special considerations of the developmental needs of youth. For first offenders who are not violent there are minimal and mandatory interventions such as police caution and extra judicial options. There are, however, very few mandatory provisions to help a girl or her family gain access to the necessary social support, economic assistance, cultural programs, or educational training except if a girl is being assessed by the courts or sentenced to custody (Hillian & Reitsma-Street, 2003). The most striking punitive change is a judge *must give an adult sentence to youths 14 years of age and older* who are convicted of serious offences (*YCJA*, Sec. 42(9); 70(1) and (2)). There are important and expensive safeguards to minimize use of adult sentences for youths, including a judicial determination of seriousness of the violence. Youths must also be provided assistance to apply for a youth sentence. Despite these safeguards, however, the punitive potential of longer sentences of the new *YCJA* is clear. Under the previous law, the onus had been on the prosecutor to justify transfer of a youth charged with a serious crime to adult court before guilt could be determined or adult sentences imposed. Now the onus is on the girl to justify the need for a youth sentence.

Charges against girls for murder, manslaughter, and attempts have been consistently low in Canada for the past decade from a low of 6 in 1996 to 17 in 2000 in a country with a population of 31,000,000. Fewer than five girls have been transferred annually in the last decade to adult court to face adult sentences. With the new law, the numbers facing adult sentences may increase significantly as the majority of the approximately 1,200 Canadian girls charged annually with crimes of murder and other serious violent crimes against the person are 14 years and older (Reitsma-Street, 1999; Canadian Centre for Justice Statistics, 1992–2000; tables available from author).

TOWARDS PROGRESSIVE POLICIES

Contemporary popular media feature an increase in the violence of girls despite years of consistently low numbers of girls charged with murder, attempted murders or other serious acts of personal violence (e.g., Chernoff & Simon, 2000; Doob & Sprott, 1998; Steffensmeier & Allan, 1996). Invisible in the media, however, are reports of overcrowded jails, inadequate services for girls, unsafe urban city streets, and the restrictive policies of the late 1990s that drastically reduce the eligibility of girls and young women to adequate educational, housing, employment, and welfare benefits. Also missing is serious debate on youth justice policies that authorize public funds for increased judicial processing of administrative charges and longer correctional sentences for girls in conflict with the law. The negative changes are particularly problematic for girls who live in poor families, impoverished neighborhoods, and in African American, First Nations, or Latino communities (Chesney-Lind, 1999; Childs, 1997; National Council of Welfare, 2000; Schissel, 1997).

It is a challenge to account for the increase in restrictive, punitive policies, and for their virtual invisibility. Feminist scholars and professionals are attempting to expose the limits of restrictive policies that benefit the minority at the expense of the majority's welfare (e.g., Cohen, 1997) while other such as Mink (1998) are questioning feminists' lukewarm attention to the concerns of poor girls and women regarding welfare cuts, compulsory work, and toxic city spaces. Pavlich (2001) argues that amplifying the deviance of individuals and their blameworthiness deflects attention away from analysis of who benefits from decisions that create damaging and violent environments. The American criminologist Anthony Platt (2001) argues that criminalizing youth and funding more police, private security, larger prisons, and longer prison sentences are aspects of law and order campaigns used to control consequences of greater inequality, desperation, and fears. Ironically, the public money needed to pay for the increased security are paid for by cuts to health, education, and welfare. The punitive justice laws, restrictive social policies, and more recently, the new anti-terrorist laws keep individuals tied to the job market or risk criminal records and removal from their communities. Platt (2001) and Childs (1997) also propose that restrictive, punitive policies hamper the efforts of social justice coalitions and economic protests to expose inequality and exploitation.

The other challenge is to put forth alternatives. Fundamental to progressive policies for girls are policies than ensure gender parity in funding so that girls obtain proportionately equivalent access to programs, whether apprenticeship training, English as a second language programs, boys and girls clubs, university education, housing, or juvenile justice programs (Hancock, 2002; Schnaffer et al., 1997; Reitsma-Street & Artz, 2000). More funding geared to prevention would also significantly decrease punitive and restrictive policies for girls in conflict with the law. Thus, the Canadian parliamentary committee and Department of Justice recommended that 80% of federal correctional funding be for non-custodial programs and services, compared to current level of 20% (House of Commons, 1997; Department of Justice, 1998).

Another approach to reversing the restrictive trends is to explore the significant variations between and within countries in responses to girls and violence. What are the policies and practices that can be amplified to promote progressive environments for youths, including poor youths and those convicted of crimes (Hackler, 2000)? Take for example the revolutionary Massachusetts policies of 1969 that closed all the correctional centers for youths. Loughran (1997, p. 177) concludes that "15 years after closing the institutions, Massachusetts was operating a system that relied less on secure confinement than any other comparable state." Moreover the community-based system supported by several secure treatment programs was surprisingly more cost effective than large training schools. Unfortunately, the trend in restrictive and punitive policies presented above also damaged this model juvenile justice system. There were cuts to Massachusetts' state services for youths in the early 1990s. Pretrial detention, community and treatment services had been cut, and some were misused. Politicians campaigning for tax cuts and punitive policies for young offenders were elected and they passed tough anticriminal legislation. Massachusetts, along with 48 other states, increased the types of offenses that may no longer be dealt with by juvenile courts, and lowered the age at which juveniles can or must be transferred to adult courts. There is also an increased use of residential commitments for youth who have breached probation. Nonetheless, despite these serious reversals, policy makers in Massachusetts and in other states, continue to pursue actively alternative policies for nonviolent youths (Longhran, 1997). For promising policy directions in Canada one could look, for example, at policy variations and practice anomalies that affect one-third of all charges laid against girls. What are the policies and practices that instruct authorities in the larger populous Canadian province of Quebec to lay far fewer administrative charges against girls than authorities in the smaller western provinces: 173 in Quebec compared to 1,036 charges were laid in British Columbia courts against girls in 1999–2000, and 1,719 in Alberta (Canadian Centre for Justice Statistics, 1999–2000).

There are several provisions within the new Canadian *Youth Criminal Justice Act* that could be used to promote positive practices and to resist the negative trends to policing girls. For example, police and justice officials are mandated by the law to use warnings, cautions, and other extrajudicial measures for girls who offend for the first time and are not violent. Section 19 encourages, although does not mandate nor fund, the use of conferences to be convened by justice officials. The conferences can include the girl, friends, family members, neighbors, and professionals who decide upon extrajudicial measures, a sentence, or reintegration plans. The most important progressive success of the new Canadian justice law, I would argue, is its refusal to lower the age of criminal responsibility. In the new law, like the old, the age of responsibility is 12 to 17 years. The exception as stated above, however, is adult sentences are now mandatory for youth 14 years and older convicted of particular serious violent crimes or patterns of violent crimes.

More radical policies and practices are those that take seriously the chronic exposure of many poor girls (and boys) to violence, as well as the opinion of youths that for them "poverty, pollution and discrimination are crimes and as problematic as abuse of drugs"(Greene, 1993; Meucci & Redmon, 1997, p. 146; Stack, 2001). One simple but significant policy that youth in Los Angeles recommended to the city authorities was an increase in the hours libraries remain open, as libraries were seen by youths, including street youths, as safe, positive places (Meucci & Redmon, 1997). There is the new American Youth Peace Movement emerging from the ghettos and reservations made up of community-based groups led by activists "who aim to end violence through constructive developments instead of repressive force." The activists negotiate cease-fires, peace settlements among gangs and safe zones (Childs, 1997, p. 250, 252).

To conclude, at the turn of the century, there is a trend to restrictive and punitive policies in U.S. and Canada that negatively affects girls. The trend is especially problematic for girls from poor and marginalized communities, making them more vulnerable to insecurity and violence within and outside their households. This restrictive trend is neither inevitable nor uniform. Everyone can contribute to the pursuit of those progressive policies mentioned above by changing their language when speaking or writing about violence and girls. Avoiding the use of abbreviated phrases such as "violent girl" or "superpredator" helps resist the intrusive policing of girls. These static adjectives and nouns are very problematic: they instruct listeners to stereotype a girl by amplifying her individual behaviors while minimizing the dynamic complexity in which she lives. Thoughtful, everyday language that does not stereotype girls helps to support policies that respond accurately and holistically to the complex interactions between individuals and their environments (Rosenberg & Garofalo, 1998; Schaffner et al., 1997).

Speaking accurately about threats posed by behaviors of both girls and by society is a challenge for each of us. Kimberly Rogers, whose story opened this chapter, could not have successfully challenged the unfair automatic suspension of welfare rights upon conviction for fraud without the ongoing, careful help of members of the local university, prisoner's aid society, and community legal clinic. These allies organized a press conference to explicate the circumstances of her death, to make submissions to the Coroner's Inquest into her death, and to launch campaigns to abolish the unfair provisions of the welfare law (Justice with Dignity, 2002). Accurate and peaceful words, spoken consistently and in concert, are the basis of protests, and the foundation for developing progressive policies and practices for youths, both girls and boys.

REFERENCES

Ackland, J. W. (1982). *Girls in care: A case study of residential treatment.* Hampshire, England: Gower.

Artz, S. (1998). *Sex, power and the violent school girl.* Toronto: Trifolium.

Bezanson, K. I., & McMurray, S. (2000). *Booming for whom? People in Ontario talk about incomes, jobs, and social programs.* Speaking Out Project Report #5. Ottawa: Caledon Institute of Social Policy.

Bhavnani, K., Kent, K. R., & Twine, R. W. (1998). Editorial on feminism and youth culture. *Signs Journal of Women in Culture and Society, 23*(3), 575–583.

Brenzel, B. (1983). *Daughters of the state: A social portrait of the first reform school for girls in North America 1856–1905.* Cambridge, MA: The MIT Press.

Brown, L. M., & Gilligan, C. (1992). *Meeting at the crossroads: Women's psychology and girls' development.* New York: Ballantine.

Cain, M. (Ed.). (1989). *Growing up good: Policing the behaviour of girls in Europe.* London: Sage.

Canadian Centre for Justice Statistics, Statistics Canada, *Youth Court Statistics,* 1992–1993; 1993–1994; 1994–1995; 1995–1996; 1996–1997; 1998–1999; 1999–2000. Ottawa: Minister for Statistics Canada and Industry, Science and Technology.

Carlen, P. (1995). Virginia, criminology, and the antisocial control of women. In T. G. Blomberg & S. Cohen (Eds.), *Punishment and social control* (pp. 211–228). New York: Aldine de Gruyter.

Chesney-Lind, M. (1999). Challenging girls' invisibility in juvenile court. *The Annals,* AAPSS, *564,* 185–202.

Chesney-Lind, M., & Sheldon, R. (1998). *Girls, delinquency and juvenile justice* (2nd ed.). Belmont, CA: Wadsworth.

Chernoff, N., & Simon, R. J. (2000). Women and crime the world over. *Gender issues 18,* 5–20.

Childs, J. B. (1997). The new Youth Peace Movement: Creating broad strategies for community renaissance in the United States. *Social Justice, 24*(4), 247–257.

Cohen, M. G. (1997). From welfare state to vampire capitalism. In P. Evans & G. Wekerle (Eds.), *Women and the Canadian welfare state* (pp. 28–70). Toronto: University of Toronto Press.

Committee to Remember Kimberly Rogers and the Sudbury Community Legal Clinic, 2002. Brief Submitted to City of Greater Sudbury, Feb. 21.

Conway, J. (1992, May). Female young offenders, 1990–1991, *Juristat Service Bulletin,* Canadian Centre for Justice Statistics, *12* (11).

Corrado, R. R., Odgers, C., & Cohen, I. M. (2000, April). The incarceration of female young offenders: Protection for whom? *Canadian Journal of Criminology, 42*(2), 189–207.

Curtis, M. (2002, April 26). "Protesters pepper-sprayed" "Protest: Broken up" *Times Colonist* (pp. A1–2).

Department of Justice Canada (1998). *A strategy for the renewal of youth justice.* Ottawa: Department of Justice Canada.

Doob, A. N. (1992). Trends in the use of custodial dispositions for young offenders. *Canadian Journal of Criminology, 34*(1), 75–84.

Doob, A. N., & Sprott, J. B. (1998). Is the "quality' of youth violence becoming more serious? *Canadian Journal of Criminology, 40*(2), 165–184.

Donzelot, J., trans. R. Hurley (1979). *The policing of families.* New York: Pantheon.

Ehrenreich, B., & Piven, F. F. (2002, June). Without a safety net. *Mother Jones,* 35–41.

Evans, P., & Wekerle, G. (Eds.) (1997). *Women and the Canadian welfare state.* Toronto: University of Toronto Press.

Ferguson, E. (1998). The child-care debate: Fading hopes and shifting sands. In C. Baines, P. Evans, & S. Neysmith (Eds.), *Women's caring* (2nd ed., pp. 191–217). Toronto: Oxford University Press.

Fetherston, D. W. (2000). The law and young offenders. In J. A. Winterdyk (Ed.), *Issues and perspectives on young offenders in Canada* (2nd ed. pp.93–118). Toronto: Harcourt.

Fournier, S., & Crey, E. (1997). *Stolen from our embrace: The abduction of First Nations children and the restoration of aboriginal communities.* Vancouver/Toronto: Douglas & McIntyre.

Friends of Women and Children in British Columbia (2002, 2003). Report Card on welfare and rent. July 15, 2000.Vol. 1(4), *www.wmst.ubc.ca* (The University of British Columbia).

Geller, G. (1987). Young women in conflict with the law. In E. Adelberg & C. Currie (Eds.), *Too few to count.* Vancouver: Press Gang.

Golderg, M., & Long, A. (2001). *Falling behind: A comparison of living costs and income assistance rates in British Columbia.* Vancouver: Social Planning and Research Council of B.C.

Greene, M. B. (1993). Chronic exposure to violence and poverty: Interventions that work for youth. *Crime and delinquency, 39*(1), 106–124.

Headey, B., Goodin, R. E., Muffels, R., & Dirven, H. (1997). Welfare over time: Three worlds of welfare capitalism in panel perspective. *Journal of Public Policy 17*(3), 329–359.

Hackler, J. (2000). International juvenile justice: Why Anglophone systems are inferior. In J. A. Winterdyk (Ed.), *Issues and perspectives on young offenders in Canada* (2nd ed., pp. 309–327). Toronto: Harcourt.

Hallett, C., & Hazel, N. (1998). *The international context: Trends in juvenile justice and child welfare* (Vol. 2). Edinburgh: The Scottish Office Central Research Unit.

Hancock, L. (2002) The care crunch: changing work, families and welfare in Australia. *Critical Social Policy, 22*(1), 119–140.

Hillian, D., & Reitsma-Street, M. (2003). Parents and youth justice. *Canadian Journal of Criminology, 45*(2), 19–42.

House of Commons (1997). *Renewing youth justice.* 13th Report Standing Committee on Justice and Legal Affairs, Shaughnessy Cohen, Chair.

Justice with Dignity. Campaign to Remember Kimberly Rogers. DAWN. Retrieved April 30, 2003 from http://dawn.thot.net/Kimberly_Rogers/.

Kearney, M. C. (1998). Essay review of *Girls, girlhood and girls' studies in transition* edited by M. de Ras & M. Lunenberg; *Girl power* by H. Carlip; *Listen up: Voices from the next feminist generation* edited by B. Findlon. *Signs, 23*(3), 844–849.

Kelly, D. (2002). Restoring common good: Reflections on a non-violent occupation. *Island Catholic News, 16* (4).

Kostash, M. (1987). *No kidding: inside the world of teenage girls.* Toronto: McClelland Stewart.

Knijn, T., & Kremer, M. (1997, Fall). Gender and the caring dimension of welfare states. *Social Politics,* 328–362.

Layton, J. (2000). *Homelessness: The making and unmaking of a crisis.* Toronto: Penguin.

Lee, K. (2220). *Urban poverty in Canada.* Ottawa: Canadian Council on Social Development.

Lindhorst, T., Mancoske, R. J., & Kemp. A. A. (2000). Is welfare reform working? A study of the effects of sanctions on families receiving temporary assistance to needy families. *Journal of Sociology and Social Welfare, XXVII*(4), 185–201.

Loughran, E. J. (1997). The Massachusetts experience: A historical review of reform in the Department of Youth Services. *Social Justice 24*(4), 170–186.

MacDonald, J. M., & Chesney-Lind, M. (2001). Gender bias and juvenile justice revisited: A multiyear analysis. *Crime and Delinquency 47*(2), 173–195.

MacKinnon, M., & Lacey, K. (2001, August 18). Bleak House: Story of Kimberly Rogers. *Globe and Mail*, p. F1.

McWatt, S., & Neysmith, S. (1998). Enter the Filipina nanny: An examination of Canada's live-in caregiver policy. In C. Baines, P. Evans, & S. Neysmith (Eds.), *Women's caring* (2nd ed., pp. 218–232). Toronto: Oxford University Press.

Meucci, S., & Redmon, J. (1997). Safe spaces: California children enter a policy debate. *Social Justice, 24(3)*, 139–151.

Mink, G. (1998). Feminists, welfare reform and welfare justice. *Social Justice 25*, 146–157.

Mosher, J. (2000). Managing the disentitlement of women: Glorified markets, the idealized family, and the undeserving other. In S. Neysmith (Ed.), *Restructuring caring labour* (pp. 30–51). Toronto: Oxford University Press.

National Council of Welfare (2000). *Justice and the poor.* Ottawa: Author.

National Council of Welfare (2001). *Child poverty profile, 1998.* Ottawa: Author

National Council of Welfare (2002). *Welfare incomes, 2000 and 2001.* Ottawa: Author.

Neysmith, S., & Reitsma-Street, M. (2000). Valuing unpaid work in the Third Sector: The case community resource centres. *Canadian Public Policy, XXVI*(3), 331–347.

Patriquin, L. (2001). The historical uniqueness of the Clinton welfare reforms: A new level of social misery? *Journal of Sociology and Social Welfare, XXVIII*(3), 71–94.

Pavlich, G. (2001) Critical genres and radical criminology in Britain. *British Journal of Criminology, 41*, 150–167.

Platt, A. (2001). Social insecurity: The transformation of American criminal justice, 1965–2000. *Social Justice, 28*(1), 138–154

Rankin, K. N. (2002). Social capital, microfinance and the politics of development. *Feminist Economics, 8*(1), 1–24.

Reitsma-Street, M. (1993, October). Canadian youth court charges and dispositions for females before and after implementation of the Young Offenders Act. *Canadian Journal of Criminology*, 437–458.

Reitsma-Street, M. (1998). Still girls learn to care: Girls policed to care. In C. Baines, P. Evans, & S. Neysmith (Eds.), *Women's caring* (2nd ed., pp. 87–113). Toronto: Oxford University Press.

Reitsma-Street, M. (1999). Justice for Canadian girls: A 1990s update. *Canadian Journal of Criminology, 41*(4), 335–363.

Reitsma-Street, M., & Artz, S. (2000). Girls and crime. In J. A. Winterdyk (Ed.), *Issues and perspectives on young offenders in Canada,* (2nd ed., pp. 61–90). Toronto: Harcourt.

Reitsma-Street, M. (2002). "A policy analysis of the proposed B.C. Employment and Assistance Law", *www.uvic.ca/spp/views.*

Rice, J. J., & Prince, M. J. (2000). *Changing politics of Canadian social policy.* Toronto: University of Toronto Press.

Rose, N. E. (1993). Gender, race, and the welfare state: Government work programs from the 1930s to the present. *Feminist Studies, 19*(3), 319–342.

Rosenberg, J., & Garofalo, G. (1998). Riot Grrrl: Revolutions from within. *Signs, 23*(3), 809–842.

Royal Commission on Aboriginal Peoples (1993). *Aboriginal peoples and the justice system.* Ottawa: Minister of Supplies and Services Canada.

Schaffner, L., Shick, S., & Stein, N. (1997). Changing policy in San Francisco: Girls in the juvenile justice system. *Social Justice* 24(4), 187–211.

Schissel, B. (1997). Youth crime, moral panics, and the news: The conspiracy against the marginalized in Canada. *Social Justice,* 24(2), 165–185.

Schlossman, S., & Wallach, S. (1978). The crime of precocious sexuality: Female juvenile delinquency in the Progressive era. *Harvard Educational Review* 48(1), 65–94.

Sharpe, S. (1994). *Just like a girl.* Harmondsworth: Penguin.

Smart, C. (1976). *Women, crime and criminology: A feminist critique.* Boston: Routledge & Kegan Paul.

Squires, P. (1990). *Anti-social policy: Welfare, ideology and the disciplinary state.* New York: Harvester Wheatsheaf.

Stack, C. (2001). Coming of age in Oakland. In J. Goode & J. Maskovsky (Eds.), *The new poverty studies* (pp. 179–200). NY: New York University Press.

Standing Committee on Justice and Legal Affairs, Canada, Parliament, House of Commons (1997). *Renewing youth justice.* 13th report. Ottawa: Queen's Printer.

Steffensmeier, D., & Allan, E. (1996) Gender and crime: Toward a gendered theory of female offending. *Annual Review of Sociology, 22,* 459–487.

Whitaker, I. P., & Time, V. (2001). Devolution and welfare: The social and legal implications of state inequalities for welfare reform in the United States. *Social Justice* 28(1), 76–90.

Walkerdine, V., Lucey, H., & Melody, J. (2001). *Growing up girl: Psychosocial explorations of gender and class.* Houndmills: Palgrave.

Winterdyk, J. A. (2000) Trends and patterns in youth crime. In J. A. Winterdyk (Ed.), *Issues and perspectives on young offenders in Canada,* (2nd ed., pp.11–35). Toronto: Harcourt.

10

Interventions for Aggressive Girls
Tailoring and Measuring the Fit

DEBRA J. PEPLER, MARGARET M. WALSH, AND KATHRYN S. LEVENE

The collection of chapters in this book heralds a burgeoning research and clinical interest in the nature of girls' aggression, its developmental course, and the outcomes experienced by aggressive girls. Girls' aggression has been shown to take somewhat different forms than that of boys, with generally lower levels of physical aggression and a higher reliance on socially directed aggression (Bjorkqvist, Osterman, & Kaukiainen, 1992; Cairns, Cairns, & Neckerman, 1989; Crick & Grotpeter, 1995; Pulkinnen, 1992; Underwood, 2003; Xie, Cairns, & Cairns, in press). Nonetheless, from a developmental perspective, the individual and family risk factors that contribute to boys' aggression appear to operate in the development of girls' aggression as well (Moffitt, Caspi, Rutter, & Silva, 2001; Pepler & Sedighdeilami, 1998). For example, troubled family contexts and ineffective parenting, which are risk factors for the development of aggressive behaviour problems in boys, also relate to the development of girls' aggression. Some outcomes are also common for aggressive girls and boys, such as conflictual peer relations, poor academic performance, school drop out, substance use, and truancy (Cairns & Cairns, 1994; Pepler, Craig,

DEBRA J. PEPLER • Department of Psychology, York University, Toronto, Ontario, Canada M3J 1P3. MARGARET M. WALSH AND KATHRYN S. LEVENE • Earlscourt Child & Family Centre, Toronto, Ontario, Canada, M6E 3V4.

Connolly, & Henderson, 2002; Pepler & Sedighdeilami, 1998), although some, such as the latter two, are particularly characteristic of girls (Robins, 1986).

The trajectories of aggressive girls and boys diverge, however, as they move through adolescence and into adulthood. Aggressive boys are more likely than girls to become involved in delinquency and violent crime (Moffitt et al., 2001). Aggressive girls experience more comorbid emotional problems such as depression (Moffitt et al., 2001; Zahn-Waxler, 1993). For both girls and boys, aggressive behavioural styles transfer to romantic relationships in which they tend to be more aggressive and more victimized by their partners than nonaggressive youths (Connolly, Pepler, Craig, & Taradash, 2000). As they reach adulthood, the prognosis for aggressive boys and girls is equally worrisome, although in somewhat different ways. A substantial proportion of aggressive boys may have accrued criminal records, whereas many aggressive girls may have entered parenthood precociously and find themselves struggling in their roles as mothers (Serbin et al., 1998).

For more than a decade, there has been a growing recognition of the differences in the way aggression is expressed by boys and girls (Bjorkqvist et al., 1992; Cairns, Cairns, Neckerman, Ferguson, & Gariepy, 1989; Crick & Grotpeter, 1995; Lagerspetz, Bjorkqvist, & Peltonen, 1988; Underwood, 2003). Given girls' propensity for intimacy and their need to belong and receive affirmation (Maccoby, 1986), girls' aggression is often expressed within the dynamics and discourses of small, same-sex groups. Girls are more likely to express social forms of aggression, such as spreading rumors, social exclusion, and manipulating others to attack or harm another socially (Lagerspetz et al., 1988; Xie et al., in press). These indirect strategies may inflict considerable harm and emotional pain on victims (Galen & Underwood, 1997). With an increased understanding of the prevalence, form, and context of girls' aggression, we believe that the time has come to direct research attention to the etiology of girls' aggression and to the types of interventions that are most appropriate and effective in addressing the problems of aggressive girls.

TAILORING AN INTERVENTION FOR AGGRESSIVE GIRLS

There is a substantial body of research on the effectiveness of a variety of treatments for aggressive behaviour problems, but these studies are almost exclusively focused on the problems of boys. Recent meta-analyses of cognitive-based problem-solving skills training (PSST) (Bennett & Gibbons, 2000) and parent management training (PMT) for antisocial children (Serketich & Dumas, 1996) found medium to large effect sizes for PSST and PMT, respectively. Kazdin (1992) found that offering concurrent PMT and PSST interventions resulted in larger effects and more stable changes in the children's antisocial and prosocial behaviours, and in parent functioning than either form of intervention alone.

Earlscourt Child and Family Centre (ECFC), a family-focused treatment centre for aggressive and antisocial children under the age of 12, incorporates both child and parent anger management and skill building interventions. Internally developed manuals guide these interventions. Prior to 1996, girls were participating in the same ECFC treatment groups as the boys. Preliminary assessments of the program indicated that the girls' inclusion in the often considered "gender-neutral" interventions were, however, found to be associated with negative outcomes. Some of the girls showed increases in aggression and others withdrew from participation in the group program. These preliminary trends motivated the development of the gender-specific intervention programme Earlscourt Girls Connection (EGC) (see chapter by Levene, Walsh, & Augimeri, this volume for a more detailed description of the development of the EGC programme).

THEORETICAL FRAMEWORK FOR
EARLSCOURT GIRLS CONNECTION

A developmental model of risk and protective factors provides the central theoretical framework for the gender-specific intervention, the Earlscourt Girls Connection. It has informed program design in three primary domains in the lives of young girls: individual behaviours, primary relationship contexts (e.g., family, parent-child), and secondary contexts (e.g., peers, school, community). According to this model, development is shaped by an interaction of risk and protective processes, which reside within the individual child and in her interactions within the family and broader social domains (Rutter, 1985). Risks are dynamic factors or processes which lead directly to a psychosocial disorder (Rutter, 1990). Protective processes, such as those associated with the level of mother's education (Werner & Smith, 1992), operate to buffer the effects of the risk processes.

At the individual level, development is influenced by predispositional risk factors (e.g., temperament) which interact with protective factors (e.g., accelerated language development). At the family level, the quality of relationships (e.g., attachment, hostility) and the interactions between the girl and her family (e.g., parenting style, conflict) shape development by placing the girl at risk for behaviour problems or by protecting her and supporting adaptive functioning. In focusing on the broader social context, the peer group and school comprise two other important domains of risk and protective processes. With this developmental-contextual framework, the EGC focuses on the impact of aggressive girls' adjustment difficulties and functioning, not only during the age period under study (under 12 years of age), but also during adolescence and into adulthood.

A range of theoretical approaches, ranging from ecological and feminist perspectives to attachment, social learning and social cognitive theories, guided development of the EGC. At this point in the evolution of the program, it is the latter three that have been most fully interpreted and implemented. A primary focus of the EGC has been on the parent-daughter relationship, guided by attachment theory, which focuses on the quality of relationships. Although the evidence for the predictive capacity of attachment classifications is mixed, there is some support for the contention that children who are insecurely attached are at greater risk for behaviour problems than those who are securely attached (Fagot & Kavanagh, 1990; Greenberg, Speltz, & DeKlyen, 1993). The purported mechanism that links attachment to the caregiver with children's subsequent behaviour problems is the development of internal working models of relationships and interactional styles. Through interactions with their caregivers, infants learn about what to expect in relationships and how to interact. If caregivers are not consistently warm and responsive, children fail to learn to trust others, to be responsive to others, and they lack motivation to respond prosocially to gain the approval of others (Shaw & Bell, 1993). There is some evidence that a troubled relationship between a girl and her mother is particularly important in the development of antisocial behaviour (Pakaslahti, Spoof, Asplun-Peltola, & Keitikangas-Javinen, 1998). An empirical question is whether these primary family relationships are more salient for girls than for boys. Fagot and Kavanagh (1990) found that attachment classifications predicted subsequent preschool behavior problems for girls, but not for boys. Given their greater propensity to play at home, girls' development may be more contingent upon family circumstances than that of boys who are more likely to play in larger groups and to roam in the broader community (Maccoby, 1986). The EGC program focuses on building positive relationships between girls and their mothers through enhancing parenting capacity, as well as through interactions in the Girls Growing Up Healthy program. By promoting positive mother-daughter relationships, the EGC aims to promote relationship capacity among the girls.

Social learning theory and the coercive model of family processes (Patterson, 1982) have informed the parenting component of the EGC. These theoretical perspectives highlight how ineffective parenting practices and coercive interactions between parents and children are mechanisms that promote the development of antisocial behaviour problems. The parent component of EGC helps parents to monitor their daughters' behaviours, provide positive reinforcement for prosocial behaviours and appropriate contingencies for negative ones, avoid hostile and coercive interactions with their daughters, and communicate positively for successful problem solving. By supporting parents to acquire effective parenting strategies, the expectation is that parents will be better equipped to set limits on their daughters' behaviours, to reduce aggressive behaviours, and to promote their daughters' development of social skills and competencies.

The child-focused interventions within the EGC derive, in part, from social cognitive theory which highlights the social information processing deficits of aggressive children and the resulting behavioural difficulties. An additional focus of the SNAP™ program is on emotion regulation and anger management. In essence, the intervention is designed to help the girls interpret social cues accurately, generate possible responses to a social dilemma, and respond prosocially in a conflict situation. Social problem solving skills and the ability to encode subtle social behaviours may be particularly relevant for girls. In her recent book, Underwood (2003) highlights the many forms of subtle behaviours that girls use to enact aggression. Although all children employ social forms of aggression in their interactions, these are particularly characteristic of aggressive girls. Attachment issues emerge in the realm of peer relationships as these girls are usually without friends and have a poor sense of connectedness to other children. Thus the treatment emphasis is on developing positive connections and social skills within the group and then outside the group.

EVALUATION OF THE EARLSCOURT GIRLS CONNECTION

We have now completed a preliminary evaluation of the effectiveness of the EGC by examining data from 98 of the 250 girls who participated in the program during its first four years of operation. Of these girls, 72 had complete data at admission and 6-month follow-up; 58 girls had both admission and 12-month follow-up data. We assessed for differential attrition in the samples by comparing the groups of girls who only had admission data, who had complete admission and 6-month data, and who had complete admission and 12-month data. There were no differences among these groups in the admission externalizing scores, suggesting no differential attrition related to participation in the research component of the program.

EGC Girls at Admission

The girls' profiles indicate that they experienced risk in a number of domains: individual social and cognitive factors, as well as in the family context. The girls who participated in the program and for whom data were available ranged in age from 5 to 11 years, with a mean age of 8.9 years. Girls were referred to the EGC for aggressive behaviour problems, which were assessed through parent reports on the Standardized Client Information System (SCIS) (Offord & Boyle, 1996). This measure, which was adapted from the Child Behavior Checklist (Achenbach & Edelbrock, 1983) is a standardized measure used to assess emotional and behavioural disorders among children 4 to 16 years old. The SCIS generates scores for overall externalizing disorders from a conduct disorder subscale (12 items), an oppositional subscale (9 items), and a hyperactivity subscale (14 items). An internalizing disorder score is generated from an overanxious subscale (11 items), a separation anxiety subscale (9 items), and a depression subscale (16 items). A social relations scale comprises three items that focus on how well the child relates to other children, teachers, and family members. Items are rated on a 3-point scale ranging from never (0) to sometimes true (1) to often or very true (2), with higher scores indicating greater impairment. For this preliminary analysis, only questionnaires completed by the parent were used due to the number of inconsistencies in follow-up data collection on the other questionnaires. Parents were typically the biological parent but in some instances involved a stepparent or guardian. Ninety-one percent of the parent forms were completed by female informants and 9% by male informants.

Parent reports confirmed that the girls experienced high levels of social and emotional difficulties. Over 85% of the girls were rated as high on interrupting, arguing with adults, not listening, being defiant, having temper tantrums, being angry and cruel, bullying, and being mean to others. At admission, 60% of the girls were rated by their parents as falling into the clinical range for externalizing behaviour problems, such as aggression and delinquency. A substantial proportion (42%) of the girls were rated by their parents as falling in the clinical range for internalizing problems, such as depression and anxiety. Consistent with this profile of aggressive and undercontrolled girls, were the parents' ratings that highlighted the girls' social problems: Over half of the girls (59%) were rated as falling within the clinical range for social relations problems. Almost a fifth (22%) of the parents indicated that they were concerned about their daughters' sexual behaviours.

The girls' problems extended to the cognitive and school domains, as well. Some of the girls were receiving support at school: 16% of the girls were in full-time learning and/or behavioural special education classes; and 23% of the girls were in part-time special education classes. The girls' academic problems were confirmed by parents' reports: 42% of parents indicated that their daughters had difficulties learning. In addition, 6% of parents indicated that their daughters experienced a developmental delay and 3% of parents indicated that their daughters experienced speech difficulties. Parents reported that 12% of their daughters had health problems that prevented or limited them from full participation in school. Ten percent of parents reported that the health problems had been present for over six months and 3% reported that the health condition had always been present for their daughter.

Family Profiles

Within their families, the girls were equally distributed across birth order positions: 28% only children, 19% first-born, 16% second born, and 24 % last born children. The family profiles of the girls show evidence of risk, which is similar in many domains to that of boys who were admitted to Earlscourt over the same time period (1996–2001). Fifty-four percent of the girls and 61% of boys lived in single-mother families, 30% of the girls and 36% of the boys lived with their two biological parents, 5% of girls and 3 % of boys lived with adoptive parents, and 2% of girls lived with grandparents (family composition data were missing for 9% of the girls). The majority of girls' and boys' families (71% and 75%, respectively) reported a low or modest family income (below $40,000). A small proportion of the girls (4%) had been separated from their parents before the age of three (this information was not available for the boys) and 7% of girls' and 11% of boys' parents reported that their children had stayed overnight in a foster or group home. For girls and boys, 16% of parents reported having been charged or arrested for a criminal offence. According to parents' reports, 10% of girls and 12% of boys had experienced physical abuse with 8% of girls and 6% of boys having experienced sexual abuse. Many of these families (34%) had been in contact with other agencies for their children's emotional and behavioural problems, with 36% of girls and 47% of boys having been in contact with the Children's Aid Society. A smaller percentage of girls (4%) than boys (57%) had contact with the police for their behaviour problems.

Preliminary Analysis of EGC over First 4 Years

For our preliminary evaluation, we have assessed changes from admission to two points in time: six months and twelve months from the time that the girls and their families began the program. Since not all girls had complete data at admission, six, and twelve months, we have maximized our numbers by examining changes for those girls with data across two of the specified time points. We have reported the general results of the evaluation in a previous publication (Walsh, Pepler, & Levene, 2002). In general, the program appears to be effective, as evidenced by changes in parents' ratings of girls' behavioural problems. We found medium effect size differences in externalizing problems from admission to both the 6- and 12-month evaluations (.42 and .49, respectively). There were medium to large effect sizes in ratings of the girls' social relations problems (.72 and .51 for the 6- and 12-month outcomes, respectively).

In this chapter, we delve into the domain of program effectiveness by examining data on clusters of behaviour problems. We conducted MANOVAs comparing admission data to 6- and 12-month follow-up data on groups of related items on the SCIS (Offord & Boyle, 1996) using age as a covariate. Given that we had a priori hypotheses of improvement in ratings of girls' behaviour problems following treatment, we also examined the univariate analyses. Parents rated their daughters on groups of items assessing anger, aggressive behaviour, defiant attitudes, and delinquency. Parents rated their daughters' sociability with two groups of items referring to peer and adult relations.

Anger Regulation

There was a multivariate main effect of time for items that assessed anger regulation for both the 6-month, F (5, 137) = 3.01, $p < .05$ and 12-month, F (5, 109) = 2.85, $p < .05$ analyses. As a covariate, age approached significance for the 6-month sample, F (5, 137) = 2.43, $p = .05$, only. An inspection of the univariate analyses indicates significant improvement over 6- and 12-month intervals on parent ratings of the girls' angry and resentful behaviour, temper tantrums, and cranky dispositions. There was no significant change over either interval on ratings of the girls' getting easily annoyed. At 6 months, there was a significant main effect of age on parent ratings of swearing. Parents of girls 10–11 years of age were more likely to report their daughters were swearing than parents of girls 4–9 years of age. Overall, parent reports of girls' swearing were generally low at admission and stayed low, with no change by 6- and 12-month follow-up.

Aggressive Behaviour

There was a significant multivariate effect of time on aggressive behaviours over the 6-month interval, F (3, 140) = 2.90, $p < .05$ and 12-month interval, F (3, 111) = 4.30, $p < .05$. The covariate of age was not significant for either time interval. Univariate analyses indicate a significant decrease in parents' ratings of cruelty and bullying, as well as of physical attacks on people for both the 6- and 12-month intervals. Only 20% of the girls were rated by their parents as being cruel to animals at admission; parents ratings of this low frequency behaviour did not change over time.

Defiant Attitudes and Behaviours

The multivariate analysis of items that describe defiant attitudes and behaviours did not reveal an overall improvement over the 6- and 12-month intervals. Age was a significant covariate at 6 months only, F (4, 138) = 3.43, $p < .05$. There was a significant univariate effect of improvement on ratings of girls' defiance and talking back over the 6-month interval. There was also a significant univariate effect in ratings of girls' arguing over the two time periods. Lying and cheating did not show improvement over time; however, it was the only behaviour that showed a significant univariate effect for age with parents of older girls reporting more lying and cheating than the parents of younger girls.

Delinquency and Vandalism

There was no significant multivariate change in ratings of the girls' delinquent behaviours and vandalism over the two time periods. Age was a significant covariate for the 6-month sample only, F (8, 134) = 2.90, $p < .01$. There was one significant difference in the expected direction on the item tapping stealing outside the home, which improved from admission to twelve-month follow-up. The items that comprise these groups of troublesome behaviours, such as carrying weapons and truancy, generally characterize the problems of older girls and boys. Evidence of this is seen in the 6-month sample, which showed significant age differences for parents' ratings of behaviours such as stealing at home, stealing outside home, running away, and truancy. The majority of girls who were reported as engaging in these particular behaviours were 10-to-11 years of age. Overall, the 5- to 11-year-old girls in the present study were seldom rated as having significant problems with delinquent behaviour and vandalism–a trend that did not change with intervention.

Prosocial Behaviours

Girls' capacities for prosocial relationships were assessed with two groups of items: peer relations and adult relations. A multivariate effect of time was found for peer relations at 6 months, F (4, 138) = 3.57, p < .01 and at 12 months, F (4, 110) = 4.13, $p < .01$; as well as for adult relations, at 6 months, F (3, 139) = 5.56, $p < .01$ and at 12 months, F (3, 111) = 3.75, $p < .05$. Age was not a significant covariate for either of the samples. For the peer items, there was a significant improvement over both time intervals in ratings of girls' abilities to wait their turn, avoid fights, and get along with friends. There was no marked improvement in reports of girls' tendencies to annoy others.

The girls' relationships with adults were rated as improved in several items differentially over the two time intervals. There were significant improvements in getting along with teachers from admission to 6 months, in getting along with parents from admission to 12 months, and in getting along with family members for the two time intervals.

TAILORING AN INTERVENTION FOR AGGRESSIVE GIRLS: HOW WELL DID IT FIT?

In trying to address the needs of aggressive girls, Earlscourt Child and Family Centre faced a dilemma. It appeared as if the standard interventions offered by the Centre, in which boys and girls participated in the same programs, were not meeting girls' needs. This dilemma emerged as a result of an exploratory internal review of data compiled in the mid 1990s in a mixed-sex group treatment program, the Outreach Project (ORP). The review revealed that the results for boys were encouraging, but the same was not true for the small group of girls. Clinicians who were involved with the ORP described the girls who attended the groups as typically subdued and unobtrusive during group sessions or, in some instances, they appeared to be imitating the boys' more direct and physical forms of aggression. Efforts to discover gender-specific approaches to augment ongoing programs were unsuccessful and in the end we determined that this would not be a useful direction to pursue. What appeared to be needed was a separate gender-specific intervention for aggressive girls and their families. With the initial evaluation, we have preliminary evidence of the effectiveness of the Earlscourt Girls Connection in addressing girlhood aggression. Comparisons of parent ratings of the girls' behaviour problems before and following treatment revealed significant improvements in a wide range of behaviour problems. Overall, there were significant decreases in parent reports of negative behaviours on anger regulation, aggressive behaviour, peer relations, and adult relations items.

The patterns of significant change in the girls' behaviour problems reflect the importance of a developmental perspective when assessing children's aggressive behaviour problems. The girls involved in the EGC and the evaluation were, on average, 9 years old and ranged from 5 to 11 years of age. Structured but adaptable, the intervention reflects the developmental levels of the two main age groups, 6–8 and 9–12 years of age. In the Girls Club manual (Levene, 2003) there is a discussion of practical ways in which the groups reflect the age grouping. The frequency with which parents reported girls' behaviour problems, in conjunction with their developmental relevance to our population of girls, appear to be associated with specific levels of change at the two time periods. The most frequently reported behaviours for the girls included temper tantrums, crankiness, being angry and resentful, being defiant, and arguing a lot. All of these behaviour problems, which were common among the school-aged girls in the program, showed a significant reduction in occurrence between admission and at 6- and 12-month follow-up points for girls of all ages. In contrast, a number of behaviour problems were seldom reported by parents of these school-aged girls including many of the items listed for delinquency, such as using weapons, vandalism, setting fires, breaking into someone's home, and running away. For the 6-month sample, the age of the girls engaging in these types of behaviours was found to differ significantly. Parents of the 10- to 11-year-old girls reported more delinquent behaviours than parents of 6- to 9-year-old girls at both admission and follow-up periods. Many of these behaviours appear to be developmentally beyond the repertoire of the majority of our under 12 antisocial girls. None of the ratings of these behaviour problems showed a significant change between admission and follow-up. The one behaviour that showed a significant decrease in frequency at twelve months was stealing outside the home. Delinquent behaviours are not as prevalent in childhood and adolescence for antisocial girls as compared to boys (Moffitt et al., 2001). The preliminary results from the EGC indicate that by intervening early in the behaviour problems and social contexts of these troubled girls, we might be able to divert them from engaging in risky and delinquent opportunities that await them as they approach adolescence.

The EGC was based on a developmental contextual perspective, which directed the focus to salient relationship contexts in the girls' lives, as well as to their developmental challenges. The quality of girls' interactions with peers and adults showed improvement following involvement in the EGC. Specifically in relationships with peers, the girls were rated as having less difficulty awaiting turns, getting along with friends, and being irritable following treatment. The girls' relationships with teachers were rated as improved at the six-month evaluation, but not at the twelve-month follow-up. The girls' relationships with parents showed a positive difference (.20) at a six-month follow-up with a significant difference (.35) reported at the 12-month follow-up. There are several possible explanations for this reported difference. Clinical staff described a pattern of heightened parent acknowledgement of difficulties that appears to emerge after an initial experience of treatment, which is then followed by growing sense of self efficacy and positive interactions. The trend of increasingly positive reports may also be indicative of the EGC's continuing care model, developed in response to the recognition that conduct problems often are chronic and require a "dental" model of service. The program is committed to supporting the girls to "stay in school and out of trouble". Services take the form of individually assessed needs, such as family sessions, individual befriending, tutoring, Girls Growing Up Healthy (GGUH)(a mother-daughter structured group course), and Leaders in Training.

EGC: THE TAILORING CONTINUES

The results of our preliminary investigation show that improvements following participation in the EGC reflect the theoretical framework used to address troubled young girls' developmental issues within multiple relationship contexts. The evidence of developmentally relevant changes among these young antisocial girls is an indication that the EGC program is on the right track to addressing the needs of these girls. Further investigations into the associations between age, frequency, and change need to be considered within the context of how other factors such as family functioning and parental disciplinary styles affect the process of change.

Through these assessments and evaluations of the program, the clinicians involved in developing the EGC continue to learn about how to address girls' aggression and related problems effectively and how to promote the development of healthy relationships. As these girls enter adolescence, new developmental problems, such as emerging sexuality will continue to challenge this group of vulnerable girls (Moffitt et al., 2001). Many of these antisocial girls are at risk for school drop out, teen pregnancy, unemployment, physical and mental health difficulties for themselves and their children. Following participation in the initial girls' and parents' group, the EGC offers ongoing support with the understanding that the changing challenges these girls face need to be recognized and addressed. The continuing support for girls is designed to reinforce the anger management and problem-solving skills that may help these girls cope with some of the unique problems and challenges they will face in their adolescence and adulthood.

The implications of the results are encouraging with regard to the decreases in externalizing behaviours and increases in prosocial behaviours at six and 12-month follow-up. Due to the limitations of our data set and the use of a single informant (parent), these results need to be interpreted with caution. This preliminary analysis shows a positive trend in change and is a promising first step in evaluating the EGC program. We are continuing with our evaluation of the EGC through a more stringent quasi-experimental design that will help us to understand more fully the individual and family factors that contribute to change in these young antisocial girls. Although EGC is designed to avert young girls from embarking on an antisocial and aggressive pathway, the findings have implications for adolescent interventions (see also Reid, Patterson, & Snyder, 2002). This cognitive-behavioural approach focuses on gender-specific issues within a relational context and these parameters would appear to apply to older troubled girls as well. Our experience indicates that conducting mother-daughter groups (GGUH) has had a powerful impact on both participants, the quality of their interactions, and potential for ongoing relationship building. Exploring approaches to implement groups for antisocial adolescent girls and their mothers (or other significant women) would be an interesting and potentially valuable direction to initiate.

At the same time as we are attempting to heighten community and professional awareness of the challenges faced by young girls and their families, we need to promote effective, well defined interventions. Examining the effectiveness of this gender specific program for young girls is underway with a two-year study, *Bridging the Gender Gap*. One of the research challenges will be to distinguish which components of the intervention, such as the mother-daughter structured intervention, are most effective. We are also examining the process of treatment to shed light on the effective components of the complicated process of intervention in the lives of troubled girls.

REFERENCES

Achenbach, T. M., & Edelbrock, D. S. (1983). *Manual for the Child Behavior Checklist and Revised Child Behavior Profile*. Burlington: University of Vermont, Department of Psychiatry.

Bennett, D. S., & Gibbons, T. A. (2000). Efficacy of child cognitive behavioral interventions for antisocial behaviors: A meta-analysis. *Child & Family Behavior Therapy, 22*, 1–15.

Bjorkqvist, K., Osterman, K., & Kaukiainen, A. (1992). The development of direct and indirect aggressive strategies in males and females. In K. Bjorkqvist & P. Niemeia (Eds.), *Of mice & women: Aspects of female aggression* (pp. 51–86). San Diego: Academic Press.

Cairns, R. B., & Cairns, B. D. (1994). *Lifelines and risks: Pathways of youth in our time*. New York: Cambridge University Press.

Cairns, R. B., Cairns, B. D., Neckerman, H. J., Ferguson, L. L., & Gariepy, J-L., (1989). Growth and aggression: I. Childhood to early adolescence. *Developmental Psychology, 25*, 320–330.

Cairns, R. B., Cairns, B. D, & Neckerman, H. (1989). Early school dropout: Configurations and determinants. *Child Development, 60*, 1437–1452.

Connolly, J., Pepler, D. J., Craig, W. M., & Taradash, A. (2000). Dating experiences of bullies in early adolescence. *Child Maltreatment, 5*, 299–310.

Crick, N. R., & Grotpeter, J. K. (1995). Relational aggression, gender, and social-psychological adjustment, *Child Development, 66,* 710–722.

Fagot, B. I., & Kavanagh, K. (1990). The prediction of antisocial behavior from avoidant attachment classifications. *Child Development, 61,* 864–873.

Galen, B. R., & Underwood, M. K. (1997). A developmental investigation of social aggression among children. *Developmental Psychology, 33,* 589–600.

Greenberg, M. T., Speltz, M. L., & DeKlyen, M. (1993). The role of attachment in the early development of disruptive behavior problems. *Development and Psychopathology, 5,* 191–213.

Kazdin, A. E. (1992). Child and adolescent dysfunction and paths toward maladjustment: Targets for intervention. *Clinical PsychologyReview, 12,* 795–817.

Lagerspetz, K., Bjorkqvist, K., & Peltonen, T. (1988). Is indirect aggression typical of females? Gender differences in aggressiveness in 11- to - 12 year-old children. *Aggressive Behavior, 14,* 403–414.

Levene, K. S. (2003). SNAP™ Girls Group Manual: The Girl's Club. Toronto: Earlscourt Child and Family Centre.

Maccoby, E. E. (1986). Social groupings in childhood: Their relationships to prosocial and antisocial behavior in boys and girls. In D. Olweus, J. Block, & M. Radke-Yarrow (Eds.), *Development of antisocial and prosocial behavior.* New York: Academic Press.

Moffitt, T., Caspi, A., Rutter, M., & Silva, P. (2001). *Sex differences in antisocial behaviour.* Cambridge: Cambridge University Press.

Offord, D., & Boyle, M. (1996). Standardized Client Information System. Toronto: Association of Children's Mental Health Centres.

Pakaslahti, L., Spoof, I., Asplun-Peltola, R., & Keitikangas-Javinen, L. (1998). Parents' social problem strategies in families with aggressive and non-aggressive girls. *Aggressive Behavior, 24,* 37–51.

Patterson, G. R. (1982). *Coercive family process: A social learning approach.* Eugene, OR: Castalia.

Pepler, D., Craig, W., Connolly, J., & Henderson, K. (2002). Bullying, sexual harassment, dating violence, and substance use among adolescents. In C. Wekerle & A. M. Wall (Eds.), *The violence and addiction equation: Theoretical and clinical issues in substance abuse and relationship violence* (pp.153–168). Philadelphia: Brunner/Mazel.

Pepler, D., & Sedighdeilami, F. (1998). *Aggressive girls in Canada* (Government Document W-98-30E): Applied Research Branch Strategic Policy Human Resources Development Canada.

Pulkkinen, L. (1992). The path to adulthood for aggressively inclined girls. In K. Bjorkqvist & P. Niemela (Eds.), *Of mice and women: Aspects of female aggression* (pp. 113–121). San Diego: Academic Press.

Rutter, M. (1985). Resilience in the face of adversity: Protective factors and resistance to psychiatric disorder. *British Journal of Psychiatry, 147,* 598–611.

Rutter, M. (1990). Psychosocial resilience and protective mechanisms. In J. Rolf, A. Masten, D. Cicchetti, S. Nuechteiein, & S. Weintraub (Eds.), *Risk and protective factors in the development of psychopathology* (pp.181–214). Cambridge: Cambridge University Press.

Serbin, L., Cooperman, J., Peters, P., Lehoux, P., Stack, D., & Schwartzman, A. (1998). Intergenerational transfer of psychosocial risk in women with childhood histories of aggression, withdrawal, or aggression and withdrawal. *Developmental Psychology, 34,* 1246–1262.

Serketich, W. J., & Dumas, J. E. (1996). The effectiveness of behavioral parent training to modify antisocial behavior in children: A meta-analysis. *Behavior Therapy, 27,* 171–186.

Shaw, D. S., & Bell, R. Q. (1993). Developmental theories of parental contributors to antisocial behavior. *Journal of Abnormal Child Psychology, 30,* 355–364.

Underwood, M. (2003). *Social aggression among girls.* New York: Guilford.

Walsh, M. M., Pepler, D. J., & Levene, K. S. (2002). A model intervention for girls with disruptive behaviour problems: The Earlscourt Girls Connection. *Canadian Journal of Counselling, 36*, 297–311.

Werner, E., & Smith, R. (1992). *Overcoming the odds: High risk children from birth to adulthood.* London: Cornell University Press.

Xie, H., Cairns, B. D., & Cairns, R. B. (in press). The development of aggressive behaviors among girls: Measurement issues, social functions, and differential trajectories. In D. Pepler, K. Madsen, K. Levene, & C. D. Webster (Eds.), *The development and treatment of girlhood aggression.* Hillsdale, NJ.: Erlbaum.

Zahn-Waxler, C. (1993). Warriors and worriers: Gender and psychopathology. *Development and Psychopathology, 5*, 79–89.

11

Linking Identification and Treatment of Early Risk Factors for Female Delinquency

KATHRYN S. LEVENE, MARGARET M. WALSH, LEENA K. AUGIMERI, AND DEBRA J. PEPLER

Increasing concern about how young girls are growing up is reflected in the scientific focus on the negative trajectories of girls (e.g., Côté, Zoccolillo, Tremblay, Nagin, & Vitaro, 2001; Moffitt, Caspi, Rutter, & Silva, 2001), and in the media attention they are receiving (Nebenzahl, 2001). The latter has largely been fueled by dramatic and tragic events that have involved girls in their early teens such as the brutal death of Reena Virk (Taffler, 1998). Correspondingly, there has been a push for answers to questions about the current state of affairs regarding incidence, onset, gender-related risk factors, and effective interventions associated with girlhood aggression. Little is known about treatment with regard to whether the same interventions apply to boys and girls and whether there is sufficient evidence to support a call for the widespread introduction of separate, gender-specific interventions. We have few answers to these questions, and the ones that we have suggest a challenging complexity. In this chapter we discuss two gender-specific initiatives that have been implemented at Earlscourt Child

KATHRYN S. LEVENE, MARGARET M. WALSH, AND LEENA K. AUGIMERI • Earlscourt Child & Family Centre, Toronto, Ontario, Canada, M6E 3V4. DEBRA J. PEPLER • Department of Psychology, York University, Toronto, Ontario, Canada, M3J163.

and Family Centre (ECFC), a family focused treatment centre for children under the age of 12 exhibiting serious aggressive and antisocial behaviors. These converging initiatives consist of a risk assessment device developed to augment and refine our understanding of the developmental pathways of aggressive and antisocial young girls and a gender-specific treatment program.

DEVELOPMENT OF A GIRLHOOD AGGRESSION RISK ASSESSMENT DEVICE: EARL-21G

BACKGROUND

Development of risk assessment tools, such as measures of psychopathology (PCL-R, Hare, 1991), adult sex offences (the SVR-20, Boer, Hart, Kropp, & Webster, 1998) and spousal assault (the SARA, Kropp, Hart, Webster, & Eaves, 1999), has become a focus of activity in the fields of psychology and criminology. Such devices have been found to be of considerable benefit to clinicians and researchers (Douglas, Cox, & Webster, 1999). As clinicians working with young conduct disordered children, we have been interested for some time in attempting to isolate those factors that place children most at risk for antisocial trajectories (Augimeri & Levene, 1997a). To this end, ECFC entered into the intense process of developing a consultation version (Augimeri, Koegl, Webster, & Levene, 1998) and, subsequently, a second version of an early risk assessment list device for boys, the EARL-20B (Augimeri, Koegl, Webster, & Levene, 2001). This risk assessment approach was derived from a device for adult psychiatric patients and prisoners with mental health and personality disorders, the HCR-20 (Webster, Douglas, Eaves & Hart, 1997). The development process was supported by a labor intensive retrospective file study of the related clinical program, the Earlscourt Outreach Project (ORP) (see Koegl, Webster, Michel, & Augimeri, 2000; Webster, Augimeri, & Koegl, 2002). The EARL-20B continues to be administered internally, for retrospective and prospective purposes, and externally for clinical and research purposes (e.g., Enebrink, Långström, Gumpert, & Hultén, 2003).

The need to expand and enhance our knowledge of the factors that place girls at risk for entering into a negative developmental trajectory is pressing, if we are to provide meaningful and effective interventions for this vulnerable population. Subsequent to the completion of the EARL-20B, we undertook the development of a consultation version of a risk assessment device for girls, the Early Assessment Risk List for Girls (EARL-21G) (Levene et al., 2001).

Overview of the EARL-21G

In initiating this project, we were aware that the developmental trajectories of conduct disordered boys and girls likely include some common risk factors. A major challenge was to unravel those factors that make particular contributions to the antisocial pathways of young girls. In creating the girls' manual, 18 of the EARL-20B risk headings were retained. Differences appear in the content of the items, the exclusion of an EARL-20B item, and the addition of two key gender-based risk factors. In its final form, the EARL-21G manual consists of 21 categories of risk associated with girls embarking on an antisocial trajectory, and items are grouped according to three constructs: family, child, and responsivity. The seven items in the Family section focus on the extent to which the girl has been nurtured, supervised, attached, encouraged, and effectively disciplined. The 12 Items in the Child section are concerned with the girl's development in behavioral, physical, academic, sexual, and social domains. The Responsivity section is comprised of two items that assess potential or actual level of family and child engagement with the program and ability to benefit from the interventions. In the EARL-21G manual, each item consists of two sections, a brief and focused overview of relevant research findings on the topic and a guide for scoring the item. The 21 items are listed in Figure 1.

In developing the EARL-2OB we were able to cull key risk factors from an extensive body of research. For the EARL-21G the best-supported risk factors needed to be identified from a very limited gender-specific literature. We extracted those factors that seemed to apply to behaviorally troubled young girls and their risk for embarking on an antisocial trajectory, and included some of the key factors that emerged from our qualitative study (Levene, Madsen, & Pepler, in press). Findings of the qualitative investigation highlighted several themes which require further study, such as the role of early constitutional problems (e.g., extensive hospitalization for kidney problems during infancy), which appeared to have some influence on the early lives of all 16 girls studied. A longing for, and sometimes an idealization of, their absent fathers was another compelling theme in the narratives of many of the girls that also requires the attention of clinicians and researchers.

As we had discovered in earlier attempts to identify childhood risk factors for future offending (Augimeri & Levene, 1997a, b), it is not

Table 1 - Items of the Early Assessment Risk List
for Girls (EARL-21G)—Version 1

Family (F) Items

F1	Household Circumstances
F2	Caregiver Continuity
F3	Supports
F4	Stressors
F5	Parenting Style
F6	Caregiver-Daughter Interaction
F7	Antisocial Values and Conduct

Child (C) Items

C1	Developmental Problems
C2	Onset of Behavioral Difficulties
C3	Abuse/Neglect/Trauma
C4	Hyperactivity/Impulsivity/Attention Deficits (HIA)
C5	Likeability
C6	Peer Socialization
C7	Academic Performance
C8	Neighbourhood
C9	Sexual Development
C10	Antisocial Attitudes
C11	Antisocial Behaviour
C12	Coping Ability

Responsivity (R) Items

R1	Family Responsivity
R2	Child Responsivity

Figure 1. EARL 21G Items

difficult to identify a large number of factors that may place young girls
at risk for antisocial behavior and aggression. The challenge has been to
distinguish well-substantiated factors from those that do not appear to
have a clear influence on antisocial outcomes. Of the gender-specific factors that have been isolated, three particularly stand out. Social forms of
aggression (Vaillancourt et al., 2002). Attention Deficit Hyperactivity Disorder (ADHD) (Bates, Bayles, Bennett, Ridge, & Brown, 1991; Loeber &
Keenan, 1994), and early sexual development represent factors that may
place girls in particular jeopardy for developing antisocial behaviors. As
discussed below, the severely detrimental effect of social forms of aggression and the negative impact of precocious sexual development had not
been widely understood or acknowledged until recently. Signs of ADHD
in young girls may tend toward the attentional end of the continuum,

(Brown, Madan-Swain, & Baldwin, 1991) and, as such, may not garner the serious attention they require. The gender-specific consequences of early ADHD in girls (Bates et al., 1991) are yet to be well understood and effectively addressed. Our examination of the literature and clinical experience suggests that there would be great benefit to heightening community and professional awareness of the symptoms and importance of these gender-specific factors. As clinicians we are trained to be alert to intimations of future problems and to weigh the impact of various ominous occurrences in the lives of young girls and their families. Without an understanding of which risk factors are best supported, we are in danger of being misled and overwhelmed by the clinical information we collect. On a broader level, refining our knowledge of the risk factors that seem to play the most important roles in the development of girls' antisocial behavior may assist us in more effectively directing limited treatment and community resources. In a subsequent section in which the Earlscourt Girls Connection (EGC) is described, we discuss in some detail how we have attempted to match risk assessment with clinical risk management.

As noted above, the EARL-21 G items parallel most of the EARL-20B headings, and it is in the content of the individual items that the differences are to be found. The research that is incorporated into the brief reviews that introduce each item is, as much as possible, informed by gender-based investigations, as are the coding guidelines. Moreover, after extensive deliberation, reviewing what we had learned from both the literature and our clinical experience, we decided to eliminate as a separate item a category that had been included in the boys' version and to add two distinct items.

Caregiver–Daughter Interaction is an added item in the Family Section (F6). The research summary for this item suggests the importance of the quality of the connection and interaction between the girl and her primary caregiver, particularly her same-sex parent. There is some evidence in the limited research literature (Funk, 1999; Osborne & Fincham, 1996; Pakaslahti, Spoof, Asplun-Peltola, & Keitikangas-Javinen, 1998) and in our clinical observations that the estrangement which exists in the relationships between problematic young girls and their mothers is an influential risk factor. Issues such as modeling, rejection, and attachment all seem to play a role in this interaction. Qualitative interviews (Levene et al., in press) have supported this item as a possible factor and suggest that the theme of mother-daughter estrangement may be intergenerational in some families. *Sexual Development* was added to the Child Section (C9) to reflect the crucial role of atypically advanced sexual development, attitudes and/or behaviors of these young girls. Researchers have begun to unravel (see

Caspi & Moffitt, 1991; Caspi, Lynam, Moffitt, & Silva, 1993; Moffitt et al., 2001) a web of associated factors and conditions. Their findings have implications for clinical practice, in particular, the need to assess the impact of early sexual development within individual contexts. Early development is only one marker; it needs to be evaluated in conjunction with the co-occurrence of factors, such as an early aggressive history and association with older males (Moffitt et al., 2001). Although contact with authority figures, such as police, firefighters, and school principals, likely has a risk quotient for all children, the frequency of such events in the lives of girls with an early aggressive history did not seem to warrant a separate section. Thus, *Authority Contact*, an EARL-20B child item, was not included in the girl's manual. The issue was incorporated into the EARL-21G item, *Antisocial Behavior (C11)*.

TRAINING AND ADMINISTRATION

As indicated on the inside cover of the EARL-21G manual, a number of cautions apply to its effective administration. These guidelines primarily relate to developing and maintaining an adequate understanding of the items and the scoring process *prior to* the evaluator administering the risk assessment procedure. Training and consultation with ECFC trainers is strongly encouraged, particularly in the initial phases. When the evaluator is sufficiently familiar with the manual and all available information on the girl and her family, she scores each item on a 0-2 range. With regard to the question of whether the girl or family meets the standards for the Item, this range represents: (0) no evidence, (1) some indication, and (2) clear evidence. This is a well-established practice, described in the previously cited risk assessment devices. As well, each item is considered for red flagging as a Critical Risk Item, one that potentially may place that girl at serious risk and requires diagnostic evaluation with regard to intervention and/or possible barriers to effective treatment. As indicated above, early ADHD in girls often goes undetected and is predictive of conduct problems at age 8 (Bates et al., 1991). Evidence of this problem is noted in Item C4, *Hyperactivity/Impulsivity/Attention Deficits*, and might be assessed as to whether it is a Critical Risk Factor. This designation also might be considered, for example, for Item C8, *Neighbourhood*, when a family relocates to a dangerous neighborhood.

Each item is rated as the ordered process of evaluation proceeds. The EARL-21G contains a one page scoring sheet, the EARL-21G Summary Sheet, with a Total Score, the maximum being 42 (see Figure 2). Each total score is assigned a rating for risk of high, moderate, or low. Combined Total Score and Critical Risk Items produce a profile of risk to which the

The EARL-21G Version 1-Consultation Edition Summary Sheet
(To be used in association with the EARL-21G Manual)

Girl s Name or ID#: _____   **Date:** _____
(First name SURNAME)   (Month Day, Year)

Assessor: _____   **Girl s DOB:** _____   **Age:** _____
(YY/MM/DD)   (YY/MM)

Family Items		Rating (0-1-2)	Critical Risk
F1	Household Circumstances		
F2	Caregiver Continuity		
F3	Supports		
F4	Stressors		
F5	Parenting Style		
F6	Caregiver-Daughter Interaction		
F7	Antisocial Values and Conduct		

Child Items		Rating (0-1-2)	Critical Risk
C1	Developmental Problems		
C2	Onset of Behavioral Difficulties		
C3	Abuse/Neglect/Trauma		
C4	HIA (Hyperactivity/Impulsivity/Attention Deficits)		
C5	Likeability		
C6	Peer Socialization		
C7	Academic Performance		
C8	Neighbourhood		
C9	Sexual Development		
C10	Antisocial Attitudes		
C11	Antisocial Behaviour		
C12	Coping Ability		

Responsivity Items		Rating (0-1-2)	Critical Risk
R1	Family		
R2	Child		

LOW   MED.   HIGH   TOTAL SCORE [   ]

Notes:

Figure 2. EARL 21G Version 1

girl has been exposed. Establishment of on-site or community workgroups is encouraged to facilitate meaningful, ongoing clinical and assessment processes.

PRELIMINARY FINDINGS

The purpose of an initial retrospective study was to assess inter-rater reliability and the association between EARL-21G scores to subsequent youth and adult court conviction data. In order to be eligible for inclusion in the study, participants had to be, at the time of follow-up, 12 years of age, the minimum age of criminal liability in Canada. The sample included 67 girls with 30 files designated as common files that were coded by three trained coders. There was a moderate-to-high level of agreement between the raters. Positive Pearson correlations of .64, .65, and .84, and intra-class correlation coefficients of .67 (single measure) and .86 (average measure) were obtained. All correlations were significant at or beyond .01. In assessing the association between the risk assessment scores and conviction, the sample was divided at the median to create two groups of equal proportion (52% and 48%). The first group was classified as "LOW" with a scoring range of 5–17 ($M = 12.7$, $SD = 3.1$), with the second group classified as "HIGH" with a scoring range of 18–30 ($M = 22.3$, $SD = 3.1$). Official conviction data showed that 18 (27%) of the girls were found guilty of committing an offence at follow-up. Of these girls there were 34% in the HIGH-risk group and 20% in the LOW-risk group. This difference did not reach statistical significance.

A small prospective study, conducted as part of internal training activities with seven members of the EGC team (clinicians and researchers), involved reviewing and rating 12 files. In this study a high rate of agreement was achieved. A mean Positive Person Correlation of .81 and intra-class correlation coefficients of .80 (single measure) and .96 (average measure) were obtained. All correlations were significant at or beyond .01.

The EARL-21G is routinely administered in the EGC at admission and is included as a measure in a 2003-4 study that the EGC is undertaking. We continue to consider the information that is emerging from ongoing EARL-21G data collection and have begun to pursue expert consultation, as we did with the consultation version of the EARL-2OB. Finally, at present we are also examining the use of the early risk assessment process for follow up purposes with both EARL-20B and the EARL-21G. As the manuals include several items derived from historical information, we have adapted the scoring procedure to reflect these items. Historical items consist of ones in which problematic occurrences, such as a birth defect (*C1 Developmental Problems*), or onset of the problems prior to the child's 6th birthday (C2 Onset of Behavioral Difficulties) is noted. Such occurrences, which had their start and at least their initial impact in the past, may or may not also have a continuing effect in the present. The historical event itself and its initial impact on the life of the child are unchangeable.

BENEFITS OF THE EARL-21G

The process of developing and administering the EARL-21G has suggested that there is a range of benefits to be gained from careful and consistent use of this device. The straightforward features of the manual and coding sheet contribute to its being consumer friendly and to the likelihood that it will be appropriately completed. Initial feedback from clinicians and researchers who have been trained to administer the EARL-21G has supported this view and indicate that it is a very useful decision enhancing tool. The process of administering the device brings scientific knowledge together with clinical practice and promotes a scientist practitioner model of service. In turn, this association between research and practice is likely to improve professional practice generally. Attuned to the levels and issues of risk overall, assessors are also encouraged to be cognizant of those items that have been assigned Critical Risk status. Risk identification underscores those issues requiring clinical risk management planning. Finally, as we explore the applications of this device, we will consider its value for research purposes, either in outcome studies and/or longitudinal research.

In the next sections, we address the issue of linking *risk identification* with *clinical risk management* in the design of the innovative multifaceted intervention, the Earlscourt Girls Connection.

DEVELOPMENT OF A GENDER-SPECIFIC TREATMENT PROGRAM: THE EARLSCOURT GIRLS CONNECTION

As has been the case in other domains of health related inquiry, the problematic trajectories of boys have overshadowed the unique issues posed by young girls (Robins, 1986; Tremblay, 1991). By virtue of sheer numbers, the strong association of boyhood conduct problems with adult criminality, and the "in your face" nature of their problems (Tremblay,

1991), boys have captured the attention of researchers and clinicians interested in the field of childhood aggression. For children's mental health services, the comparatively small population of young conduct disordered girls has received scant notice; they have typically been admitted to mixed gender programs that seem to have been considered to be "gender neutral".

Earlscourt Child and Family Centre (ECFC) paralleled similar facilities in not having gender-specific programming. The guiding ECFC therapeutic approach, SNAP™(STOP NOW AND PLAN), a cognitive–behavioral self-control and problem-solving technique, was applied similarly to boys and girls in our mixed treatment groups. In the mid-1990s an increasing awareness of the inadequacy of male dominated groups for girls, led to a search for a literature that would inform us about the etiology and treatment of girlhood aggression. We soon discovered that the literature was sparse and effectively in its infancy. Incorporating what was known about girlhood aggression, particularly its trajectory (e.g., Zoccolillo & Rogers, 1991; Moffitt et al., 2001), and evidence-based interventions conducted with boys such as the SNAP™ Children's Group (*Earlscourt Child and Family Centre*, 2001), we crafted a unique gender-specific treatment model designed for girls with disruptive behavior disorders: the Earlscourt Girls Connection (EGC). This program was launched in late 1996 with two staff (B.A. level Family and Child Workers) and a researcher. Since then over 350 girls and their families have been engaged in this cognitive-behavioral program consisting of three core and several adjunctive treatment components.

Overview of the EGC

The core treatment components are three structured groups: concurrent parent and child groups, and a mother-daughter group. Based on the assessment of each girl and her family, other components, such as family counseling, tutoring, advocacy and a 'special friend' (staff or volunteer), are added to individualized treatment plans. As well, an elevated admission score in the attention deficit area typically leads to an assessment by the consulting psychiatrist. The design of the group courses was informed by a range of theoretical perspectives, including cognitive, behavioral, feminist, ecological, attachment, and social learning theories. The key psychoeducational strategies used in each of the groups are modeling, role-playing, and generalization activities such as homework and joint practice sessions. One benefit of having concurrent parent and girls groups is the scheduling of three joint sessions which allows parents and daughters opportunities to practice their skill acquisition in a safe environment in which they can receive coaching and support. In the following brief descriptions of the core groups, examples of links between risk identification and risk management are highlighted:

1. SNAP™ Parenting (SNAPP) Group is a 12-session cognitive behavioral parent training group, which is informed by psychoeducational principles (see Levene, 2001). It focuses on parents acquiring effective parenting (Patterson, 1982), and anger management skills. The course was designed to address the unique challenges posed by their daughters by matching interventions with known risk factors. Extrapolating from what we know about the prominence of social forms of aggression (e.g., exclusion, verbal cruelty) in the lives of young, behaviorally disordered girls, for example, the course pays special attention to these forms of aggression. Researchers and clinicians have begun to highlight their potentially damaging consequences, such as isolation, rejection, and psychosocial maladjustment (Vaillancourt et al., 2002). In the group sessions, parents are coached to attend to and find effective ways to ameliorate such problems, regardless of whether their daughters assume the roles of onlooker, target, protagonist, or any of these roles at different times. Not doing so has led to dire consequences (Spears, 2002). The course also addresses and fosters awareness of the parents' own use of social aggression (e.g., sarcasm, mean teasing, verbal abuse). Group participants are trained and have opportunities to practice more effective approaches to parenting to counter this maladaptive modeling, particularly problematic same sex modeling (Johnson & O'Leary, 1987).

2. The Girls' Club is a 12 session SNAP™ intervention which focuses on girls learning effective self-regulation and problem-solving strategies. The manual (Levene, 2003), which is modeled after other such cognitive behavioral programs (see, *Earlscourt Child and Family Centre*, 2001), incorporates gender-specific elements into a structured group program. It has been our experience, for example, that the principal "triggers" for group participants are often related to appearance (e.g., girls being labeled as fat or ugly) and their social status within their peer group (e.g., unpopularity, exclusion); these catalysts are anticipated in the course content, role plays, and activities. In a session devoted to cognitive distortions, for example, a cartoon of an ambiguous scenario of a group of girls whispering is reviewed and the girls are encouraged to imagine themselves being on the margins of the group. This exercise typically elicits immediate negative attributions and cognitive distortions (e.g., "Just like always, everyone is making fun of me. They think I look like a boy!") that contribute to aggressive and antisocial behaviors (e.g., "I am going to punch them out for making fun of me"). Such difficulties are evident in

discussions that occur during Girls Club sessions, as reflected in the following example of problematic interactions reported by a 10-year-old EGC participant:

> I got really mad and didn't use SNAP™. And then I got into a lot of trouble with everyone—my Mom, my teacher and the whole school knows about it. Whenever there are no adults around, Jane always pretends to hold her nose when she sees me. I feel like such a loser, sad and mad both. I couldn't stand it anymore. I tossed Jane's desk when I thought that no one was around.

Although social forms of aggression seem to be more characteristic of girls than boys (Vaillancourt et al., 2002), physical aggression is also evident in the profiles of girls referred to this program. The program works with each girl to identify the events ("triggers") and cues (feelings and thoughts) that precede her aggressive behavior and to develop effective coping responses. Ignoring displays of physical aggression, perhaps because they figure less prominently in girls' interactions than is the case for boys, may contribute to these displays becoming more strongly linked with the problems that trigger their very challenging behaviors. At the beginning of the session each participant reviews a "Hassle Log" about a problem she has experienced since the last meeting, and how she evaluates herself in terms of "making my problem bigger or smaller". In the following example, Tanika reports to her Girls Club group about a serious hassle she had at school.

> I got suspended from school for three days and it's all Josie's fault. Her desk is right behind mine. One day she whispered to me that she was starting an "I Hate Tanika Club". I got mad—felt like my head was a volcano. I thought to myself "Why does everybody always pick on me?" Then I made my problem really bigger. I had a pencil in my hand and I scratched her face with it. My teacher yelled at me and sent *me* to the principal's office, and took Josie to the nurse.

Following Tanika's reporting of her problem scenario, she and the group brainstorm how she might have made her problem 'smaller'. Using the feedback that she thought would work best for her, Tanika and another girl practice a corrective role-play for the group, and check out with a group member, who has the role of "reality judge", how real the role-played interaction was. Role-plays are typically videotaped, and this teaching aid is used to facilitate a meaningful group debriefing process when the group observes the videotape. If needed, the role-players may incorporate the reality feedback in the practice of an even more refined role-play.

3. A structured 8-session mother-daughter group, Girls Growing Up Healthy (GGUH), has relationship building as the objective of the therapeutic process. The content addresses physical and sexual health issues, such

as nutrition, models of women and girls in the media, puberty, and intimate relationships. One session is devoted to a narrative exploration of the mother's biography and a beginning story of the girl's life, supported by "My Life" workbook. Each session begins with the group considering a topic, which is usually followed by a related mother–daughter activity, such as in assessing a list of possible sexual harassment scenarios to determine the salient issues and whether they represented a sexual harassment interaction. Homework assignments, reviewed at the end of each session, also involve a joint mother–daughter activity. Risk factors that informed program design include the role of mother daughter connection and same sex modeling in the lives of girls who are growing up angry (Johnson & O'Leary, 1987; Sprott & Doob, 1998). Sessions are also designed to open mother daughter communication about the hazards the girls encounter as they begin to develop sexually, especially those vulnerable young girls who experience precocious sexual maturity (Moffitt et al., 2001).

STAFFING

Female staff conduct each of the program components because of the importance of positive same sex modeling. It has been of particular benefit to have Peer Mentors, girls who have graduated from the program, as Girls Club group co-leaders. We have found that these mentors, perhaps because of their age and experience, have a great deal of credibility with the participants. Parent graduates usually assume the role of co-leader with SNAP^{TM} Parenting Groups and their views and directions are given considerable weight. Their credibility seems to come from both their experience in dealing with challenging daughters and their parenting accomplishments, having applied SNAPP skills with these daughters.

RESEARCH

Fundamental to the ECFC approach to clinical practice has been the integration of research into each program. As referred to above, a qualitative study, *Girls growing up angry: A qualitative investigation* (Levene, Madsen, & Pepler, in press), the first EGC study, was initiated in 1997. This exploratory study was aimed at expanding our limited understanding of the salient factors in the lives of behaviorally troubled young girls by listening to and extracting common key themes from the narratives of members of recently admitted families. The findings of that inquiry, a recent retrospective study, and other girlhood aggression research, in conjunction with feedback from staff and families, inform ongoing program development. In another chapter included in this volume (Walsh, Pepler, & Levene, 2004), preliminary program evaluation findings of the EGC are discussed as well as their implications for possible enhancements of program design. The next phase of our research plan began in January 2003 when EGC initiated a two-year evaluation of the core treatment program, *A quasi-experimental study of a multifaceted intervention for young girls with behaviour problems*. Using four cohorts, a randomized-control group design will be utilized to examine program effectiveness. Given the high level of community and professional interest in the intervention, this investigation is crucial if we are to participate in dissemination of the program.

FUTURE DIRECTIONS

The EARL-21G has proved to be a useful addition to the assessment process for the EGC, a recently developed treatment program that continues to evolve, guided by many sources including the application of the manual. We are extremely grateful to Dr. David Farrington and Dr. Rolf Loeber who reviewed this consultation version with ECFC in January 2003. Gathering feedback from others who specialize in this field will continue until late 2004 when a final version of the EARL-21G will be produced, integrating the information we have gleaned from feedback and formal consultations. We encourage clinicians and researchers who are administering this device to engage with us in this process by letting us know what they are experiencing in its application. In particular, we are interested in strengthening the items and approaches that are effective and in adapting those that have displayed various levels of problems. At least initially, it has assisted in the formulation of EGC treatment plans that match salient assessment points, so that limited resources can be directed in an increasingly informed manner. Our experience with the EARL-21G has led us to reflect on other issues that require further study. The predictive utility of the number of Critical Risk items and negative scoring on the Responsivity items for negative outcomes (e.g., criminal convictions, severity) requires close investigation. As well as examining the influence of particular risk factors, the field of girlhood aggression would benefit from investigation into the clusters and interactions of risk items may predict different forms of problematic trajectories such as teen pregnancy.

The EGC, as noted, is currently being scrutinized in a two-year study. Initial results emerging from descriptive studies (Walsh, Pepler, & Levene, 2002) have been encouraging and informative, and have contributed to development of the program. Of particular note, for example, is the co-morbid assessment profile (depression and externalizing problems) that appears to be linked with poor outcomes for girls who have participated in the program. This speaks to program development with a greater stress on addressing the overlapping symptoms and behaviors of girls who often describe themselves as "mad" and "sad". The convergence of the EGC and the EARL-21G as gender-specific developments for young girls embarking on an aggressive and antisocial pathway represents a promising approach to grounding evidence-based practice. Much remains to be done to understand the effects of various risk factors on the lives of girls how they may contribute to negative trajectories, and how to intervene most effectively.

REFERENCES

Augimeri, L. K., Koegl, C., Webster, C., & Levene, K. (1998). *Early assessment risk list for boys, EARL-20B (Version 1).* Toronto, ON: Earlscourt Child and Family Centre.

Augimeri, L. K., Koegl, C. J., Webster, C. D., & Levene, K. S. (2001). *Early assessment risk list for boys, EARL-20B (Version 2).* Toronto, ON: Earlscourt Child and Family Centre.

Augimeri, L. K., & Levene, K. S. (1997a). *Outreach Programme: Risk factors associate with possible conduct disorders and non-responders.* Toronto, ON: Earlscourt Child and Family Centre.

Augimeri, L. K., & Levene, K. S. (1997b). *Earlscourt Girls Connection: Risk factors associated with possible conduct disorders and non-responders.* Toronto, ON: Earlscourt Child and Family Centre.

Bates, J. E., Bayles, K., Bennett, D. S., Ridge, B., & Brown, M. (1991). Origins of externalizing behavior: Problems at eight years of age. In D. Pepler & K. H. Rubin (Eds.), *The development and treatment of childhood aggression* (pp. 93–120). Hillsdale, NJ: Erlbaum.

Boer, D .P., Hart, S. D., Kropp, P. R., & Webster, C. D. (1998). *SVR-20. Manual for the sexual violence risk—20. Professional Guidelines for Assessing Risk of Sexual Violence.* Burnaby: The Mental Health, Law, and Police Institute, Simon Fraser University.

Brown, R., Madan-Swain, A., & Baldwin, K. (1991). Gender differences in a clinic-referred sample of attention deficit disordered children. *Child Psychiatry and Human Development. 22,* 111–128.

Caspi, A., Lynam, D., Moffitt, T. E., & Silva, P. A. (1993). Unraveling girls' delinquency: Biological, dispositional, and contextual contributions to adolescent misbehavior. *Developmental Psychology, 29,* 19–30.

Caspi, A., & Moffitt, T. E. (1991). Individual differences are accentuated during periods of social change: The sample case of girls at puberty. *Journal of Personality and Social Psychology, 61,* 157–168.

Côté, S., Zoccolillo, M., Tremblay, R. E., Nagin, D. S., & Vitaro, F. (2001). Predicting girls' conduct disorder in adolescence from childhood trajectories of disruptive behaviors. *Journal of the American Academy of Child and Adolescent Psychiatry, 40,* 678–688.

Douglas, K. S., Cox, D. N., & Webster, C. D. (1999). Violence risk assessment: Science and practice. *Legal and Criminological Psychology, 4,* 149–184.

Earlscourt Child and Family Centre (2001). *SNAP^{TM}Children's Group Manual.* Toronto, ON: Earlscourt Child and Family Centre.

Enebrink, P., Långström, N., Gumpert, C. H., & Hultén, A. (2003). *Evaluating risk for antisocial behavior: Properties of the Early Assessment Risk List for Boys (EARL-20B).* Sweden: Karolinska Institutet.

Funk, S. (1999). Risk assessment for juveniles on probation: A focus on gender. *Criminal Justice and Behavior, 26,* 44–68.

Hare, R. D. (1991). *Manual for the Hare Psychopathy Checklist—Revised.* Toronto, ON: Multi-Health Systems.

Johnson, P., & O'Leary, D. (1987). Parental behavior patterns and conduct disorder in girls. *Journal of Abnormal Child Psychology, 15,* 573–581.

Koegl, C. J., Webster, C. D., Michel, M., & Augimeri, L. K. (2000). Coding raw data: Toward understanding raw life. *Child and Youth Care Forum, 29,* 229–246.

Kropp, P. R., Hart, S. D., Webster, C. D., & Eaves, D. (1999). *Spousal Assault Risk Assessment Guide—User's Manual.* Toronto, ON: Multi-Health Systems.

Levene, K. S. (2001). *SNAPP Stop-Now-And-Plan Parenting: Parenting Children with Behavior Problems Manual.* Toronto, ON: Earlscourt Child and Family Centre.

Levene, K. S. (2003). *SNAP™ Stop-Now-And-Plan: Girls Club Manual.* Toronto, ON: Earlscourt Child and Family Centre.

Levene, K. S., Augimeri, L. K., Pepler, D. J., Walsh, M. M., Webster, C. D., & Koegl, C. J. (2001). *Early assessment risk list for girls, EARL-21G (Version 1).* Toronto, ON: Earlscourt Child and Family Centre.

Levene, K., Madsen, K., & Pepler, D., (in press). Girls growing up angry: A qualitative study. In D. Pepler, K. Madsen, K. Levene, & C. Webster (Eds.), *The development and treatment of girlhood aggression.* Hillsdale, NJ: Erlbaum.

Loeber, R., & Keenan, K. (1994). Interaction between conduct disorder and its comorbid conditions: Effects of age and gender. *Clinical Psychology Review, 14,* 497–523.

Moffitt, T. E., Caspi, A., Rutter, M., & Silva, P. A. (2001). *Sex differences in antisocial behaviour.* Cambridge: Cambridge University Press.

Nebenzahl, D. (2001, April 3). 'A lot of anger: Bullying and physical aggression are growing problems among girls. Montreal Gazette, A1, A4.

Osborne, L., & Fincham, F. (1996). Marital conflict, parent-child relationships, and child adjustment: Does gender matter? *Merrill-Palmer Quarterly, 42,* 48–75.

Pakaslahti, L., Spoof, I., Asplun-Peltola, R., & Keitikangas-Javinen, L. (1998). Parents' social problem solving strategies in families with aggressive and non-aggressive girls. *Aggressive Behavior, 24,* 37–51.

Patterson, G. R. (1982). *Coercive family process: A social learning approach.* Eugene, OR: Castalia.

Robins, L., N. (1986). *The consequences of conduct disorder in girls.* Orlando, FL: Academic Press.

Spears, B. (2002, July). Indirect aggression as bullying? A precursor to girls' suicide attempt. *The Development of Aggression among Canadian Children. Part II: Indirect Aggression.* Meeting of the International Society for Research on Aggression, Montreal.

Sprott, J., & Doob, A. (1998). *Who are the most violent ten and eleven year olds?* (W-98-29E): Applied Research Branch of Strategic Policy Human Resources Development Canada.

Taffler, S. (1998). The lonely death of Reena Virk. [Electronic version]. *The Reading Room,* Retrieved October 4, 2002, from www.islandnet.com/pwacvic/tafler04.

Tremblay, R. (1991) Aggression, prosocial behavior, and gender : Three magic words but no magic wand. In D. Pepler & K. Rubin (Eds.), *The development and treatment of childhoood aggression* (pp. 71–78). Hillsdale NJ : Erlbaum.

Vaillancourt, T., Cote, S., Farhat, A., Boulerice, B., Leblanc, J., Boivin, M. et al. (2002). *The development of aggression among Canadian children. Part II Indirect Aggression.* Paper presented at the meeting of the International Society for Research on Aggression, Montreal.

Walsh, M. M., Pepler, D. J., & Levene, K. S. (2002). A model intervention for girls with disruptive behavior problems: The Earlscourt Girls Connection. *Canadian Journal of Counseling, 36,* 297–311.

Webster, C. D., Augimeri, L. K., & Koegl, C. J. (2002). The under 12 outreach project for antisocial boys: A research based clinical program. In R. R. Corrado, R. Roesch, S. D. Hart, & J.K. Gierowski (Eds.), *Multi-problem violent youth: A foundation for comparative research on needs, interventions and outcomes.* Amsterdam: IOS Press.

Webster, C. D., Douglas, K. S., Eaves, D., & Hart, S. D. (1997). HGB-20: *Assessing risk for violence, Version 2.* Burnaby, BC: Mental Health, Law, and Policy Institute, Simon Fraser University.

Webster, C. D., Douglas, K. S., Belfrage, H., & Link, B. G. (2000). Capturing change: An approach to managing violence and improving mental health. In S. Hodgins (Ed.), *Violence among the mentally ill: Effective strategies* (pp. 119–144). Norwell, MA: Kluwer.

Zoccolillo, M., & Rogers, K. (1991). Characteristics and outcomes of hospitalized adolescent girls with conduct disorder. *Journal of the American Academy of Child and Adolescent Psychiatry, 30,* 973–981.

12

Girls in the Justice System
Treatment and Intervention

JILL ANTONISHAK, N. DICKON REPPUCCI, AND CARRIE FRIED MULFORD

Girls' rates of arrest and adjudication, although still far below those of boys, have been rising for the past 15 years. In the United States, arrest rates for girls increased 35% from 1991 to 2000, while the rates for boys decreased 11% (Snyder, 2002). Accompanying this rise in arrest rates has been a 65% increase of girls in juvenile detention facilities (Porter, 2000). The U.S. Juvenile Justice and Delinquency Prevention (JJDP) Act Reauthorization of 1992 acknowledged the increasing number of girls in the juvenile justice system and mandated that states investigate treatment options for girls and gender disparity within the justice system (Budnick & Sheilds-Fletcher, 1998; OJJDP, 1998). The subsequent generation of intervention programs focusing on gender-specific issues appears promising as they emphasize a comprehensive approach to treatment. However, gender specific programs may be overly focused on self-esteem and empowerment issues, without addressing other important problems, such as mental health needs. Unfortunately, research on treatment options that work for justice-involved youth is limited, and the paucity of research on what works for girls is particularly striking. In this chapter, we use the term "justice-involved" to represent youths experiencing various degrees of involvement in the justice system, ranging from those who have gone to court for committing minor delinquent acts to those who have been placed in state custody. As

JILL ANTONISHAK, N. DICKON REPPUCCI, AND CARRIE FRIED MULFORD • Department of Psychology, University of Virginia, Charlottesville, Virginia, United States, 22901.

such, we do not examine prevention programs per se, although in some instances, we do discuss the efficacy of school- or community-based programs because they may serve as exemplars for programs in the justice system. We focus on four key questions related to justice-based intervention efforts for girls: 1) What are the outcomes for justice-involved girls? 2) Are the intervention needs of girls the same as those for boys? 3) Are interventions designed for boys appropriate for girls? 4) Should programs be developed specifically for girls? We conclude with recommendations for developing interventions for girls.

WHAT ARE THE OUTCOMES FOR JUSTICE-INVOLVED GIRLS?

Currently, we lack appropriate prospective and longitudinal data to determine what interventions work for girls, yet it is imperative that we undertake such research in order to determine which girls may experience negative adult outcomes, which girls will naturally desist, and what services are the most effective in helping justice-involved girls.

Researchers have demonstrated that former female delinquents without intervention experience considerable social impairments as adults (Lewis et al., 1991). Silverthorn and Frick (1999) and Pajer (1998) reviewed studies of girls with conduct problems in adolescence and found that they often experience poor outcomes in adulthood, including increased likelihood of substance abuse, adult arrests, and/or diagnosis of psychiatric disorders. Pajer (1998) also found that antisocial girls were likely to experience dysfunctional interpersonal relationships and poor educational advancement. Werner and Smith (1992), in their 25-year longitudinal study of high risk youth, reported that mothers who had been delinquent as girls had higher rates of family court records than other women. They also had more psychiatric problems compared to adults who had been male delinquents or non-delinquent girls. One explanation, advocated by Chamberlain and Moore (2002), focuses on the intergenerational transmission of mental health problems. These investigators found that mothers with significant mental health problems provide poor parenting and become involved with men who also have severe mental health problems, thereby putting their children at risk and perpetuating a cycle of aggression and abuse. For serious and chronic female offenders, the justice system may mark a meaningful point of intervention to break this cycle. Intervention efforts targeting justice-involved girls have opportunities to affect rehabilitative gains in multiple problem domains, not just criminal recidivism.

It is important to note that 73% of justice-involved girls do not return to the justice system, which at first glance appears to be a relatively positive outcome, particularly given that 54% of males return to the system (Snyder & Sickmund, 1999). However, although these girls may desist from anti-social and delinquent behaviors as reflected in official criminal recidivism rates, we know that many have continued contact with the social service system, and that rates of interpersonal violence, domestic assault, and substance use remain high within these populations. Given these realities, we clearly need research to assess developmental processes that support or counter females' deviant behaviors.

Although theoretical debate is ongoing regarding the similarities of boys' and girls' trajectories of offending (Moffitt, Caspi, Rutter, & Silva, 2001; Silverthorn & Frick, 1999), there is evidence to suggest that a sizeable number of girls who enter the justice system as adolescents will not return to either the justice or the social service system. Lanctôt and Le Blanc (2002) have identified three trajectories in a prospective study which included a sample of 150 delinquent girls: 1) little involvement in deviance throughout adolescence, with a very late initiation into deviance with little variety in problem behaviors (39%); 2) high involvement in deviant behaviors until mid-adolescence, which then sharply declines, as girls became more attached to parents and significant others and less attached to delinquent peers (42%); and 3) high and persistent involvement in deviance throughout adolescence (19%). These results suggest that interventions focused specifically on criminal recidivism reduction may be short-sighted and that more gender-specific interventions for multiple problems are needed.

ARE THE INTERVENTION NEEDS OF GIRLS THE SAME AS THOSE OF BOYS?

Research regarding the similarity of risk factors for boys and girls is conflicting, and while some researchers have proposed a different set of risk factors for each gender (e.g., Chesney-Lind & Shelden, 1992; Storvoll & Wichstrom, 2002), others suggest that the same set of risk factors predicts involvement in the justice system for both genders (e.g., Odgers & Moretti, 2002; Moffitt et al., 2001). Regardless of these inconsistencies, once youths enter the justice system, boys and girls often present different profiles for intervention and have different clusters of needs. Specifically, girls are more likely than boys to have increased mental health needs, histories of victimization and chaotic family lives, and a tendency to engage in relational forms of aggression. Arguably, these needs are important considerations for any girls' intervention programming.

Mental Health Needs

Estimates of rates of mental disorders in the justice system vary based on diagnostic criteria, ranging from 20% for serious mental health disorders (Otto, Greenstein, Johnson, & Friedman, 1992) to 80% including conduct disorder and substance abuse (see Kazdin, 2000). Girls exhibit strikingly high rates, and although the degree of difference varies based on sampling characteristics and diagnostic criteria, researchers have consistently found differences in the types and degree of mental health problems between girls and boys (Cauffman, 2001; Veysey & Hirschinger, in press; Teplin, Abram, McClelland, Dulcan, & Mericle, 2002). For example, Timmons-Mitchell and colleagues (1997) found that in a sample of 173 incarcerated youths, 27% of males and 84% of females exhibited mental health needs. Teplin et al. (2002) examined the rates of mental disorders in a detained sample (657 girls and 1,172 boys) and found that, of 20 categories of disorders, girls were more likely than boys to be diagnosed in 16 of them. Although girls are stereotypically viewed as having more internalizing problems (e.g., depression), Cauffman (2001) found higher rates of *both* internalizing and externalizing (e.g., conduct disorder) mental health problems among incarcerated girls than incarcerated boys.

Not only are the rates of mental disorders substantially higher for girls, but the types of mental health problems differ. Particularly prevalent among girls are post-traumatic stress disorder (PTSD), depression, and attention-deficit hyperactivity disorder (ADHD). Cauffman, Feldman, and Waterman (1998) found 65% of girls in the custody of the California Youth Authority, compared to 11% of girls in the general adolescent female population exhibited PTSD symptoms. This high rate is the likely result of many incarcerated girls' traumatic experiences with family and community violence, and sexual victimization. Another important link for girls in the justice system is the prevalence of depression. Obeidallah and Earls (1999) theorize that depression may be a central pathway for the development of girls' antisocial behaviors. Depression may weaken girls' bonds to prosocial institutions or increase their indifference to personal safety, leading to greater participation in risky activities. Female delinquents are more likely than male delinquents and non-delinquents to attempt to commit suicide (Lewis et al., 1991; Silverthorn & Frick, 1999). Furthermore, delinquent girls have higher rates of ADHD than delinquent boys (although in the general population, boys have much higher rates of ADHD) (Zoccolillo, 1993).

Both boys and girls often have substance abuse problems, and researchers have found contradictory findings regarding differences in the prevalence rates of substance abuse. For example, Teplin et al. (2002) and Timmons-Mitchell et al. (1997) found higher prevalence rates of substance abuse for boys, while Jasper, Smith, and Bailey (1998) found higher rates for girls. Regardless, the problem is widespread for both justice-involved boys and girls.

Many youth involved in the justice system meet the criteria for conduct disorder as delinquent behaviors are one of the symptoms for this diagnosis (Veysey & Hirschinger, in press). Note, however, that not all youths with conduct disorder become involved with the justice system. Conduct disorder diagnoses differ for boys and girls, as the criteria includes maladaptive social norm violations. Since these norms differ for boys and girls, several researchers have questioned the utility of this diagnosis (Odgers & Moretti, 2002; Veysey & Hirschinger, in press), and suggest that comorbidity of mental health disorders may be a more important consideration (for a review, see Odgers and Moretti, 2002). Loeber and Keenan (1994) found that girls were more likely than boys to have comorbid diagnoses, including ADHD, depression, and substance abuse. According to Katoaka et al. (2001), 80% of incarcerated girls exhibit symptoms of an emotional disorder and/or a substance use problem, with high rates of comorbidity.

The high prevalence of mental disorders among girls in the justice system may be an artifact resulting from a shortage of mental health resources in the community. Prescott (1998) reports that non-secure placements for adolescents have declined by 25% over a 10-year period, and many have argued that the justice system has become a clearinghouse for those in need of mental health treatment (Cocozza & Scowyra, 2000; Prescott, 1998). Given the lack of available community services, many girls are being channeled into the justice system, even though access to mental health services in the justice system is limited (Bialchik, 1998). In addition, girls may be less likely to receive the services that do exist. Zahn-Waxler (1993) points out that boys' aggressive and externalizing behaviors make them more likely to receive treatment. In the justice system, referrals for mental health services are often reserved for those charged with violent or sexual offenses. Since girls are less likely than boys to be charged with these types of offenses, they may be less likely to be referred for mental health services (Prescott, 1997). The high rates of mental health problems and the lack of available services in the community highlight the importance of providing mental health services as central components in justice system interventions.

HISTORY OF VICTIMIZATION AND CHAOTIC ENVIRONMENTS

Girls' problem behaviors are strongly related to their experiences with abusive and traumatic home lives (Chamberlain & Moore, 2002; Chesney-Lind & Shelden, 1992). Dembo et al. (1998) suggest that while boys' antisocial behaviors often reflect involvement in a delinquent lifestyle, heavily influenced by delinquent peers, girls' problem behaviors frequently appear to be related to a history of victimization. Researchers have consistently cited physical and sexual victimization as a significant factor contributing to girls' involvement in the justice system (Prescott, 1997; Veysey & Hirschinger, in press). Viale-Val and Sylvester (1993) reviewed studies of incarcerated youth and found that 50% of girls, compared to 2% of boys, had been sexually abused, and 42% of girls, compared to 22% of boys reported physical abuse. In Silverthorn and Frick's (1999) review, the number of antisocial girls who have been sexually abused ranged from 43% to 75%, compared to the general population rate of 12%. Of youths who experience abuse, girls are more likely than boys to be arrested for property offenses, selling drugs, and violent crimes and to become substance abusers (Rhodes & Fischer, 1993; Widom & White, 1997).

   In addition to experiencing higher rates of sexual and physical abuse, delinquent girls may also come from more dysfunctional family backgrounds than boys, with highly conflictual parental relationships (Dembo et al., 1998; Viale-Val & Sylvester, 1993; Henggeler, Edwards, & Borduin, 1987; Silverthorn & Frick, 1999). Henggeler et al. (1987) studied two-parent families of female delinquents and found that girls experience high levels of conflict and hostilities with their mothers. Additionally, fathers of female delinquents are more neurotic and exhibit less familial control than those of male delinquents. Chesney-Lind (1987) suggested that the total effect of family conflict affects girls more strongly than boys, but that this effect may be indirect through reduced parental supervision, reduced identification with parents, and increased exposure to delinquency. Henggeler et al. (1987) contend that because of the exceptionally strong social sanctions and gender role stereotypes that do not support female delinquency, it takes a very dysfunctional family environment to promote delinquency. These researchers also proposed that because girls place such value on interpersonal relationships, they may become more involved in conflictual family relations than boys, and are therefore more strongly affected.

   Girls in the justice system have greater rates of familial mental illness and criminality than their male counterparts (Dembo et al. 1998; Offord, Abrams, Allen, & Poushinsky, 1979; Rosenbaum, 1989). Chamberlain and Moore (2002), examining data from the Oregon Social Learning Center, found significant differences between boys' and girls' parental contact with the justice system, with 43% of girls' mothers and 63% of girls' fathers having contact, compared to 22% of boys' mothers and 22% of boys' fathers. Antisocial girls are also more likely than antisocial boys to have delinquent siblings (Jones, Offord, & Abrams, 1980). Research on girls' chaotic, and often victimizing, experiences in the home and community emphasizes the need for intervention components that assist girls and their families in building stable and safe environments.

RELATIONAL AGGRESSION

Researchers have recently begun to examine non-physical forms of aggression that may be especially common for girls, such as relational aggression (see Crick et al., present volume). Girls who are highly relationally aggressive are likely to have difficulties with social adjustment. Wolke, Woods, Bloomfield, and Karstadt (2000) found that children who reported using relational strategies to bully other children showed increased conduct problems and fewer prosocial behaviors than non-bullies. Crick and Grotpeter (1995) found relational aggression was highly associated with externalizing and internalizing adjustment problems, such as loneliness and depression. Crick et al. (1999) also suggested that in addition to many of the same maladjustments of physically aggressive children, relationally aggressive children have added difficulties, such as borderline personality features and eating disorders. Justice-involved girls report encountering high levels of interpersonal conflict and relational aggression in their daily lives, with 72% of girls in Chamberlain and Moore's (2002) study reporting having committed some form of relational aggression in the previous 24 hours. Moretti and Odgers (2002) have suggested that severe forms of relational aggression may be a "marker" or predictor of other types of aggression. Targeting relationally aggressive behaviors may help girls find other ways to deal with interpersonal conflicts and prevent them from escalating into physical conflicts.

In summary, girls in the justice system do present with different needs than boys. Girls have an increased likelihood of mental health problems, greater experiences of victimization, and manifest aggression differently than boys. These differences suggest that girls have distinct intervention needs that are not always the same as boys.

ARE INTERVENTIONS DESIGNED FOR BOYS APPROPRIATE FOR GIRLS?

The majority of current intervention programs are designed to serve boys. For many jurisdictions, limited funding and small numbers of female delinquents make it difficult to justify separate programs for girls. However, the increasing number of girls in the justice system has drawn greater attention to consideration of their intervention needs. In many cases, interventions designed to serve boys are simply expanded to include girls. These programs are usually adopted wholesale for girls, with little attention to whether they are equally appropriate. When programs which include girls are evaluated, the number of girls participating is frequently too small to make any definitive conclusions regarding the effects of the programs for girls or to examine differential effects for boys and girls. Often, girls may be excluded from evaluations, or when they are included, they are combined with the male participants to determine an overall programmatic effect. This omission has made it difficult to discover if traditional intervention programs work for girls, particularly for justice-involved youths. Some examples from school- or community-based programs demonstrate the difficulty of translating programs designed to serve boys to a population of girls. For example, Brestan and Eyberg (1998) reviewed 82 studies on the treatment of conduct disorders in children and adolescents and concluded that since interventions primarily used samples of boys, it was impossible to determine the effect of these programs for girls.

When girls are included in adequate numbers, there is some compelling evidence to support the differential effects of programs on boys and girls. In fact, in some instances, the programs may have iatrogenic effects on girls. Farrell and Meyer (1997) evaluated a school-based intervention designed to teach social problem-solving skills and reduce aggressive behaviors for 6th graders. Although boys in the intervention group reported fewer problem behaviors than those in the control group, the opposite was true for the girls who participated in the intervention. Farrell and Meyer suggest that the girls may not have fared as well because the problem solving techniques may not have addressed forms of aggressive behaviors that are more common in girls. The effect of the program for the girls may also have been influenced by the mixed-gender group format and the male leadership of these groups.

Despite the dearth of information and the pessimistic findings of Farrell and Meyer (1997), effective evaluation designs may provide some guidance as to how programs can be modified to serve girls appropriately. Chamberlain and Moore's (2002) Therapeutic Foster Care (TFC) program, based on social learning theory and targeting adolescents involved in the court system, is notable. Adolescents are placed in individual foster homes, with foster parents who are trained and supported by a case worker. The program is comprehensive in its approach, focusing not only on the individual child, but also helping the birth/adoptive parents with child management skills. A case worker coordinates the child's treatment plan, which includes individual and family therapy, and monitors school performance. The program was originally designed for boys, and later, at the request of service providers, was expanded to serve girls. Chamberlain and Moore (2002) evaluated the program and found that boys began with higher rates of problems that decreased over time. In comparison, girls reported fewer problem behaviors but unexpectedly, these behaviors increased over time. Chamberlain and Moore hypothesized that they had failed to include components in the program to address the social/relational forms of aggression, which were affecting girls' relationships with parents and support staff in the TFC program. As a result, they restructured the intervention to address girls' needs and help them maintain positive relationships with the supportive adults. Although evaluation of the program is still in the early stages, the investigators have found a positive effect on girls, which they attribute to the consideration of the unique needs of girls involved with the justice system.

In summary, it would appear that programs for boys may serve as a potential basis for girls' programs, but they may need to be modified and adapted to meet the unique needs of girls in the system. Researchers should include specific evaluation components to determine the efficacy of these programs for girls and examine the programs within the justice system. Programs such as TFC, which includes components to serve the needs of girls, are promising interventions. Other widespread interventions currently targeting boys may be effective for girls (e.g., multisystemic therapy, family functioning therapy), but sparse evaluation data prevent any definitive conclusions regarding the efficacy of these programs for girls.

SHOULD PROGRAMS BE DEVELOPED SPECIFICALLY FOR GIRLS?

In response to the increasing numbers of girls in the justice system, policymakers have begun to develop gender-specific programming guidelines. In 1998, the United States' Office of Juvenile Justice and Delinquency Prevention (OJJDP) issued recommendations for gender specific programs. Although many of these recommendations should be universally applied (i.e., respectful staff, safe supportive environment, educational services) (Chesney-Lind, 2001), OJJDP (1998) suggested special service provisions for girls that aim to improve self-esteem, body image, feelings of empowerment, and interpersonal relationships. These programs are compelling because they advocate for strong staff training on girls' development and emphasize the importance of cultural diversity. While gender specific efforts appear promising, several challenges exist in the design and implementation of such programs.

Much of the theoretical framework for gender specific programming is based on normative female adolescent development. The OJJDP report primarily used research on female adolescent development as a basis for their gender-specific program recommendations, but perhaps indicative of the lack of research on female delinquency, provided little information to differentiate the experiences of delinquent girls from either the normative development of adolescent girls or the experiences of delinquent boys. The emphasis on normative development alone may be misguided unless careful consideration is given to the unique needs of female offenders. For example, although gender specific programming that emphasizes increasing girls' self-esteem and feelings of empowerment may be important, for many girls these components will have limited effects without meaningful change in an abusive environment or assistance with their mental health needs.

Advocates of gender specific programs suggest a strong relationship building component for interventions, based on normative research on the importance of relationships for girls (OJJDP, 1998). The cautionary note of applying research on delinquent boys to delinquent girls may also apply to the application of research on non-delinquent girls to delinquent girls. Gender specific program advocates emphasize the need for girls to build peer relationships, but evaluation data are needed to determine the viability of this approach as an intervention strategy. As a caution, Poulin, Dishion, and Burraston (2001) have found that interventions for delinquent boys, which they call "deviancy training," may undesirably strengthen their cohesion to other delinquent youth through group treatments. Whether these iatrogenic effects would hold for girls, and under what circumstances, is unclear.

Gender specific theorists advocate a comprehensive approach to intervention, but in practice, with limited resources, programs for girls may be too narrowly focused and result in one-size fits all. Chesney-Lind (2001) found that some programs that exclusively targeted girls were overly focused on one specific gender stereotyped issue, such as pregnancy or sexual abuse. Gender specific programs may also be weakened if intervention efforts are cast too broadly, without regard for the specific type of offense. Justice-involved girls do not represent a homogeneous group, and programs should consider such factors as cultural diversity and the pathways which bring girls into the justice system. Treatment programs for boys often work best when tailored to the type of offense and target the underlying problems that led to the delinquent behavior (Mulvey, Arthur, & Reppucci, 1993); the same is likely true for girls. The most promising gender-specific programs are those that are individualized and comprehensive. For example, a focus on developing healthy relationships may be important for a relationally aggressive girl, while a focus on family issues and victimization may be important for runaways.

In summary, the new generation of gender-specific programs for girls appear promising, especially if they include components based on both normative development and female delinquency. However, it is too early in their development to have determined their short- or long-term efficacy. Moreover, most gender-specific programs are small and, unfortunately, lack sufficient resources to conduct comprehensive evaluations. As a result, in most cases, resources have been focused exclusively on service provision, so it is difficult to judge their effectiveness (Acoca, 1999).

RECOMMENDATIONS

Researchers have determined several factors that contribute to program effectiveness for interventions targeting justice-involved boys, including goodness of fit of the treatment options, consideration of multiple contexts, and implementation of community based-interventions. These factors are particularly important for interventions targeting girls. For example, one of the most important factors related to amenability to treatment is the goodness of fit between the juvenile and treatment option (Fried, Mulvey, Portwood, Woolard, & Reppucci, in press; Kruh & Brodsky, 1991). Dowden and Andrews (1999) examined the effectiveness of interventions for adult female offenders and emphasized the importance of an intervention's responsivity—the style of the program should be matched to the offender. As already noted, the limited spectrum of treatments for girls has resulted in similar treatment options regardless of the girls' background or offense type. The recent attention and allocation of resources to girls programming should broaden the types of interventions available so that girls cease to be seen as a homogenous group, without regard to the diversity of their experiences.

Effective programs should also look beyond girls as isolated individuals and consider the multiple contexts that influence them. Interventions tend to focus on the individual or the individual in the correctional peer group, but evidence regarding high rates of victimization and conflictual home environments highlight the importance of addressing ecological factors in any intervention for girls. Without appropriate transitional services, they may be returning to unsafe, damaging environments that may have instigated the behaviors for which the girls were incarcerated and the need for services in the first place. Tate, Reppucci, and Mulvey (1995), in their review of interventions for serious and violent juveniles, found that the community-based services were the most effective, but most of these programs served only boys. Such services seem equally, or even more important, for girls as they return to potentially stressful home and neighborhood environments and regain daily contact with their families and peers. Interventions that provide support for girls and their families and involve the coordination of services in the community to assist girls with coping in the home, school, and peer group appear more likely to prevent future justice system contact.

In summary, to determine what interventions work for girls, the most important component is rigorous evaluation. Although many programs targeting girls are small and have limited resources, evaluations are essential in order to hone in on effective components of programming. To conduct effective evaluations, several methodological considerations are essential: a) evaluators should include process measures to check for program fidelity and to determine what components of the program work well; b) researchers should utilize experimental research design to determine the relationship between the program and outcomes for girls; and c) program participants should be followed longitudinally to determine if the intervention has a long-term impact (Muehrer & Koretz, 1992).

Specific recommendations for interventions with girls include:

1. Interventions should consider the mental health problems that are common for justice-involved girls. Programs should pay particular attention to the needs of girls affected by substance abuse, ADHD, post-traumatic stress disorder, and depression.
2. Intervention programs should address a) the family and home lives of girls and b) problems at a larger systemic level by providing services for families and communities.
3. Programs originally designed to serve boys should not be considered equally effective or ineffective for girls without rigorous process and outcome evaluations. These programs may provide the foundation for interventions, but may need to be modified to fit the unique needs of girls by addressing mental health needs, histories of victimization, and family issues.
4. A gender-specific approach to programming may be promising if research on delinquent girls and the specific needs of offenders are included in program components. Empowerment models usually should be coupled with intensive mental health and family-based services.
5. Girls come to the attention of the justice system through various pathways, and they do not represent a homogenous group. Interventions should be tailored to the needs of different types of girls.
6. Girls need assistance and support as they return to their communities to ensure they return to safe homes and continue to receive services.

7. In addition to research on girls' natural desistance, evaluations are desperately needed to determine what works for girls.

Throughout this chapter, we have focused on areas in which research on justice-involved girls is needed. We echo the call for more prospective studies, longitudinal follow-ups, and control-group evaluations. Although development of interventions for girls remains in the early stages, we are hopeful that a new generation of programs will conduct evaluations to determine what works and what doesn't work for them. By incorporating the needs of girls into *comprehensive* and *appropriate* treatment plans, contact with the justice system could serve as an important gateway to help girls with safety, security, and health.

REFERENCES

Acoca, L. (1999). Investing in girls: A 21st century strategy. *Juvenile Justice Journal, 6,* Washington DC: OJJDP.

Bialchik, S. (1998). Mental health disorders and substance abuse problems among juveniles. OJJDP Fact Sheet. Washington, DC: US Department of Justice.

Brestan, E. V., & Eyberg, S. M. (1998). Effective psychosocial treatments of conduct-disordered children and adolescents: 29 years, 82 studies, and 5,272 kids. *Journal of Clinical Child Psychology, 27,* 180–189.

Budnick, K. J., & Shields-Fletcher, E. (1998). What about girls? *OJJDP Fact Sheet, 48.* Washington. DC: Office of Juvenile Justice and Delinquency Prevention.

Cauffman, E. (2001, March). Delinquent girls: Developmental considerations and public policy implications. In C. Odgers (Chair), *Serious and violent offending among girls: Current research and public policy implications.* Symposium conducted at the biennial meeting of the American Psychology-Law Society, Austin, TX.

Cauffman, E., Feldman, S. S., Waterman, J., & Steiner, H. (1998). Posttraumatic stress disorder among female juvenile offenders. *Journal of the American Academy of Child & Adolescent Psychiatry, 37,* 1209–1216.

Chamberlain, P., & Reid, J. B. (1994). Differences in risk factors and adjustment for male and female delinquents in treatment foster care. *Journal of Child & Family Studies, 3,* 23–39.

Chamberlain, P., & Moore, K. J. (2002). Chaos and trauma in the lives of adolescent females with antisocial behavior and delinquency. *Journal of Aggression, Maltreatment & Trauma, 6,* 79–108.

Chesney-Lind, M., & Shelden, R. (1992). *Girls, delinquency, and juvenile justice* (2nd ed.). Pacific Grove, CA: Brooks/Cole.

Chesney-Lind, M. (1987). Girls and violence: An exploration of the gender gap in serious delinquent behavior. In D. H. Crowell and I. M. Evans (Eds.), *Childhood aggression and violence: Sources of influence, prevention, and control* (pp. 207–229). New York: Plenum Press.

Chesney-Lind, M. (2001). What about girls? Delinquency programming as if gender mattered. *Corrections Today, 63,* 38–41.

Cocozza, J. J., & Scowyra, K. R. (2000). Youth with mental health disorders: Issues and emerging responses. *Juvenile Justice, 7,* 3–13.

Crick, N. R., Werner, N. E., Casas, J. F., O'Brien, K. M., Nelson, D. A., Grotpeter, J. K., & Markon, K. (1999). Childhood aggression and gender: A new look at an old problem. In D. Bernstein (Ed.), *Nebraska Symposium on Motivation* (vol. 45, pp. 75–141). Lincoln: University of Nebraska Press.

Crick, N. & Grotpeter, J. (1995). Relational aggression, gender, and social-psychological adjustment. *Child Development, 66*, 710–722.

Dembo, R., Pacheco, K., Schmeidler, J., Ramirez-Garmica, G., Guida, J., & Rahman, A. (1998). A further study of gender differences in service needs among youths entering a juvenile assessment center. *Journal of Child and Adolescent Substance Abuse, 7*, 49–77.

Dembo, R., Williams, L., & Schmeidler, J. (1993). Gender differences in mental health service needs among youths entering a juvenile detention center. *Journal of Prison and Jail Health, 12*, 73–101.

Dowden, C., & Andrews, D. A. (1999). What works for female offenders: A meta-analytic review. *Crime & Delinquency 45*, 438–452.

Farrell, A. D., & Meyer, A. L. (1997). The effectiveness of a school-based curriculum for reducing violence among urban sixth-grade students. *American Journal of Public Health, 87*, 979–984.

Fried, C. S., Mulvey, E. P., Portwood, S. L., Woolard, J. L., & Reppucci, N. D. (in press) Legal issues affecting youth with mental health disorders in the juvenile justice system. In J. J. Cocozza (Ed.), *Responding to the mental health needs of youth offenders: A comprehensive review.*

Henggeler, S. W., Edwards, J., & Borduin, C. (1987). The family relations of female juvenile delinquents. *Journal of Abnormal Child Psychology, 15*, 199–209.

Hoyt, S., & Scherer, D. G. (1998). Female juvenile delinquency: Misunderstood by the juvenile justice system, neglected by social science. *Law and Human Behavior, 22*, 81–107.

Jasper, A., Smith, C., & Bailey, S. (1998). One hundred girls in care referred to an adolescent forensic mental health service. *Journal of Adolescence, 21*, 555–568.

Jones, M. B., Offord, D. R., & Adams N. (1980). Brothers, sisters and antisocial behaviour. *British Journal of Psychiatry, 136*, 139–145.

Katoaka, S. H., Zima, B. T., Dupre, D. A., Moreno, K. A., Yank, X., & Mccracken, J. T. (2001). Mental health problems and service use among female juvenile offenders: Their relationship to criminal history. *Journal of the American Academy of Child & Adolescent Psychiatry, 40*, 549–555.

Kazdin, A. (2000). Adolescent development, mental disorders, and decision making of delinquent youths. In T. Grisso & R. G. Schwartz (Eds.), *Youth on trial: A developmental perspective on juvenile justice* (pp. 33–65). Chicago, IL: University of Chicago Press.

Kruh, I. P., & Brodsky, S. L. (1997). Clinical evaluations for transfer of juveniles to criminal court: Current practices and future research. *Behavioral Sciences and the Law, 15*, 151–165.

Lanctot, N., & Le Blanc, M. (2002). Explaining deviance by adolescent females. *Crime and Justice, 29*, 113–202.

Lewis, D. O., Yeager, C. A., Cobham-Portorreal, C. S., Klein, N., Showalter, C., & Anthony, A. (1991). A follow-up of female delinquents: maternal contributions to the perpetuation of deviance. *Journal of the American Academy of Child and Adolescent Psychiatry, 30*, 197–201.

Loeber, R., & Keenan, K. (1994). Interaction between conduct disorder and its comorbid conditions: Effects of age and gender. *Clinical Psychology Review, 14*, 497–523.

Moffitt, T. E. (1993). Adolescence-limited and life-course-persistent antisocial behavior: A developmental taxonomy. *Psychological Review, 100*, 674–701.

Moffitt, T. E., Caspi, A., Rutter, M., & Silva, P. A. (2001). *Sex differences in antisocial behavior: Conduct disorder, delinquency, and violence in the Dunedin Longitudinal Study.* Cambridge: Cambridge University Press.

Moretti, M., & Odgers, C. (2002). Aggressive and violent girls: Prevalence, profiles, and contributing factors. In R. R. Corrado, R. Roesch, & S. D. Hart (Eds.), *Multi-problem youth: A foundation for comparative research on needs, interventions, and outcomes* (pp. 302–329). Amsterdam: IOS Press.

Muehrer, P., & Koretz, D. S. (1992). Issues in preventive intervention research. *Current Directions in Psychological Science, 1*, 109–112.

Mulvey, E. P., Arthur, M. W., & Reppucci, N. D. (1993). The prevention and treatment of juvenile delinquency: A review of the research. *Clinical Psychology Review, 13*, 133–176.

Obeidallah, D. A., & Earls, F. J. (1999). Adolescent girls: The role of depression in the development of delinquency. *National Institute of Justice Research Preview*. Washington, DC: National Institute of Justice.

Odgers, C., & Moretti, M. (2002). Aggressive and antisocial girls: Research updates and future research challenges. *International Journal of Forensic and Mental Health, 2*, 17–33.

Office of Juvenile Justice and Delinquency Prevention (OJJDP). (1998). *Guiding principles for promising female programming: An inventory of best practices*. Washington, DC: Author.

Offord, D. R., Abrams, N., Allen, N., & Poushinsky, M. (1979). Broken homes, parental psychiatric illness, and female delinquency. *American Journal of Orthopsychiatry, 49*, 252–264.

Otto, R. K., Greenstein, J. J., Johnson, M. K., & Friedman, R. M. (1992). Prevalence of mental disorders among youth in the juvenile justice system. In J. J. Cocozza (Ed.), *Responding to the mental health needs of youth in the juvenile justice system* (pp. 7–48). Seattle, WA: The National Coalition for the Mentally Ill in the Criminal Justice System.

Pajer, K. A. (1998). What happens to 'bad' girls? A review of the adult outcomes of antisocial adolescent girls. *American Journal of Psychiatry, 155*, 862–870.

Porter, G. (2000). Detention and delinquency cases, 1988–1997. Washington, DC: Office of Juvenile Justice and Delinquency Prevention.

Poulin, A. B. (1996). Female delinquents: Defining their place in the justice system. *Wisconsin Law Review, 541*, 1–33.

Poulin, F., Dishion, T. J., & Burraston, B. (2001). 3-Year iatrogenic effects associated with aggregating high-risk adolescents in cognitive-behavioral preventive interventions. *Applied Developmental Science, 5*, 214–224

Prescott, L. (1997). *Adolescent girls with co-occurring disorders in the juvenile justice system*. Delmar, NY: GAINS Center.

Prescott, L. (1998). *Improving policy and practice for adolescent girls with co-occurring disorders in the juvenile justice system*. Delmar, NY: GAINS Center.

Rhodes, J., & Fischer, K. (1993). Spanning the gender gap: Gender differences in delinquency among inner-city adolescents. *Adolescence, 28*, 879–890.

Rosenbaum, J. L. (1989). Family dysfunction and female delinquency. *Crime and Delinquency, 35*, 31–44.

Silverthorn, P., & Frick, P. (1999). Developmental pathways to antisocial behavior: The delayed-onset pathway in girls. *Development and Psychopathology, 11*, 101–126.

Snyder, H. (2002). Juvenile arrests, 2000. *Juvenile Justice Bulletin*. Washington, DC: OJJDP.

Snyder, H., & Sickmund, M. (1999). *Juvenile offenders and victims: 1999 national report*. Washington D.C.: Office of Juvenile Justice and Delinquency Prevention.

Storvall, E. E., & Wichstrom, L. (2002). Do the risk factors associated with conduct problems in adolescents vary according to gender? *Journal of Adolescence, 25*, 182–202.

Tate, D. C., Reppucci, N. D., & Mulvey, E. P. (1995). Violent juvenile delinquents: Treatment effectiveness and implications for future action. *American Psychologist, 50*, 777–781.

Teplin, L. A., Abram, K. M., McClelland, G. M., Dulcan, M. K., & Mericle, A. A. (2002). Psychiatric disorders in youth in juvenile detention. *Archives of General Psychiatry, 59*, 1133–1143.

Timmons-Mitchell, J., Brown, C., Schulz, S. C., Webster, S. E., Underwood, L. A., & Semple, W.E. (1997). Comparing the mental health needs of female and male incarcerated juvenile delinquents. *Behavioral Sciences and the Law, 15*, 195–202.

Veysey, B. M., & Hirschinger, N. (in press). Adolescent girls with mental health disorders in the juvenile justice system. In J. J. Cocozza (Ed.), *Responding to the mental health needs of youth offenders: A comprehensive review.*

Viale-Val, G., & Sylvester, C. (1993). Female delinquency. In M. Sugar (Ed.), *Female development* (2nd ed., pp. 169–187). New York: Brunner/Mazel.

Werner, E. E. & Smith, R. S. (1992). *Overcoming the odds: High risk children from birth to adulthood.* Ithaca, NY: Cornell University Press.

Widom, C. S., & White. H. R. (1997). Problem behaviors in abused and neglected children grown up: Prevalence and co-occurrence of substance abuse, crime, and violence. *Criminal Behaviour and Mental Health, 7*, 287–310.

Wolke, D., Woods, S., Bloomfield, L., & Karstadt, L. (2000). The association between direct and relational bullying and behavioral problems among primary school children. *Journal of Child Psychology and Psychiatry, 41*, 989–1002.

Zahn-Waxler, C. (1993). Warriors and worriers: Gender and psychopathology. *Development and Psychopathology, 5*, 79–89.

Zoccolilo, M. (1993). Gender and the development of conduct disorder. *Development and Psychopathology, 5*, 65–78.

Prediction and Prevention of Peer Victimization in Early Elementary School
How Does Gender Matter?

BONNIE J. LEADBEATER, MANDEEP K. DHAMI,
WENDY L. HOGLUND, AND
ERIN M. BOONE

While all children engage in physical aggression (e.g., pushing and hitting) and relational aggression (e.g., spreading rumors and social exclusion), past research suggests that the former is more prevalent among boys, and the latter is typically more frequent among girls (Björkqvist, Lagerspetz, & Kuakiainen, 1992; Cairns, Cairns, Neckerman, Ferguson, & Gariepy, 1989; Crick, 1997; Crick & Grotpeter, 1995; Lagerspetz, Bjorkqvist, & Peltonen, 1988; Owens, 1996; Smith & Sharp, 1994). Furthermore, the fact that children often interact with same-sex peers suggests these differences are also reflected in their victimization experiences, with boys generally reporting more physical and girls reporting more relational victimization (Crick et al., 2001). However, few gender differences in levels of physical victimization are evident for boys and girls in early school grades (Kochenderfer & Ladd, 1997). Moreover, while some studies suggest that boys are more likely to

BONNIE J. LEADBEATER, MANDEEP K. DHAMI, WENDY L. HOGLUND, AND ERIN M. BOONE • Department of Psychology, University of Victoria, Victoria, British Columbia, Canada, V8P 5C2.

experience victimization than girls (e.g., Cleary, 2000; Dhami, Leadbeater, Hoglund, & Boone, 2003; Olweus, 1994; Whitney & Smith, 1993), others have found no significant gender differences in victimization of third to sixth graders (Crick & Grotpeter, 1996) and adolescents (Paquette & Underwood, 1999). These mixed findings suggest that we need to look beyond gender per se for explanations of gender differences that have been observed in risks for aggression and victimization.

Understanding the development of aggression and victimization in girls has become particularly urgent given the widespread public acceptance of the idea that girls exhibit increasingly more dangerous, relational aggression than boys do. Indeed, two highly publicized court cases in 2002 in British Columbia and Nova Scotia, Canada resulted in the first convictions to girls for "uttering threats" that were deemed to contribute to the suicides of their peers. A better understanding of the mechanisms that link gender differences to subtypes of victimization or aggression for subgroups of girls and boys would help to determine appropriate program, school policy, and even legal responses to these problems.

Although there is little empirical research to illuminate these mechanisms, possible explanations for how gender matters are beginning to emerge. First, gender differences in types of victimization may be unstable in elementary-school children, but become more differentiated in early adolescence as individual differences in gender-linked risk and protective factors intensify (e.g., behavior problems, internalizing symptoms; see review in Leadbeater, Blatt, & Quinlan, 1995), or as gender-appropriate behaviors are increasingly enforced by peers (Maccoby, 2002). For example, Schwartz, McFadyen-Ketchum, Dodge, Pettit, and Bates (1999) demonstrated that risks for victimization were greater for children who violated gender stereotyped norms, (i.e., victimization was higher for girls who showed hyperactive-impulsive behaviors and for boys who showed immature-dependent behaviors). Friendships reduced risks for victimization, particularly for the immature-dependent boys.

A second explanation for inconsistent findings of gender differences in victimization is that these differences may be observed in high-risk youths, but be negligible in youths with few behavioral or peer problems. For example, Vaillancourt, Hymel, and McDougall (2002) found that adolescent girls who were identified as bullies by their peers were more relationally aggressive than male bullies. Finally, context differences (e.g., levels of aggressive children grouped together in one classroom) may have different implications for aggression and victimization in boys and girls. Kellam, Ling, Merisca, Brown, and Ialongo (1998) found that boys (but not girls) exposed to first grade classrooms with high concentrations of aggressive children were more aggressive in sixth grade than boys in first grade classrooms with low concentrations of aggressive children.

Our own program of ongoing longitudinal research at the University of Victoria, British Columbia, The W.I.T.S. Longitudinal Study, is investigating the individual and context level differences (in classrooms and schools) that contribute to peer victimization in the early elementary school years (Dhami et al., 2003; Hoglund & Leadbeater, 2003; Leadbeater, Hoglund, & Woods, 2003). In this chapter, we hope to add to the understanding of how gender matters in predicting peer victimization by addressing the following questions: 1) Do gender differences in the levels and changes in peer victimization emerge in early elementary school? 2) Does gender moderate the effects of a school-wide prevention program on relational and physical victimization? 3) Does gender interact with individual differences in social competence or emotional and behavioral problems in predicting relational and physical victimization?

PEER VICTIMIZATION IN ELEMENTARY SCHOOL: THE W.I.T.S. LONGITUDINAL STUDY

We have assessed children's reports of their experiences of peer relational and physical victimization, as well as predictors of these problems at three time points; namely, the beginning and end of first grade, and the end of second grade. Teacher and parent reports of the children's social competence and emotional and behavioral problems were obtained at each time point. We focus on the teacher reports in this chapter.

Details of the sample, procedure and methods are presented in Leadbeater et al. (2003). Briefly, the initial sample consisted of 432 children (49% girls, mean age = six years and three months) with parent consent. The overall participation rate was 64%, and 92% ($N = 397$) participated at the third wave of data collection. Attrition was generally due to children moving out of the school district. Parent reports indicated that 32% of the children lived in a household with a total annual income of less than $30,000. Sixty-one per cent of children lived with both parents. The median level of mothers' education was "some college or technical training beyond high school" (range = eighth grade or less to graduate degree). Seventy-three percent of the parents identified themselves as Caucasian, and 73% of parents reported that English was the only language spoken at home.

Forty-four classrooms, in 17 elementary schools in a local school district are participating in the W.I.T.S. Longitudinal Study. Initially, 290 of the children in the W.I.T.S. Longitudinal Study were in one of the 11 program schools, whereas 142 were in one of the 6 control programs. Program schools were chosen based on an initial implementation assessment showing that the school had adequately implemented a school-wide, peer violence prevention program, called *The W.I T.S. Rock Solid Foundation Primary Program* (*www.youth.society.uvic.ca*). This is a school-wide peer victimization prevention program that was developed through a community-school-university partnership between the Rock Solid Foundation (a community-based police group), the Greater Victoria School District 61, and the Centre for Youth and Society at the University of Victoria. The W.I.T.S. acronym stands for "Walk away," "Ignore," "Talk it out," and "Seek help." Using your "W.I.T.S." easily becomes a code-word with school-wide visibility, and parent and community support.

The W.I.T.S. program is implemented through a collaboration among police school-liaison officers, classroom teachers, playground supervisors, librarians, parents, and older students. The curriculum directs teachers to early childhood literature and activities that reinforce the W.I.T.S. messages. Uniformed police officers visit the school on a regular basis to deputize the children (as W.I.T.S. special constables) and encourage them to use their W.I.T.S.. Similarly, student athletes from the University of Victoria regularly visit the school and act as positive role models, and remind children to use their W.I.T.S.. A playground program enlists and trains older children in the school as peer helpers, so that they may intervene in conflicts and remind children to use their W.I.T.S.. A siblings program takes the W.I.T.S. message into the child's home via a pamphlet that informs parents of the program, and guides them to use the W.I.T.S. approach when dealing with sibling conflicts. A stuffed walrus (called WITSUP), activity books, and gifts (bookmarks, pens, pencils) are used to reinforce the W.I.T.S. messages and help take them home.

Measures: Children's *social competence* (e.g., "gets along with other children," "shares toys or materials"), *emotional problems* (e.g., "appears unhappy or depressed," "is withdrawn, shy, or bashful"), and *behavioral problems* (e.g., "appears unhappy or depressed," "is shy or bashful") were assessed using teacher reports of children's behaviors on the Early School Behavior Rating Scale (ESBS; Caldwell & Pianta, 1991). The Social Experiences Questionnaire (SEQ; Crick & Grotpeter, 1996) was used to assess children's experiences of *prosocial acts* (e.g., "How often does another kid help you when you need it?"), *relational victimization* (e.g., "How often do other kids leave you out on purpose when it is time to play or do an activity?"), and *physical victimization* (e.g., "How often do you get hit by another kid at school?"). Children rated how often the events occurred on a 3-point scale.

1) Do Gender Differences in the Levels and Changes in Victimization Emerge in Early Elementary School?

Mean levels over first and second grade and gender differences in children's reports of their experiences of prosocial acts and relational and physical victimization are displayed in Table 1. The average levels of prosocial acts reported by the children increased significantly, while average levels of relational and physical victimization decreased significantly over the three time points for both boys and girls. Girls consistently reported higher average levels of prosocial acts, F (1, 393) = 24.25, $p < .001$, and relational victimization, F (1, 393) = 5.28, $p < .05$, across the three assessments compared to boys. Gender differences in mean levels of physical victimization were not statistically significant. Because the children in this study came from schools with or without a victimization program it is important to assess whether program effects dampened the expected gender differences.

2) Does Gender Moderate the Effect of the W.I.T.S. Program on Victimization?

Recent evaluations suggest that there are gender differences in responsiveness to some school-based interventions for peer victimization. Some

TABLE 1. Repeated Measures Analyses of Mean Level (and Standard Deviations) Changes in Peer Prosocial Acts and Victimization by Gender

	Time 1	Time 2	Time 3
1) *Prosocial Acts*			
Girls	6.63 (.19)	7.19 (.17)	7.16 (.16)
Boys	5.97 (.19)	6.23 (.16)	6.13 (.16)
Total	6.30 (.13)	6.71 (.12)	6.66 (.11)
Multivariate F (2, 392) = 0.73, $p = .48$. Time, Univariate $F = 4.88$, $p < .01$.			
2) *Relational Victimization*			
Girls	2.84 (.18)	2.69 (.17)	2.61 (.15)
Boys	2.48 (.17)	2.45 (.16)	1.96 (.15)
Total	2.66 (.12)	2.59 (.12)	2.29 (.11)
Multivariate F (2, 392) = 1.59, $p = .21$. Time, Univariate $F = 4.43$, $p < .01$.			
3) *Physical Victimization*			
Girls	2.78 (.18)	2.47 (.17)	2.22 (.14)
Boys	2.74 (.18)	2.73 (.16)	2.13 (.14)
Total	2.75 (.13)	2.59 (.12)	2.16 (.10)
Multivariate F (2, 393) = 1.19, $p = .31$. Time, Univariate $F = 10.39$, $p < .001$.			

prevention programs mainly affect aggression in boys (Farrell & Meyer, 1997; Kellam et al., 1998), while others show similar effects on boys' and girls' aggression (Aber, Brown, & Jones, 2003), and still others have primary effects for girls' attitudes and prosocial behaviors (Artz & Riecken, 1997). Moreover, focusing on classroom-level factors, Kellam et al. (1998) found that aggressive boys (but not girls) in aggressive classroom groupings in first grade (assessed by average levels of teacher-rated aggression of all children in a classroom) showed higher levels of aggression in sixth grade than aggressive boys in less aggressive first grade classrooms. Gender did not interact with classroom characteristics (levels of aggression, emotional problems, and social competence) in predicting changes in levels of victimization from first to second grade in the W.I.T.S. Longitudinal Study (Leadbeater et al., 2003).

We examined gender differences in changes in mean levels of prosocial behaviors, and relational and physical victimization, separately for program and control children from entry to first grade to the end of first and second grade (see Table 2). Gender differences in program effects were small and not statistically significant. This could be explained by the reduced power for these analyses, although some patterns in the results suggest that changes in receipt of prosocial acts and reports of physical victimization did differ slightly for boys and girls in schools that were not part of the intervention. Boys and girls in the program schools and girls in the control schools reported increases in their experiences of *prosocial behaviors* from their peers, while boys in control schools reported fewer prosocial behaviors over time. Boys and girls in the program schools reported declines in *relational victimization* by the end of second grade, while boys and girls in control schools reported similar levels of relational victimization at each time point. Boys and girls in the program schools and boys in the control schools reported declines in *physical victimization* over time; however, girls in the control schools reported similar levels at each assessment. Overall, however, these gender differences for prosocial behaviors and physical victimization were slight and should not be over interpreted.

While gender is not a strong predictor of the W.I.T.S. program effects, previous research with this sample (Leadbeater et al., 2003) has drawn attention to the importance of context differences in classroom contexts that may have importance in helping us to understand how gender matters in understanding victimization as we continue to follow this sample. We investigated whether *classroom characteristics* (i. e., average levels of social competence, emotional problems, and behavioral problems) in first grade influenced changes in children's reports of relational and physical victimization by the end of second grade. Findings showed that classroom levels

TABLE 2. Repeated Measures Analyses of Mean Level (And Standard Deviations) Changes in Peer Prosocial Acts and Victimization by Gender and Intervention Group.

	Time 1		Time 2		Time 3	
	Program	Control	Program	Control	Program	Control
1) Prosocial Acts						
Girls	6.45 (.24)	7.20 (.37)	7.21 (.20)	7.29 (.32)	7.15 (.19)	7.33 (.31)
Boys	5.95 (.23)	6.07 (.35)	6.34 (.20)	6.16 (.31)	6.42 (.19)	5.67 (.29)
Total	6.20 (.17)	6.63 (.26)	6.77 (.14)	6.72 (.22)	6.78 (.14)	6.49 (.21)
Multivariate $F_{(2, 368)} = 0.75$, $p = .47$.						
2) Relational Victimization						
Girls	2.98 (.22)	2.63 (.34)	2.75 (.21)	2.62 (.33)	2.47 (.18)	2.81 (.28)
Boys	2.63 (.21)	2.19 (.32)	2.59 (.21)	2.41 (.32)	1.87 (.18)	2.14 (.27)
Total	2.81 (.15)	2.41 (.23)	2.67 (.15)	2.52 (.23)	2.17 (.13)	2.48 (.19)
Multivariate $F_{(2, 368)} = 0.00$, $p = .99$.						
3) Physical Victimization						
Girls	2.92 (.22)	2.53 (.35)	2.37 (.21)	2.77 (.32)	1.95 (.17)	2.77 (.27)
Boys	2.82 (.22)	2.71 (.33)	2.99 (.20)	2.45 (.31)	2.13 (.17)	2.24 (.26)
Total	2.87 (.16)	2.62 (.24)	2.68 (.14)	2.61 (.22)	2.04 (.12)	2.51 (.19)
Multivariate $F_{(2, 369)} = 2.31$, $p = .10$.						

of emotional problems predicted increases in relational victimization (beyond individual differences in emotional and behavioral problems). Classroom levels of behavioral problems predicted increases in physical victimization (beyond individual differences). Since past research has demonstrated that, by mid-adolescence, girls show higher levels of emotional problems and boys show higher levels of behavioral problems (see Leadbeater et al. 1995), it is possible that stability in emotional or behavioral problems from the early grades could set in motion gender differences in victimization and that its consequences may not be detectable until later grades. Longitudinal research is needed to clarify the component risk and protective factors that make gender matter.

3) Does Gender Interact with Individual Differences in Social Competence or Emotional and Behavioral Problems in Predicting Relational and Physical Victimization?

Past research indicates that peer victimization is linked to an array of emotional, behavioral, and social problems that typically differ in their frequencies of occurrence for boys and girls by adolescence (Leadbeater et al., 1995). Compared to boys, girls demonstrate higher levels of *emotional problems* such as depression, anxiety, withdrawal, and low self-esteem by adolescence, and these problems have also been associated with peer victimization in several studies (Boulton & Underwood, 1992; Hanish & Guerra, 2000; Hodges, Boivin, Vitaro, & Bukowski, 1999; Kochenderfer & Ladd, 1997; Kumpulainen et al., 1998; Schwartz et al., 1999). Victimized children may also develop feelings of social rejection, loneliness (Hodges & Perry, 1999; Kumpulainen et al., 1998), social anxiety, and social avoidance (Crick & Grotpeter, 1995, 1996). Studies have also found that girls experience more anxiety than boys in response to victimization (Crick et al., 2001; Grills & Ollendick, 2002). Given this past research, we would expect that girls would be more likely to display emotional problems and that these girls would be more vulnerable to victimization. However, Gazelle and Ladd (2003) found that anxious-solitary children, particularly boys, experienced higher levels of peer exclusion (one aspect of relational victimization) and that children who had both risk factors (anxious-solitary and peer exclusion) in early grades showed the most elevated depressive symptoms over time. They argue that socially anxious boys may have greater problems in the large peer group contexts that typify boys' play compared to the more normative dyadic contexts for girls. It may be that as risks for emotional problems in girls increase in frequency they similarly experience greater peer exclusion and depressive symptoms.

Behavioral problems, like aggression, also appear to play a role in victimization. Boys in preschool (LaFreniere & Dumas, 1996), elementary school (Hanish & Guerra, 2000; Hodges & Perry, 1999; Hoglund & Leadbeater, 2003), and middle school (Leadbeater, Kuperminc, Blatt, & Hertzog, 1999) have been shown to be significantly more aggressive than girls. Studies (mainly of older children) have revealed that the propensity to be victimized increases if a child lacks social skills and friends (e.g., Hodges & Perry, 1999) and demonstrates behavioral problems (e.g., Kumpulainen et al., 1998). Moreover, these risks may be interactive. Schwartz et al. (1999) found that the relations between early behavioral problems (in kindergarten and first grade) and peer nominations of victimization three years later were related to peer rejection and friendships.

Gender differences in *social competence* also appear at an early age and may affect victimization. Girls in preschool (LaFreniere & Dumas, 1996), childhood (Hodges & Perry, 1999; Hoglund & Leadbeater, 2002) and adolescence (Paquette & Underwood, 1999) have been found to be more socially competent. A common sense assumption would be that increased social competence would lead to reduced aggression and victimization. However, the role of social competence in victimization may be more complex than previously thought. In a study of 3 to 6 year olds, Hawley (2002) observed that more socially dominant boys and girls achieved their personal goals in controlling resources through a combination of both coercive strategies (e.g., aggressive and demanding) and prosocial strategies (e.g., helping and demonstrating). Moreover, both types of strategies were associated with parent ratings of social competence. Pepler, Craig, and Roberts (1998) also observed that aggressive elementary school children exhibited more prosocial acts in the playground than non-aggressive children. Other studies of preschoolers and elementary school children report that increases in social understanding with age do not guarantee that these skills will be used to reduce conflict or enhance prosocial behavior, rather than to get one's own way or to bully others (Dunn, Cutting, & Fisher, 2002; Sutton, Smith, & Swettenham, 1999). Highly competent children may also interact more with other children in both aggressive and prosocial ways, thus exposing themselves to greater levels of relational and physical victimization than their less competent counterparts.

In the W.I.T.S. Longitudinal Study, we investigated whether gender and individual differences in social competence, and emotional and behavioral problems predicted increases in children's relational and physical victimization across first grade (i.e., controlling for baseline levels of victimization in multiple regression analyses; see Dhami et al., 2003). First grade data for the program and control sample are combined given the non-significant gender differences in program effects on victimization. Difference scores were used to reflect changes in levels of social competence and emotional and behavioral problem from the beginning to end of first grade. Increases in *physical victimization* were greater for boys than girls. Gender also interacted with individual differences in predicting physical victimization. Boys (but not girls) who demonstrated increases in social competence ($p < .05$) or increases in behavioral problems ($p = .06$) tended to be at risk for physical victimization. Girls (but not boys), who showed increased emotional problems, tended to be at greater risk for physical victimization ($p = .06$). Predictors of increases in *relational victimization* were not significant, however, boys reported greater increases than girls in victimization ($p = .09$).

The association of increases in behavioral problems with children's reports of receiving higher levels of victimization is consistent with past research showing that bullies are also at risk for victimization (Pepler et al., 1998). The gender differences reflected in these findings are also expected given the greater socialization of young boys for rough and tumble play and the greater acceptance of aggression in boys' relationships with their peers. In addition, more competent boys may be more vulnerable to victimization both because they interact more with others and because they may be skilled at using both prosocial and coercive strategies to obtain desired resources (Hawley, 2002; Sutton et al., 1999). The use of coercive strategies may be more likely to provoke aggressive responses from their peers. Parents and teachers need to cooperate in identifying boys (and girls) who show problems limiting aggression in first grade. It is possible that these behaviors reflect social learning problems that could be considered, much like other learning disabilities, in need of early remediation efforts (rather than behaviors in need of punitive or disciplinary actions).

It is also evident that girls do not escape victimization either and indeed, as shown in the longitudinal data presented in Table 1, girls report higher levels of relational victimization than boys and levels of physical victimization that are similar to boys. Girls also showed only slightly lower levels of behavioral problems at each assessment point in this study (means for the beginning and end of first grade were 11 [$SD = .30$] and 13 [$SD = .29$] for girls and boys, respectively, and at the end of second grade were 11.6 [$SD = .31$] and 14 [$SD = .29$], respectively). Nevertheless, our findings indicate that it is the shy, withdrawn, or anxious girls who are at greater risk for victimization. This held despite the fact that boys and girls had similar levels of emotional problems at each assessment (means for the beginning and end of first grade were both close to 25 [$SD = .44$] for girls and boys and at the end of second grade means were both 26 [$SD = .45$]). Girls with emotional problems may be less able to defend themselves or to create the kinds of supportive friendships that are protective. It may be that, if identified, these girls would respond to targeted training in resolving interpersonal conflicts assertively, group entry skills, and knowing when to get help from adults. It is also possible that more depressed, withdrawn, anxious children internalize negative peer assessments of themselves, setting in place negative trajectories of self isolation and peer exclusion that are exaggerated in adolescence (Gazelle & Ladd, 2003).

SUMMARY AND CONCLUSIONS

The findings from the W.I.T.S. Longitudinal Study, suggest that the role of gender in the prediction of relational and physical victimization is complex. Gender, alone, cannot be thought of as a direct explanation of the etiology of victimization. Rather, observations of gender differences in relational and physical victimization point to the need to investigate the individual or contextual risks and protective factors that interact with gender to give rise to or serve to maintain differences in the experiences of girls and boys.

Consistent with past research, the W.I.T.S. Longitudinal Study shows that individual differences matter in determining which children are targeted for physical victimization by their peers. Boys (but not girls) who showed increases in social competence or increases in behavioral problems tended to be at greater risk for physical victimization. On the other hand, girls (but not boys) who showed increases in emotional problems were at greater risk for physical victimization. Few predictors of increases in relational victimization were found, although, the boys tended to report greater increases in relational victimization than girls.

There is a need to examine changes in both levels and predictors of victimization as children age and progress through elementary school. In the middle school years, gender differences emerge in risk factors such as aggression (which is higher in boys) and depression (which is higher in girls) and these may create gender-linked risks for specific forms of peer victimization. A better understanding of how contexts (e.g., class, school, or neighborhood levels of aggression) influence girls' and boys' risks for victimization across the school years is also needed in order to identify gender specific targets for school policies and programs (Aber et al., 2003; Leadbeater et al., 2003). Emotional or behavioral problems need to be identified early and parents' and teachers' cooperation may be necessary to reduce their negative effects on children's development.

In order to actually understand the nature of gender differences in aggression and victimization, researchers need to go beyond controlling for gender or collecting data from samples that focus exclusively on either boys or girls. Rather, we must continue to ask the more challenging question of *how* does gender matter and *how* does this change over time.

REFERENCES

Aber, J. L., Brown, J. L., & Jones, S. M. (2003). Developmental trajectories toward violence in middle childhood: Course, demographic differences and response to school-based intervention. *Developmental Psychology, 39,* 324–348.

Artz, S., & Riecken, T. (1997). What, so what, then what?: The gender gap in school-based violence and its implications for child and youth care practice. *Child and Youth Care Forum, 26,* 291–303.

Björkqvist, K., Lagerspetz, K., & Kuakiainen, M. (2003). Do girls manipulate and boys fight? Developmental trends in regard to direct and indirect aggression. *Aggressive Behavior, 18,* 117–127.

Boulton, M. J., & Underwood, K. (1992). Bully/victim problems among middle school children. *British Journal of Educational Psychology, 62,* 73–87.

Cairns, R. B., Cairns, B. D., Neckerman, H. J., Ferguson, L. L., & Gariepy, J. L. (1989). Growth and aggression: I. Childhood to early adolescence. *Developmental Psychology, 25,* 320–330.

Caldwell, C. B., & Pianta, R. C. (1991). A measure of young children's problem and competence behaviors: The Early School Behavior Scale. *Journal of Psychoeducational Assessment, 9,* 32–44.

Cleary, S. D. (2000). Adolescent victimization and associated suicidal and violent behaviors. *Adolescence, 35,* 671–682.

Crick, N. R. (1997). Engagement in gender normative versus nonnormative forms of aggression: Links to social-psychological adjustment. *Developmental Psychology, 33,* 610–617.

Crick, N. R., & Grotpeter, J. K. (1995). Relational aggression, gender, and social-psychological adjustment. *Child Development, 66,* 710–722.

Crick, N. R., & Grotpeter, J. K. (1996). Children's treatment by peers: Victims of relational and overt aggression. *Development and Psychopathology, 8,* 367–380.

Crick, N. R., Nelson, D. A., Morales, J. R., Cullerton-Sen, C., Casas, J. F., & Hickman, S. E. (2001). Relational victimization in childhood and aggression: I hurt you through the grapevine. In J. Juvonen, & S. Graham (Eds.), *Peer harassment in school: The plight of the vulnerable and victimized* (pp. 196–214). NY: Guilford.

Dhami, M. K., Leadbeater, B., Hoglund, W., & Boone, E. (2003). The moderating effects of gender and school level poverty on changes in risks for peer victimization in first grade. Available from the authors, Department of Psychology, University of Victoria, B.C. Canada.

Dunn, J., Cutting, A. L., & Fisher, N. (2002). Old friends, new friends: Predictors of children's perspective on their friends at school. *Child Development, 73,* 621–635.

Farrell, A. D., & Meyer, A. L. (1997). The effectiveness of a school-based curriculum for reducing violence among urban sixth-grade students. *American Journal of Public Health, 87,* 979–984.

Gazelle, H. & Ladd, G. W. (2003). Anxious solitude and peer exclusion: A diathesis-stress model of internalizing trajectories in childhood. *Child Development, 74,* 257–279.

Grills, A. E., & Ollendick, T. H. (2002). Peer victimization, global self-worth, and anxiety in middle school children. *Journal of Clinical Child and Adolescent Psychology, 31,* 59–68.

Hanish, L. D., & Guerra, N. G. (2000). Predictors of peer victimization among urban youth. *Social Development, 9,* 521–543.

Hawley, P. H. (2002). Social dominance and prosocial and coercive strategies of resource control in preschoolers. *International Journal of Behavioral Development, 26*, 167–176.

Hodges, E. V. E., Boivin, M., Vitaro, F., & Bukowski, W. M. (1999). The power of friendship: Protection against an escalating cycle of peer victimization. *Developmental Psychology, 35*, 94–101.

Hodges, E. V. E., & Perry, D. G. (1999). Personal and interpersonal antecedents and consequences of victimization by peers. *Journal of Personality and Social Psychology, 76*, 677–685.

Hoglund, W. L., & Leadbeater, B. J. (2003). The effects of family, school, and classroom ecologies on changes in children's social competence and emotional and behavioral problems during first grade. Available from the authors, Department of Psychology, University of Victoria, B.C. Canada.

Kellam, S. G., Ling, X., Merisca, R., Brown, C. H., & Ialongo, N. (1998). The effect of the level of aggression in the first grade classroom on the course and malleability of aggressive behavior into middle school. *Development and Psychopathology, 10*, 165–185.

Kochenderfer, B. J., & Ladd, G. W. (1997). Victimized children's responses to peers' aggression: Behaviors associated with reduced versus continued victimization. *Development and Psychopathology, 9*, 59–73.

Kumpulainen, K., Rasanen, E., Henttonen, I., Almqvist, F., Kresanov, K., Linna, S. et al., (1998). Bullying and psychiatric symptoms among elementary school-age children. *Child Abuse & Neglect, 22*, 705–717.

LaFreniere, P. J., & Dumas, J. E. (1996). Social competence and behavior evaluation in children ages 3 to 6 years: The short form (SCBE-30). *Psychological Assessment, 8*, 369–377.

Lagerspetz, K., Björkqvist, K., & Peltonen, T. (1988). Is indirect aggression more typical of females? Gender differences in aggressiveness in 11- to 12-year-old children. *Aggressive Behavior, 14*, 403–414.

Leadbeater, B., Blatt, S. J., & Quinlan, D. M. (1995). Gender-linked vulnerabilities to depressive symptoms, stress, and problem behaviors in adolescents. *Journal of Research on Adolescence, 5*, 1–29.

Leadbeater, B. J., Hoglund, W., & Woods, T. (2003). Changing contexts? The effects of a primary prevention program on classroom levels of peer relational and physical victimization. *Journal of Community Psychology, 31*, 1–22.

Leadbeater, B. J., Kuperminc, G. P. Blatt, S. J., & Hertzog, C. (1999). A Multivariate model of gender differences in adolescents' internalizing and externalizing problems. *Developmental Psychology, 35*, 1268–1282.

Maccoby, E. (2002). Perspectives on gender development. In W. Hartup & R. Silbereisen (Eds.), *Growing points in developmental science* (pp. 202–222). NY: Psychology Press.

Olweus, D. (1994). Bullying at school: Long-term outcomes for the victims and an effective school-based intervention program. In L. R. Huesmann (Ed.), *Aggressive behavior: Current perspectives*. NY: Plenum.

Owens, L. D. (1996). Sticks and stones and sugar and spice: girls' and boys' aggression in schools. *Australian Journal of Guidance Counseling, 6*, 45–55.

Paquette, J. A., & Underwood, M. K. (1999). Gender differences in young adolescents' experiences of peer victimization: Social and physical aggression. *Merrill-Palmer Quarterly, 45*, 242–266.

Pepler, D. J., Craig, W. M., & Roberts, W. L. (1998). Observations of aggressive and nonaggressive children on the school playground. *Merrill-Palmer Quarterly, 44*, 55–76.

Schwartz, D., McFadyen-Ketchum, S., Dodge, K. A., Pettit, G. S., & Bates, J. E. (1999). Early behavior problems as a predictor of later peer group victimization: Moderators and mediators in the pathways of social risk. *Journal of Abnormal Child Psychology, 27*, 191–201.

Smith, P. K., & Sharp, S. (1994). *School bullying: Insights and perspectives*. London: Routledge.

Sutton, J., Smith, P., & Swettenham, J. (1999). Social cognition and bullying: Social inadequacy or skilled manipulation? *British Journal of Developmental Psychology, 17*, 435–450.

Vaillancourt, T., Hymel, S., & McDougall, P. (2002). Bullying is power: Implications for school-based intervention strategies. Unpublished manuscript available from author, Department of Psychology, McMaster University, ON, Canada.

Whitney, I., & Smith, P. K. (1993). A survey of the nature and extent of bullying in junior/middle and secondary schools. *Educational Research, 35*, 3–25.

——————14——————

Reframing Violence Risk Assessment for Female Juvenile Offenders

CANDICE L. ODGERS, MELINDA G. SCHMIDT, AND N. DICKON REPPUCCI

The assessment of risk for future violence is a task that clinicians and criminal justice practitioners are faced with on a daily basis. Recent advances in risk assessment research have led to an increased understanding of the empirical relationships between risk factors and violent outcomes among adult male populations (see Borum, 1996; Douglas & Ogloff, 2003; Monahan & Steadman, 1994). Simultaneously, a plethora of risk assessment instruments, such as the Violence Risk Appraisal Guide (VRAG; Harris, Rice, & Quinsey, 1993) Psychopathy Checklist-Revised (PCL-R; Hare, 1991), Psychopathy Checklist-Screening Version (PCL-SV; Hart, Cox, & Hare, 1995) and Historical and Clinical Risk Guide (HCR-20; Webster, Douglas, Eaves, & Hart, 1997) have been developed and tested widely among adult male forensic populations.

Research indicates that, when consistently applied, the use of structured violence risk assessment systems increase case management efficiency and produce predictions of future violence that surpass those of unstructured clinical judgments and, in many cases, actuarial schemes (Kropp, Hart, Webster, & Eaves, 1999; Monahan et al., 2001; Otto, 2000).

CANDICE L. ODGERS, MELINDA G. SCHMIDT, AND N. DICKON REPPUCCI • Department of Psychology, University of Virginia, Charlottesville, Virginia, United States, 22901.

Consequently, structured assessment tools are now accepted as an integral part of violence risk assessments, and are considered by some to be a *necessary* component (Nicholls, Hemphill, Boer, Kropp, & Zapf, 2001).

While the field of violence risk assessment among adult males has rapidly progressed, there remain unanswered questions regarding the generalizability of these instruments to other populations. In particular, the validity of violence risk instruments within minority, adolescent, and female populations has been questioned (Monahan, 1995; Nichols et al., 2001; Vitale & Newman, 2001; Vincent, 2002). In this chapter, we outline the challenges of assessing risk for violence among adolescent and female samples. Particular attention is paid to the application of risk assessment schemes to female juvenile offender populations. Future directions for research and assessment are outlined.

VIOLENCE RISK ASSESSMENT IN ADOLESCENTS

There are a number of contexts where the assessment of future violence among adolescents is relevant. For example, within juvenile justice systems, risk assessments are often employed when making decisions related to transfer to adult court and treatment placements. Mental health professionals are also required to consider future violence when determining the risk that adolescents pose to themselves and others in civil commitment and treatment settings. Finally, recent acts of school violence have led to demands for tools designed to identify youths who may become violent within educational venues. Although risk assessment is not a legal requirement across these contexts, professionals are often called upon, and in some cases are obliged, to conduct such assessments (*Tarasoff v. Regents of the University of California*, 1976).

While many of the threats to the validity of assessments among adolescents are similar to those that exist with adults (e.g., inadequate inclusion and access to information, rater bias, failure to consider dynamic and contextual factors), a number of unique challenges have been noted. Specifically, behaviors that are normative during adolescence may appear pathological from a risk assessment perspective (Seagrave & Grisso, 2002). For example, Vincent (2002) reported differential item functioning between adolescents and adults on interpersonal and behavioral items of the Psychopathy Checklist (PCL). In this case, adolescents who were rated as psychopathic needed higher levels of the latent trait of psychopathy in order to receive ratings as high as adults on items such as irresponsibility and impulsivity (Vincent, 2002).

It is also the case that the majority of youths engage in some form of antisocial behavior during adolescence, however this behavior is largely transient and desists as youths enter young adulthood (Cauffman & Steinberg, 2000; Farrington, 1989; Moffitt, 1993). Due to this state of rapid change, the presentation of disorders and traits are likely to vary significantly with the adolescents' stage of emotional and psychosocial development. As such, adolescents have been described as moving targets that are difficult to assess based on single observations (Grisso, 1998).

The instability that characterizes adolescence is particularly important in light of the assumption that many of the traits that comprise risk assessment instruments are stable within the individual and can be assessed *reliably* over time. There is considerable debate, however, regarding whether adolescent personality development has stabilized sufficiently to extract the information required to conduct such evaluations. For example, although psychopathy, as measured by the PCL-R (Hare, 1991) is the gold standard in the prediction of both violent and general criminal recidivism in adults (Hare, 1991; Hare, McPherson, & Forth, 1988; Harris, Rice, & Cormier, 1991), it is unclear to what extent this disorder exists or can be assessed prior to early adulthood (Vincent & Hart, 2002). Moreover, the relative weight that should be given to various risk factors developmentally has not been established. For example, there are a number of behaviors, such as aggression, that are normative in preschool children, yet at an undefined moment in development become an important marker of pathology or risk of future violence.

In sum, despite the demands for the development and use of violence risk assessment tools with adolescent populations, the nature of adolescence poses unique barriers to conducting valid assessments. Nonetheless, there are a number of tools that have been developed specifically to assess risk among adolescents (for a review see Office of Juvenile Justice and Delinquency Prevention, 1995). While there are promising developments in this area (e.g., SAVRY: Borum, Bartel, & Forth, 2002), for the most part, instruments designed for use with adult offenders are either directly applied to, or adapted slightly for use with, adolescents. Developmental considerations have not been factored into the majority of current risk assessment schemes and prospective studies that would support the use of such instruments during this period are lacking.

VIOLENCE RISK ASSESSMENT IN ADULT WOMEN

One of the most consistent findings in criminological research is that males are far more likely than females to engage in serious physical forms of violence (Duffy, 1996). Perhaps it is no surprise, then, that females have been ignored in violence research (Heimer & DeCoster, 1999). Historically, studies of women who engage in violent crime have been limited to the context of family violence (Sommers & Baskin, 1994). Males are also more likely than females to be the victims of violent crime and to cause serious physical injury when they engage in violence (MacArthur Violence Risk Assessment Study, 2001; Straus & Gelles, 1986). A synthesis of studies that examined differences in the level of risk factors across gender concluded that female offenders are more likely to have a history of abuse and mental health problems, including a history of suicide attempts and substance abuse disorders (Shaw & Dubois, 1995). Moreover, there is a growing body of evidence supporting the existence of unique relational and contextual risk factors among female offender populations. For example, research has demonstrated a linkage between specific attachment styles and the development of aggression in women and girls, that may form the context in which aggression occurs, and the selection of targets (see Moretti & DaSilva, this edition). In addition, qualitative research has reaffirmed the importance of understanding the intersection between gender, ethnicity, and socio-economic status when examining violence among females (Jackson, this edition).

Until recently, violence risk assessment has also ignored gender (Gendreau, Little, & Goggin, 1996; Funk, 1999). As a result, risk assessment tools for females have *not* evolved alongside the field of assessment in adult male populations. Despite this fact, we do know some things about risk assessment in females from studies that compare male and female offenders on factors related to criminal offending. In a recent review, Nicholls (2003) concluded that despite the lower base rate among women, psychopathy appears to have a similar relationship to violence as that observed in men. Although the lack of validation studies calls into question whether the construct of psychopathy is actually being measured by these instruments, support was found for the use of the PCL as risk assessment tool with women. Nichols et al. (2001) have also reported that the HCR-20 and PCL-SV generalize well to female civil psychiatric patients. These findings are consistent with previous claims made by experts in the risk assessment field that male based instruments are likely to function similarly within female populations (Hare, 1991). It is important to note, however, that the present findings are tentative due to the limited and small body of research that has included women subjects.

Some researchers have argued that a greater understanding of the differences that exist between male and female populations would most likely increase the accuracy of future predictions of violent behavior (Uggen & Kruttschnitt, 1998). Brennan and Austin (1997) charge that gender neutral classification tools tend to over-classify females, while others (Coontz, Lidz, & Mulvey, 1994) assert that the bias functions in the opposite direction, producing an under-prediction in females. Coulson, Flacqua, Nutbrown, Giulekas, and Cudjoe (1996) concluded that current risk cut-off thresholds that have been normed on samples of men (LSI-OR) are not appropriate for female offenders. While the consideration of other methodological issues, such as a heavy reliance on file information and behavior observations within institutional settings, suggests that further research could improve the predictive validity for all groups (Griffiths & Cunningham, 2000).

In sum, the limited amount of research that has been conducted to date with adult women has focused on domestic forms of violence. When non-domestic forms of violence have been studied, the highly select nature of the samples (e.g., incarcerated) makes it difficult to speak confidently regarding gender differences in risk factors that are related to violence. Similarly, although researchers have started to examine the application of risk assessment instruments with women the incongruent research findings and limited sample sizes make it difficult to make conclusive statements in this field. Finally, if violence risk prediction is the goal, the low base rate of the types of violence that are recorded in traditional risk assessment studies among women makes accurate prediction difficult if not impossible. In contrast, if case management is the primary objective, several key factors related to the types of relationally based violence that women are more likely to engage in are missing from current assessment schemes.

ASSESSING VIOLENCE RISK IN FEMALE ADOLESCENTS

Although researchers have begun to test the utility of violence risk assessment with male adolescents (Vincent, 2002) and adult women (Forth, 1996; Rutherford, Cacciola, Alterman, & McKay, 1996: Salekin, Rogers, Ustad, & Sewell, 1998) there are virtually no studies that have focused specifically on adolescent female populations. Similar to the situation with adult women, it is likely that female youths have been neglected in large part due to their absence within the violence arena. The vast majority of research on juvenile offenders has focused exclusively on boys and men (Chesney-Lind & Sheldon, 1998; Horowitz & Pottieger, 1991; Hoyt & Scherer, 1998). From a gender perspective, unless we assume that the relationships between risk factors and violence are invariant across gender, there are significant limitations in the research base necessary to construct valid assessment tools for girls.

Despite the lack of empirical information, the demand for gender specific risk assessment tools is increasing. Over the last decade, female youths are the only population that has continued to experience an increase in official rates of violent crime (FBI Uniform Crime Report, 2002; Puzzanchera, Stahl, Finnegan, Tierney, & Snyder, 2003; Statistics Canada, 2001) and practitioners are increasingly being called upon to conduct assessments for the growing number of girls who are entering into mental health and criminal justice settings.

What Unique Challenges Do Adolescent Girls Pose to Violence Risk Assessments?

Presently, very little is known regarding risk assessment with adolescent females. In fact, the empirical data that are necessary to directly address this issue do not exist. The following discussion, therefore, relies on evidence drawn from the more general domain of research on female juvenile offenders in order to outline what we view as the primary barriers to conducting violence risk assessments with adolescent females.

1. *Female juvenile offenders are a marginalized and highly victimized group.* Data from juvenile justice centers indicate that incarcerated girls are more likely than boys to have a broad array of mental health problems (e.g. high rates of suicidal ideation, suicide attempts, substance abuse, depression, and post traumatic stress disorder diagnoses); experience more severe maltreatment and trauma; experience high levels of distress and preoccupation related to their involvement in abusive and highly conflictual relationships, and come from homes that are characterized by high levels of dysfunction (Bergsmann, 1989; Lewis, Yeager, Cobham-Portorreal, & Klein, 1991; Moretti, Holland, & McKay, 2001; Odgers & Moretti, 2002; Odgers & Reppucci, 2002; Rosenbaum, 1989; Viale–Val & Sylvester, 1993). Female juvenile offenders are also more likely to belong to an ethnic minority group. Although racial over-representation exists for all populations of offenders, documented rates of over-representation among female juvenile offenders are among the highest, ranging from 45–90%, across North American institutions (Chesney-Lind & Sheldon, 1998; Corrado, Odgers, & Cohen, 2001; Teplin, 2003). In sum, the majority of these girls live on the margins of society and are likely to be exposed to a number of unique risk factors.

How do the characteristics of female juvenile offenders impact violence risk assessment? First, within the adult literature co-morbidity of mental disorders and racial bias have both been cited as a threat to the validity of current risk assessment schemes. Arguably, our current lack of understanding regarding the developmental course and manifestation of co-morbid disorders presents unique challenges for assessments. For example, two disorders may share common risk factors, or one disorder can create conditions that increase the probability of other conditions developing—where the presence of one disorder will alter developmental trajectories toward increasing pathology (Gottlieb & Halpern, 2002; Sroufe, 1990). In the case of high risk adolescent females, who are characterized by extremely high levels of co-morbidity, it is plausible that the more development is skewed by the presence of multiple risk factors and emergent disorders over time, the more likely development will continue to proceed along a pathological course. In other words, once these young women cross a threshold of risk their probability of engaging in future violence may increase exponentially.

With respect to racial bias, very few assessment schemes take into consideration the influence of ethnicity and culture on the presentation and weighting of various risk factors. For example, traits such as empathy and remorse may be expressed differently within Native American individuals due to a greater reliance on collective values and the stigma that is associated with violating cultural norms. Similarly, contextual factors such as poverty and marginalization may warrant more weight than individual factors in understanding violence among ethnic minority youth. The high prevalence of both co-morbidity and ethnic minority status in female juvenile offender populations, therefore, has the potential to greatly increase challenges for assessment.

Second, there has been a tendency to de-emphasize the role of maltreatment/abuse as a relevant risk factor for violence. Recent meta-analyses and reviews of abuse literature point to a weak relationship between exposure to abuse and later violence (Lipsey & Derzon, 1998; Odgers & Busch, 2003). In addition, the majority of studies relying on normative populations have *not* shown that aggressive girls and boys differ in exposure to such risk factors as physical maltreatment (Moffitt, Caspi, Rutter, & Silva, 2001; Pepler & Sedighdeilami, 1998). Yet research conducted within forensic and clinical samples consistently show that, compared to boys, girls in these populations are significantly more likely to have experienced severe victimization, particularly sexual abuse (Bergsmann, 1989; Corrado, Odgers, & Cohen, 2000; U.S Bureau of Justice Statistics, 1997; Viale–Val & Sylvester, 1993) and that this risk factor may be especially relevant for girls (Rivera & Widom, 1990). Arguably, a greater emphasis on victimization factors may improve both the prediction and management of future violence among girls. For instance, in some cases, it may be useful to consider girls who are exposed to higher levels of marginalization and abuse as less of a risk for future instrumental violence due to the fact that their behavior represents an attempt to survive in extraordinary conditions, as opposed to being motivated by thrill seeking or hedonistic goals. Perhaps more importantly, abuse experiences should be given special emphasis in risk management in order to encourage treatment that is designed to assist in formation of healthy romantic relationships and adaptive parenting skills—both of which form the context for the majority of violence that is committed by adult women.

2. *Violence among adolescent girls may be a qualitatively different phenomenon.* It is well established that the rates of violence differ significantly across gender. There is also a growing body of evidence that the contextual and individual factors that characterize violent acts committed by females may be unique. For example, research with adult women has shown that *when* females engage in physical forms of violence they are more likely to assault a partner or family member, less likely to cause injuries that result in medical attention, and more likely to be suffering from depression and/or be under the influence of substances (Shaw & Dubois, 1995).

In addition to the growing body of qualitative data that describes the different manifestations and motivations for female violence (Artz, 1998; Chesney–Lind & Sheldon, 1998), recent quantitative analyses provide support for these differences. For example, Odgers, Moretti and Pepler (2003) reported a different underlying structure of aggression among high risk girls as compared to the structure for girls in normative settings and boys from both normative and high risk settings. Here, even when the same instrument was used, the Youth Self Report (Achenbach, 1991), a different latent underlying construct of aggression was being measured within a subgroup of females.

Researchers have also pointed to the greater tendency for females to rely on alternative forms of violence—such as relational and social aggression. Studies have shown that relational forms of aggression may be equally as harmful as overt forms (Crick & Bigbee, 1998; Paquette & Underwood, 1999) and are more common in young women than previously believed (Bjorkgvist & Niemela, 1992; Crick & Grotepeter, 1995; Moretti et al., 2001). These findings reaffirm the need to re-examine how violence manifests itself across and within gender.

How does the definition and measurement of violence impact violence risk assessment? From a quantitative perspective, if equivalent measurement is *not* obtained across gender the potential for misinterpreting research findings is high. At best, results could be misconstrued through a reporting of inaccurate estimates in the size of the relationships between various risk factors and violent outcomes, and at worst, researchers may be reporting the wrong size and direction of the effects. In other words, we cannot assume that, just because we use the same measure for males and females, we are measuring the same thing. For example, studies that compare mean values between males and females on scales such as the Youth Self Report or other indices of aggression may be comparing "apples and oranges". Similarly when the weight of various predictors of aggression are then evaluated using these outcomes the results that are obtained may not be directly comparable due to the fact that the outcome measure is qualitatively different. Thus, at a fundamental level, until we establish that we are measuring the same construct of aggression within males and females conclusions regarding the comparison of risk factors across gender remain tentative.

As noted, the high levels of relationship dysfunction that are evident in the lives of these young women often form the context in which their future violence occurs. For example, female youths are most likely to aggress against family members, romantic partners, and members of their peer group. These girls are also likely to rely on alternative forms of aggression that may operate as markers of concurrent and future overt violence, as well as form the interpersonal context in which acts of severe physical aggression may be perpetrated (Moretti & Odgers, 2002).Yet, very few risk assessment schemes have included the types of factors that would capture the interpersonal and context dependent nature of violence among girls.

3. *The adult outcomes for aggressive and violent girls differ.* Research has demonstrated a pervasive pattern of negative adult outcomes among adolescent girls who exhibit severe forms of antisocial behavior (Moffitt et al., 2001; Robins, 1986; Zoccolillo & Rogers, 1991). For example, in the Dunedin longitudinal study, Moffitt and colleagues (2001) found that 21 year old women diagnosed with conduct disorder (CD) in childhood or adolescence were significantly more likely to show mental health symptoms (anxiety, depression, psychosis, mania, and suicidality), suffer from more medical problems, require social assistance, be victimized by their partners, and perpetrate physical abuse against them in return than were girls not diagnosed with CD. Similar negative outcomes have been found for female juvenile offenders with respect to mental health symptoms of depression, substance abuse, and suicidality (Lewis et al., 1991) and social and economic marginalization in young adulthood (Lanctot, 2002). Female juvenile offenders are also more likely than their male counterparts to fall off the radar of the criminal justice system and desist with respect to their rates of official violent offending (Lanctot, 2002). The lack of official recidivism among this group, however, should not be interpreted to mean that these young women have made a positive transition into early adulthood. Instead, they are likely to surface in other systems—e.g., requiring mental health, medical, welfare, and social assistance. There is also a growing body of evidence to suggest that these young women continue to be highly aggressive in their intimate relations with romantic partners and against their children—within contexts where official reporting of the violent incident is less likely.

How do different adult outcomes for girls impact violence risk assessment? First, there is a low probability that these girls will go on to commit the types of non-familial violence that traditional risk assessment instruments were designed to predict. The low base rate of future serious and violent official offending among female adolescents makes accurate prediction difficult if not impossible. Second, violence risk assessment among girls may be governed by a unique set of assumptions and priorities. In other words, the use of violence among female adolescents may be more accurately conceptualized as a risk marker for a wide spectrum of negative adult outcomes as opposed to a specific risk factor for future violence.

Arguably, the differing conceptualizations and manifestations of violence in girls create the need to *reframe risk* with this population. In the case of female juveniles, the relevant societal costs include the high likelihood that these young women will suffer from psychological and mental health problems, engage in violence against children, partners, and themselves, be dependent on social and economic systems, and become victims of violent crime (Moffitt et al., 2001). Here, the risk paradigm shifts for young women from one that is guided by a concern for the welfare and safety of others to one that is centered on concerns for the safety and welfare of the girls themselves, their intimate partners, and their children. This sentiment is supported by views of criminal justice practitioners who often view female juvenile offenders as a vulnerable population in need of protection from hostile family, street, and social environments (Chesney-Lind & Sheldon, 1998; Corrado, et al., 2000; Moretti et al., 2001).

FUTURE DIRECTIONS IN VIOLENCE RISK ASSESSMENT FOR FEMALE JUVENILE OFFENDERS

Regardless of whether the primary purpose of the violence assessment is risk prediction or management there are a number of areas that require a re-examination prior to applying adult–male based instruments to female juvenile offenders.

1. *Inclusion of gender specific risk and protective factors.* Only recently have researchers begun to investigate empirically the form and predictive utility of gender-specific risk factors (Levene, Augimeri, & Pepler, 2001). Although studies of normative samples provide little empirical evidence to support the need for gender specific risk factors (Moffitt et al., 2001; Pepler & Sedighdeilami, 1998; Fergusson & Horwood, 2002; Rowe, Vazsonyi, & Flannery, 1995; Simourd & Andrews, 1994), several researchers have advocated for their consideration (Chesney-Lind & Sheldon, 1998; Reitsma-Street, 1999; Totten, 2000). It should be noted that the majority of research

to date has included only small numbers of girls and has tended to include risk factors identified and tested within male-only samples

A literature review of 46 published studies focusing on gender and aggression (Leschied, Cummings, Van Brunschot, Cunningham, & Saunders, 2000) found that regardless of the form of aggression that was displayed, there was remarkable similarity in the risk factors associated with violence behavior for males and females (e.g., antisocial peers, academic problems, and antisocial parental behavior). Differences that did exist included higher rates of sexual abuse and depression for females. Cunningham et al. (2000) have argued that while adolescent women share several risk markers with their male counterparts, there are others that are unique to females that are not generally considered in most instruments. For example, they argued for the inclusion of variables such as history of attempted suicide and depression.

It is also likely that current risk assessment instruments could better predict adult outcomes for adolescent girls if they took into account factors that are associated with a *decreased* probability of violence as well. According to Farrington (1998), "protective factors may have more implications than risk factors for prevention and treatment" (p. 451). As noted earlier the majority of aggressive adolescent girls do not go on to commit non-domestic acts of violence as adults. Careful examination of the ways aggressive girls are socialized during adolescence and early adulthood could offer important clues as to why the majority of these girls desist from "detectable" forms of violent offending. For example, girls are more likely than boys to have empathy modeled for them (Zahn-Waxler, Cole, & Barrett, 1991), which is associated with lower levels of aggressive behavior (Miller & Eisenberg, 1988); it is also a key element of the psychopathy risk assessment (Hare, 1991). Another factor influencing aggressive girls' desistance from violent behavior may be their relationships with male partners who are themselves adolescence-limited aggressors/delinquents. Initial research suggests that having a boyfriend, who is at least moderately prosocial during adolescence, can be a protective factor for highly aggressive and antisocial girls (Bender & Losel, 1997); this may also be the case for young women entering adulthood. In sum, risk assessment tools could be improved by heeding Farrington's call for a more careful consideration of the role of protective factors.

2. Re-defining our terms. The outcome measure of violence within both basic and applied research settings should be expanded beyond official acts of recidivism. While this may be true for all populations, it is especially relevant for female youths who are unlikely to engage in violence that is detected by the criminal justice system. The use of collateral informants to assess the nature and the extent of the damage that is caused by the violence that these women go on to commit against their children, spouses, and themselves will be crucial in completing the complex picture of the developmental course of aggression among females. There is also a need for qualitative research that examines the phenotypic pattern of violence committed by adolescent and adult females.

The establishment of equivalent measurement of aggression across males and females requires advancements in both qualitative and quantitative research designs. Although the same measures of violence may be used across gender, there is a growing body of research suggesting that measurement equivalence cannot be assumed. Exploratory research is required in order to modify existing violence measures and coding schemes to account for the diverse nature and patterns of violence among females. Greater attention should also be paid to the contextual and relational factors in which violent acts committed by girls are embedded.

4. Careful evaluation of current risk assessment schemes. At the most basic level, young women need to be included in risk assessment research. In the absence of empirical data it cannot be assumed that current risk assessment schemes apply to this population.

The increasing number of young women who are participating in serious violent acts (e.g., robbery, assault) has increased the demand for assessment tools for girls who were once the *violent few.* As a result, there is pressure to apply adult and male-based instruments to girls within mental health and forensic settings. The question, therefore, is not whether violent risk assessment instruments should be used with young women, rather, the key issue is *how* current risk assessment practices can be improved in order to maximize their utility when they are applied. At present, however, we cannot empirically or ethically justify their use due to the obvious limitations in our knowledge regarding risk assessment for girls and the serious decisions that may be made based on these assessments.

REFERENCES

Achenbach, T. M. (1991). Manual for the Youth Self-Report and 1991 profile. Burlington: University of Vermont, Department of Psychiatry.

Artz, S. (1998). *Sex, power, and the violent school girl.* Toronto: Trifolium.

Bender, D., & Losel, F. (1997). Protective and risk effects of peer relations and social support on antisocial behaviour in adolescents from multi-problem milieus. *Journal of Adolescence, 20,* 661–678.

Bergsmann, I. R. (1989). The forgotten few: Juvenile female offenders. *Federal Probation, 12,* 73–78.

Bjorkqvist, K., & Niemela, P. (1992). *Of mice and women: Aspects of female aggression.* San Diego: Academic Press.

Borum, R., Bartel, P., & Forth, A. (2002). *Manual for the structured assessment of violence risk in youth (SAVRY)*. University of South Florida.

Borum, R. (1996). Improving the clinical practice of violence risk assessment: Technology, guidelines, and training. *American Psychologist, 51*, 945–956.

Brennan, T., & Austin, J. (1997). *Women in jail: Classification issues*. Washington, DC: U.S. Department of Justice, National Institute of Corrections.

Cauffman, E., & Steinberg, L. (2000). The cognitive and affective influences of adolescent decision making. *Temple Law Review, 68*, 1763–1789.

Chesney-Lind, M., & Sheldon, R. (1998). *Girls, delinquency, and juvenile justice* (2nd ed.). Pacific Grove, CA: Brooks/Cole.

Coontz, P., Lidz, C., & Mulvey, E. (1994). Gender and the assessment of dangerousness in the psychiatric emergency room. *International Journal of Law and Psychiatry, 17(4)*, 369–376.

Corrado, R., Odgers, C., & Cohen, I. (2001). The use of incarceration for female youth: Protection for whom? *Canadian Journal of Criminology, 42*, 189–206.

Corrado, R., Cohen, I., & Odgers, C. (2000). Teen violence in Canada. In A. M. Hoffman & R. W. Summers (Eds.), *Teen violence: A global view*. Westport, CT: Greenwood Press.

Coulson, G., Flacqua, G., Nutbrown, V. Giulekas, D., & Cudjoe, F. (1996). Predictive utility of the LSI for incarcerated female offenders. *Criminal Justice and Behavior, 23*, 427–439.

Crick, N. R., & Bigbee, M. A. (1998). Relational and overt forms of peer victimization: A multiinformant approach. *Journal of Consulting and Clinical Psychology, 66*, 337–347.

Crick, N. R., & Grotpeter, J. K. (1995). Relational aggression, gender, and social-psychological adjustment. *Child Development, 66*, 710–722.

Cunningham, A., Baker, L., Mazaheri, N., Ashbourne, L., VanBrunschot, M., & Currie, M. (2000), *Best practice programming for phase II young offenders: A literature review*. London: Centre for Children and Families in the Justice System.

Douglas, K. S., & Ogloff, R. P. (2003). Multiple facets of risk for violence: The impact of judgmental specificity on structured decisions about risk. *International Journal of Forensic Mental Health, 2*, 19–34.

Duffy, A. (1996). Bad girls in hard times: Canadian female juvenile offenders. In G. O'Bireck (Ed.), *Not a kid anymore* (pp. 203–220). Scarborough, ON: Nelson Canada.

Farrington, D. P. (1989). Predictors, causes, and correlates of male youth violence. In M. Tonry & M. H. Moore (Eds.), *Crime and justice: A review of research: Vol. 24. Youth violence* (pp. 421–476). Chicago: University of Chicago Press.

FBI Uniform Crime Report. (September 2002). Online. Available at: http://www.fbi.gov/ucr/ucr. htm

Fergusson, D. M., & Horwood, J. H. (2002). Male and female offending trajectories. *Development and Psychopathology, 14*, 159–177.

Forth, A. E. (1996). Psychopathy in adolescent offenders: Assessment, family background, and violence. In D. J. Cooke, A. E. Forth, J. P. Newman, & R. D. Hare (Eds.), *Issues in criminological and legal psychology: No. 24, International perspectives on psychopathy* (pp. 42–44). Leicester, UK: British Psychological Society.

Funk, S. (1999). Risk assessment for juveniles on probation: A focus on gender. *Criminal Justice and Behavior, 26*, 44–68.

Gendreau, P., Little, T., & Goggin, C. (1996). A meta-analysis of the predictors of adult offender recidivism: What works! *Criminology, 34*, 574–607.

Gottlieb, G., & Halpern, C. T. (2002). A relational view of causality in normal and abnormal development. *Development and Psychopathology, 14*, 421–535.

Griffiths, C. T., & A. Cunningham (2000). *Canadian corrections*. Toronto: ITP Nelson.

Grisso, T. (1998). *Forensic evaluation of juveniles*. Sarasota, FL.: Professional Resource Press/Professional Resource Exchange, Inc.

Hare, R. D. (1991). *The Hare Psychopathy Checklist—Revised.* Toronto: MultiHealth Systems.

Hare, R. D., McPherson, L. E., & Forth, A. E. (1988). Male psychopaths and their criminal careers. *Journal of Consulting and Clinical Psychology, 56,* 710–714.

Harris, G. T., Rice, M. E., & Cormier, C. (1991). Psychopathy and violent recidivism. *Law and Human Behavior, 26,* 377–394.

Harris, G. T., Rice, M. E., & Quinsey, V. L. (1993). Violent recidivism of mentally disordered offenders: The development of a statistical prediction instrument. *Criminal Justice and Behavior, 20,* 315–335.

Hart, S. D., Cox, D. N., & Hare, R. D. (1995). *Manual for the Psychopathy Checklist: Screening Version (PCL: SV).* Toronto: Multi-Health Systems.

Hart, S. D. (1998). The role of psychopathy in assessing risk for violence: Conceptual and methodological issues. *Legal and Criminological Psychology, 3,* 121–137.

Heimer, K., & DeCoster, S. (1999). The gendering of violent delinquency. *Criminology, 37,* 277–317.

Horowitz, R., & Pottieger, A. E. (1991). Gender bias in juvenile justice handling of seriously crime-involved youths. *Journal of Research in Crime and Delinquency, 28,* 75–100.

Hoyt, S., & Scherer, D. G. (1998). Female juvenile delinquency: Misunderstood by the juvenile justice system, neglected by social science. *Law and Human Behavior, 22,* 81–107.

Kropp, R., Hart, S., Webster, C. & Eaves, D. (1999). *Manual for the Spousal Risk Assessment Guide* (3rd ed.). Toronto: Multi-Health Systems.

Lanctot, N. (2002, May). *Violence among females from adolescence to adulthood: Results from a longitudinal study.* Paper presented at the Vancouver Conference on Aggressive and Violent Girls, Vancouver, Canada.

Leschied, A., Cummings, A., Van Brunschot, M., Cunningham, A., & Saunders, A. (2000). *Female adolescent aggression: A review of the literature and the correlates of aggression* (User Report No. 2000–04). Ottawa: Solicitor General of Canada.

Lewis, D. O., Yeager, C. A., Cobham-Portorreal, C. S., & Klein, N. (1991). A follow-up of female delinquents: Maternal contributions to the perpetuation of deviance. *Journal of the American Academy of Child and Adolescent Psychiatry, 30,* 197–201.

Levene, K. S., Augimeri, L. K., Pepler., D. J., Walsh, M. M., Webster, C. D., & Koegl, C. J. (2001). *Early Assessment Risk List for Girls (EARL-21G).* Toronto: Earlscourt Child and Family Centre.

Lipsey, M. W., & Derzon, J. H. (1998). Predictors of violence and serious delinquency in adolescence and early adulthood: A synthesis of longitudinal research. In R. Loeber & D. P. Farrington (Eds.), *Serious and violent juvenile offenders: Risk factors and successful interventions* (pp. 86–105). Thousand Oaks, CA: Sage.

MacArthur Violence Risk Assessment Study: Executive Summary. Retrieved December 2, 2001 from the MacArthur Research Network on Mental Health and the Law Web site. *http://www.macarthur.virginia.edu/risk.html*

Miller, P. A., & Eisenberg, N. (1988). The relation of empathy to aggressive and externalizing/ antisocial behavior. *Psychological Bulletin, 103,* 324–344.

Moffitt, T. E. (1993). Adolescence-limited and life course-persistent antisocial behavior developmental taxonomy. *Psychological Review, 100,* 674–701.

Moffitt, T. E., Caspi, A., Rutter, M., & Silva, P. A. (2001). *Sex differences in antisocial behavior: Conduct disorder, delinquency, and violence in the Dunedin Longitudinal Study.* Cambridge: Cambridge University Press.

Monahan, J. (1995). The violence prediction scheme: Assessing dangerousness in high-risk men. *Criminal Justice and Behavior, 22,* 446–455.

Monahan, J., & Steadman, H. (1994). *Violence and mental disorder: Developments in risk assessment.* Chicago: University of Chicago Press.

Monahan, J., Steadman, H., Silver, E., Appelbaum, P., Robbins, P., Mulvey, E., Roth, L., Grisso, T., & Banks, S. (2001). *Rethinking risk assessment: The MacArthur study of mental disorder and violence*. New York: Oxford University Press.

Moretti, M. M., Holland, R., & McKay, S. (2001). Self-other representations and relational and overt aggression in adolescent girls and boys. *Behavioral Sciences and the Law, 19,* 109–126.

Moretti, M. M., & Odgers, C. L. (2002). Aggressive and violent girls: Prevalence, profiles and contributing factors. In R. R. Corrado, R. Roesch, S. D. Hart, & J. Gierowski (Eds.), *Multi-problem violent youth: A foundation for comparative research on needs, interventions and outcomes* (pp. 302–329). Amsterdam: IOS Press.

Nicholls, T. L., Hemphill, J. F., Boer, D. A., Kropp, P. R., & Zapf, P., (2001). Offenders: Assessment and treatment in special populations. In R. Schuller & J. R. P. Ogloff (Eds.), *Introduction to psychology and law: Canadian perspectives.* (pp. 248–282). Toronto, ON: University of Toronto Press.

Nicholls, T. L., Logan, C., Webster, C. D., & Ogloff, J. R. P. (2003, April) Assessing violence risk in women: A review and critique. *Society for Research on Child Development Annual Meetings.* Tampa, FL.

Odgers, C. L., & Busch, J. (2003, April). The impact of physical and sexual victimization on violent behavior in adolescence: A meta-analytic approach. *Society for Research on Child Development Annual Meetings.* Tampa, FL.

Odgers, C. L., & Moretti, M. M. (2002). Aggressive and antisocial girls: Research update and future challenges. *International Journal of Forensic and Mental Health, 2,* 17–33.

Odgers, C. L., Moretti, M. M., & Pepler, D. J. (2003, April). Antisocial and aggressive behavior in girls: Are we measuring the same construct? *International Association of Forensic Mental Health Services.* Miami, FL.

Odgers, C. L., & Reppucci, N. D. (2002, May). *Female young offenders: A meta-analytic approach.* Paper presented at the Vancouver Conference on Aggressive and Violent Girls: Contributing Factors and Intervention Strategies, Vancouver, Canada.

Office of Juvenile Justice and Delinquency Prevention. (1995). *Guide for implementing the comprehensive strategy for serious, violent, and chronic juvenile offenders.* Washington, D.C.: Office of Juvenile Justice and Delinquency Prevention, Department of Justice.

Otto, R. (2000). Assessing and managing violence risk in outpatient settings. *Journal of Clinical Psychology, 56,* 1239–1262.

Paquette, J. A., & Underwood, M. K. (1999). Gender differences in young adolescents' experiences of peer victimization: Social and physical aggression. *Merrill-Palmer Quarterly, 45,* 242–266.

Pepler, D. J., & Sedighdeilami, F. (1998). *Aggressive girls in Canada.* Ottawa: Applied Research Branch, Strategic Policy Human Resources Development Canada.

Puzzanchera, C., Stahl, A. L., Finnegan, T. A., Tierney, N., & Snyder, H. N. (2003). *Juvenile Court Statistics 1998.* Washington, DC: Office of Juvenile Justice and Delinquency Prevention.

Reitsma-Street, M. (1999). Justice for Canadian girls: A 1990s update. *Canadian Journal of Criminology, 41,* 335–364.

Rivera, B., & Spatz Widom, C. (1990). Childhood victimization and violent offending. *Violence & Victims, 5,* 19–35.

Robins, L. N. (1986). The consequence of conduct disorder in girls. In D. Olweus, J. Block, & M. Radke-Yarrow (Eds.), *Development of antisocial and prosocial behavior* (pp. 385–414). New York: Harcourt Brace Jovanovich.

Rosenbaum, J. L. (1989). Family dysfunction and female delinquency. *Crime & Delinquency, 35,* 31–44.

Rowe, D., Vazsonyi, A., & Flannery, D. (1995). Sex differences: Do means and within-sex variation have similar causes? *Journal of Research in Crime and Delinquency, 32,* 84–100.

Rutherford, M. J., Alterman, A. I., & Cacciola, J. S. (1995). Reliability and validity of the Revised-Psychopathy Checklist in opiate and cocaine addicted women. *Issues in Criminological and Legal Psychology, 24*, 136–141.

Salekin, R., Rogers, R., & Sewell, K. (1998). Psychopathy and recidivism among female inmates. *Law and Human Behavior, 22*, 109–128.

Seagrave, D., & Grisso, T. (2002). Adolescent development and the measurement of juvenile psychopathy. *Law and Human Behavior, 26*, 219–239.

Shaw, M., & Dubois, S. (1995). *Understanding violence by women: A review of the literature*. Ottawa: Correctional Service of Canada.

Simourd, L., & Andrews, D. A. (1994). Correlates of delinquency: A look at the gender differences. *Women in Prison, 6*, 28–44.

Sommers, I., & Baskin, D. (1994). Factors related to female adolescent initiation into violent street crime. *Youth and Society, 25*, 468–489.

Sroufe, L. A. (1990). Considering normal and abnormal together: The essence of developmental psychopathology. *Development and Psychopathology, 2*, 335–347.

Straus, M., & Gelles, R. J. (1986). Societal change and change in family violence from 1975 to 1985 as revealed by two national surveys. *Journal of Marriage & the Family, 48*, 465–479.

Tarasoff v. the Regents of the University of California, et al, 551 P.2d 334 (Cal. 1976).

Teplin, L. A. (2003, April). Psychiatric disorders in detained youth: Implication for treatment and public health policy. *Plenary address at the 3rd annual International Association of Forensic Mental Health Services conference*, Miami, FL.

Statistics Canada. (2001). *Canadian dimensions: Youth and adult crime rates*. Online. Available: http://www. statcan/english/Pgdb/State/Justice/legal .

Totten, M. (2000). *The special needs of females in Canada's youth justice system: An account of some young women's experiences and views*. Ottawa: Department of Justice Canada.

Uggen C., & Kruttschnitt C. (1998). Crime in the breaking: Gender differences in desistance. *Law & Society Review, 32*, 339–366.

U. S. Bureau of Justice Statistics. (1997). *Privacy and juvenile justice records: A mid-decade status report*. Annapolis Junction, MD: Bureau of Justice.

Viale-Val, G., & Sylvester, C. (1993). Female delinquency. In M. Sugar (Ed.), *Female adolescent development* (pp. 169–191). New York: Brunner-Mazel.

Vincent, G. M. (2002). Investigating the legitimacy of adolescent psychopathy assessment: Contributions of item response theory. Unpublished dissertation, Simon Fraser University.

Vincent, G. M., & Hart, S. (2002). Psychopathy and youth. In R. R. Corrado, R. Roesch, S. D. Hart, & J. Gierowski (Eds.), *Multi-problem violent youth: A foundation for comparative research on needs, interventions and outcomes* (pp. 302–329). Amsterdam: IOS Press.

Vitale, J. E., & Newman, J. P. (2001). Using the Psychopathy Checklist-Revised with female samples: Reliability, validity, and implications for clinical utility. *Clinical Psychology: Science & Practice, 8*, 117–132.

Webster, C. D, Douglas, K. S., Eaves, D., & Hart, S. D. (1997). *HCR-20 assessing risk for violence: Version 2*. Burnaby, British Columbia: Mental Health, Law, and Policy Institute, Simon Fraser University.

Zahn-Waxler, C., Cole, P. M., & Barrett, K. C. (1991). Guilt and empathy: Sex differences and implications for the development of depression. In J. Garber & K. A. Dodge (Eds.), *The development of emotion regulation and dysregulation* (pp. 243–272). Cambridge, UK: Cambridge University Press.

Zoccolillo M., & Rogers K. (1991). Characteristics and outcome of conduct disorder in hospitalized adolescent girls. *Journal of the American Academy of Child and Adolescent Psychiatry, 30*, 973–981.

15

From Crime Control to Welfare and Back Again
*(R)Evolving Youth Criminal Justice Policy and Its Possible Effect on Young Female Offenders**

DEBORAH A. CONNOLLY, TRISTIN M.WAYTE, AND ZINA LEE

"Just desserts," "crime control," and "public protection" are common phrases used to describe contemporary policy and legislation that govern young people who commit serious crimes. In Canada (Anand, 1999a; Campbell, Dufresne, & Maclure, 2001; Hylton, 1994; Micucci, 1998), as well as the United States (Feld, 1993, 1999a, b), Britain and Wales (Goldson, 1999; Loveday, 1999), Sweden (Von Hofer, 2000), Australia, Japan, and South Africa (Butts & Harrell, 1998) sanctions for serious offences committed by young people are becoming more severe. This represents a significant shift from the welfare-based model of youth justice that prevailed during most of the twentieth century. One possible consequence of this policy shift is that the youth criminal justice system loses its distinctiveness and becomes more like the adult system of criminal justice (also known as "adultification," Steinberg & Schwartz, 2000: see also Grisso, 1996; Salekin, Rogers, & Ustad, 2001; Scott, 2000; Steinberg & Cauffman, 1999). It is also possible that this kind of policy shift could result in continued differentiation of the youth justice system, thereby entrenching its distinctiveness.

* This work was supported in part by a SSHRC operating grant to the first author.

DEBORAH A. CONNOLLY, TRISTIN M.WAYTE, AND ZINA LEE • Department of Psychology, Simon Fraser University, Burnaby, British Columbia, Canada, V5A 1S6.

Changes enacted in Britain and Wales under the *Crime and Disorder Act* (1998) aim to maintain the distinctiveness of adult and youth justice systems.[1] Adultification, Feld (1993, 1998, 1999a, b) argued, is precisely the course embraced in the United States: Policy and legal changes continue to blur the boundaries between the adult and juvenile justice systems. In this chapter we argue that Canada's crime control measures also have the effect of adultifying the youth criminal justice system. We consider implications of this trend with special emphasis on young female offenders. To serve as a contrast to the current system, we begin with a brief history of youth justice policy and law. We then discuss Canada's new *Youth Criminal Justice Act* (hereinafter "YCJA"). In the final section we argue that, notwithstanding the current trend, a separate system of youth justice is advisable.

HISTORY OF JUVENILE JUSTICE

Prior to the 1300s all persons convicted of crimes, regardless of age, were held to the same standard of liability and subject to the same punishment. By the early 1300s, English Common Law recognized that young children and adults should not be held to the same level of responsibility. However, prior to 1602 there was no universal system of birth registration and so it was impossible to establish a child's age reliably. Accordingly, children were held to an adult standard of liability only if a physical examination revealed the onset of puberty. If the process of puberty had not begun, the child would only be held criminally liable if the Crown could prove malice. By the early 1600s it was accepted that children under the age of 7 were not criminally liable for their actions and those between the ages of 7 and 14 were criminally responsible only if the Crown could prove malice. Together, these two concepts became known as the doctrine of *doli incapax* (Anand, 1999b).

By the late 1800s, there were radical changes in attitudes and beliefs concerning the causes of delinquent behavior. Deviance was seen as symptomatic of a condition or disease caused by external forces over which youth had no control. In particular, social evils and/or deficient parenting were thought to cause juvenile delinquency. These beliefs and attitudes were the catalysts for fundamental changes in youth criminal justice policy at the turn of the last century. The development of a welfare-based model of youth criminal justice had begun.

---

[1] For instance, under the *Crime and Disorder Act*, 1998, parents may be required to attend counselling and guidance sessions to help them to learn to control their children, children under the age of 10 who are "at risk" of becoming offenders may be subject to restrictions, and children who are truant from school may be returned to school or some other designated location.

There were four important characteristics of this welfare-based system of criminal justice (Anand, 1999b; Feld, 1998, 1999a, b). First, youthful offending was seen as a symptom of a larger societal and/or familial problem. Symptoms of delinquency, all of which could be subject to state intervention, included criminal activities and/or other potentially harmful activities such as truancy, sexual promiscuity, and/or incorrigibility. Second, young persons were denied many of the procedural rights guaranteed to adults. Under this system, the welfare of youths was the primary concern and procedural rights impeded the process of helping young people. For example, the right to counsel was thought to be unnecessary because the court was assumed to know the youths' best interests. Third, indeterminate sentences were permitted. When young persons were found to be delinquent, dispositions were passed to treat and cure the youths. Because the appropriate length of treatment varied from case to case and could not be known in advance, indeterminate sentences were passed. Fourth, the new system of youth justice established separate courts and correctional facilities. This system was to be staffed with specially trained judges and court personnel, such as social service personnel, clinicians, and probation officers, who understood developmental issues, were sensitive to the special needs of delinquents, and were qualified to make appropriate therapeutic decisions.

By the mid 1960s, concerns about possible injustices in the North American youth justice system began to emerge. These concerns focused on problems with limited due process rights, the inequity of trying and holding youths for non-criminal behaviors, the efficacy of treatment programs, and the need to hold youths accountable for their criminal behavior (Anand, 1999b; Bolton et al., 1993; Feld, 1999b; Maxim & Whitehead, 2000). Consequent changes in law in Canada (the Young Offender's Act, 1984) and the United States provided youths with some due process rights, implemented determinate sentences, eliminated the offence of delinquency, established that young people could only be charged with criminal offences, and increased the emphasis on accountability and responsibility. Changes over the following several decades continued to transform the youth justice system from a welfare-based model to a crime-control model of justice (Feld, 1993, 1998, 1999).

On April 1, 2003 the *Youth Criminal Justice Act* came into force. It continues Canada's trend towards a crime-control model of youth justice that began in the 1960s. To illustrate this trend, we analyze the YCJA in the context of Feld's (1998, 1999) indicators of "adultification": (a) diversion of some youths from the juvenile justice system into alternative social service systems or into the adult criminal justice system, (b) enhancing procedural rights, (c) de-emphasizing the offender, and (d) emphasizing the rule of law over judicial discretion. We also consider the effect of some of these changes on male and female offenders. We use the YCJA to illustrate "adultification" measures because it is the most recent manifestation of this shift in policy that is prevalent in North America. We argue that similar trends, measures, and effects are operative in the United States.

THE YOUTH CRIMINAL JUSTICE ACT

To consider whether the YCJA may differentially treat and manage young male and female offenders, we first examine gender differences in the pattern of juvenile offending. The following information is based on statistics of juvenile crime in Canada for the year 2000, although the pattern is also found in 1999 and 1998, which suggests a trend. First, it is important to note that the majority of crime committed by juveniles is property crime and males are much more likely than females to commit crime (Canadian Centre for Justice Statistics, 2001). In the year 2000, of all youths recommended for a charge in Canada, 77% were males and 23% were females. Statistics from the United States reflect a similar pattern: Of all youths arrested in the United States in 2000, 72% were males and 28% were females (Uniform Crime Reports, 2000).

DIVERSION

There are two ways that youths can be diverted out of the youth sentencing system. First, several provisions encourage diversion of less serious offenders to community or mental health services. Diversion out of the criminal justice system is to be considered by police as well as Crown counsel (the prosecution). Less serious offences may include theft under $5000, possession of stolen property, mischief, and bail violations. The most recent statistics illustrate that a greater percentage of the females are recommended for charges of this nature. In Canada, 62% of females and 50% of males who were recommended for a charge were recommended for a charge of a less serious nature (see Figure 1). This suggests that a higher proportion of female than male offenders will be dealt with in the community or in the mental health system.

A second method of diversion is to impose an adult sentence on the youths. Under the YCJA, young offenders will not be transferred to adult court (currently possible in the United States and possible in Canada until April 1, 2003). They may, however, be given adult sentences in certain circumstances. As discussed below, under the YCJA there is a broader range of circumstances under which an adult sentence is presumed to be

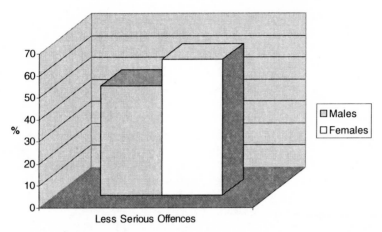

Figure 1. Percentage of males and females recommended for less serious offence charges.

appropriate. Moreover, as discussed below, this broader range of circumstances may impact a higher proportion of female than male offenders.

PROCEDURAL RIGHTS

Under the YCJA, whenever a young person is at risk of receiving an adult sentence she obtains additional procedural rights. In particular, she gains the right to a preliminary inquiry and the right to be tried by a judge and jury. If she exercises either of these rights then the trial cannot proceed in provincial court—the court that has been designated a youth court. In such circumstances the trial must proceed in superior court—the court that has been designated an adult court. The superior court judge will be "deemed" a youth court judge for the purposes of that trial and will hear the case under the YCJA. If the prosecution routinely notifies youths who could be subject to adult sentences, that it intends to apply for one and if notified youths routinely elect to have a preliminary inquiry and/or a jury trial, many more youths will have their cases heard in superior court. If this is the case, we could also see more youths in courtrooms that were previously the near-exclusive domain of adult justice.

An important question is whether notified male and female young offenders will differentially exercise their procedural rights. It is possible, for instance, that sympathetic-looking young female offenders will be more likely than young male offenders to elect to be tried by a judge and jury. If this is the case, there may be a higher proportion of female offenders being tried in superior court. Of course, research is needed to examine the impact of proceeding in superior court and of proceeding before a jury on the outcome of such cases and the treatment of these juveniles in the adult system.

DE-EMPHASIZE THE OFFENDER

Public protection is the guiding principle in the YCJA and all other principles, including rehabilitation and reintegration, are subject to that guiding principle. Certainly, a court may take the needs and circumstances of the young offender into consideration, but it can do so only to the extent that such deliberation does not compromise the essential principle of public protection. Consistent with this principle and the crime-control model, the YCJA creates a new presumptive offence.

When a young person is convicted of certain offences, he or she is presumptively subject to an adult sentence unless it can be proven that a youth sentence is appropriate in the circumstances (these are called "presumptive offences"). Presumptive offences include first- and second-degree murder, manslaughter, attempted murder, and aggravated sexual assault. By definition, presumptive offences de-emphasize the offender because it is the nature of the offence rather than the offender that triggers the presumption. The YCJA creates a new presumptive offence: The third conviction for a "serious violent offence" (serious violent offence is undefined in the Act). For reasons discussed below, this new presumptive offence may lead to a substantial increase in the number of youths who receive adult sentences.

Although it is unclear how this new presumptive offence will be defined, it is likely to include the following: sexual offences, assault with a weapon, assault causing bodily harm, robbery, abduction, and kidnapping. In Canada, 10% of males and 6% of females who were recommended for a charge were recommended for a charge of this nature. Contrast this with statistics for the same year wherein less than 1% of youths who were recommended for a charge were recommended for charges that would have been presumptive under the old Act. Clearly the addition of this presumptive offence, the third conviction for a serious violent offence, has the potential to substantially increase in the percentage of youths presumptively subject to an adult sentence.

It is possible that some provinces will classify common assault as a serious violent offences, especially in regions where a more punitive stance on young offending is taken. In the year 2000, a greater percentage of females than males who were recommended for a charge in 2000, were recommended for a charge of common assault, 19% and 22% for males and females, respectively (see Figure 2). If courts include common

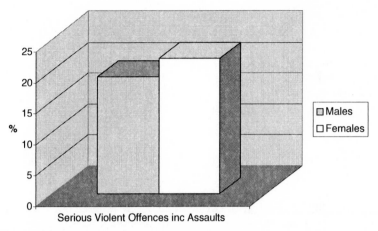

Figure 2. Percentage of males and females recommended for serious violent offences including assault charges.

assault in the definition of serious violent offence, the introduction of this new presumptive offence will have a greater impact on female than male young offenders. Of course, the offence is presumptive only if there were two prior convictions for serious violent offences and so the absolute impact will depend on recidivism rates for these kinds of offences.

Under the YCJA, provinces may opt to lower the age at which a youth convicted of a presumptive offense is subject to an adult sentence, from 16 to 14 years. The emphasis here is on age and nature of the offence rather than relevant characteristics of the offender. This change may well differentially affect female and male offenders. Canadian statistics show that girls' offending peaks at about the age of 15, whereas boys' offending increases between 12 and 17 (Carrington & Moyer, 1998; Juristat, 2000, 2001, 2002). The fact that girls' offending peaks earlier than boys, and the possibility that common assaults could fall under the serious violent offences legislation (discussed above), mean that the new legislation may have a differential impact on girls. That is, if an assault is treated as a serious violent offence, then a girl would face the first of the three offences earlier, on average, compared to boys. If a particular girl remains in the penal system, then by age 17 she would have had longer to garner the three offences over the course of adolescence, compared to a particular boy. While boys are over-represented in other offences that fall under the three strikes parameters (e.g., sexual assault), and recidivate at a greater rate (Juristat, 2000, 2001, 2002), the particular combination of age, offence, and frequency factors that differentiate adult and youth sentencing parameters may have a differential impact on girls. The differential impact of this legislative change is uncertain until outcome studies provide empirical support.

Compared to young male offenders, there is a broader range of mental health outcomes for young female offenders (for a review see Odgers & Moretti, 2002). Accordingly, the continuing trend in North America to de-emphasize the young offender may have a greater impact on serious female offenders because of their poorer prognosis.

RULE OF LAW

With the YCJA, young people will be subject to more of the legal rules that apply in the adult system. For instance, youth sentences are not to be longer than the sentence that would be imposed on a similarly situated adult. Also, mandatory release will occur when the offender has served 2/3 of her sentence, unless there is a good reason to detain her for the full length of the sentence. And, the YCJA is bringing the law with respect to the admissibility of confession evidence closer to the law that applies to adults: A "technical irregularity" in obtaining self-incriminating evidence will not necessarily render the evidence inadmissible (s. 146(5)).

The "adultification" of the youth criminal justice system in North America has been progressing at least since the mid 1980s. The YCJA gives provinces the power to accelerate the process and to create a system of youth criminal justice that differs very little from the adult system. Although we focused on the YCJA, for three reasons discussed above, the implications of such measures are not unique to Canada. First, the offending patterns of female offenders are similar in Canada and the United States. Second, the transformation of the juvenile justice system from one based on welfare to one based on crime control is similar in the two countries. Third, Canada and the United States share particular strategies to achieve the goal of crime control—namely adultification of the youth criminal justice system. Given these striking similarities, the experience in one jurisdiction is informative and applicable in the other jurisdiction. In other words, the implications and analysis of the YCJA in Canada can inform policy-makers in the United States, both those who have similar provisions and those considering new laws that would be similar to the YCJA.

A SYSTEM OF YOUTH JUSTICE

Maintaining a separate criminal justice is meant to respond to the unique needs of young people who commit crimes. These policies reflect assumptions that adolescents are still in the process of developing adult-like decisional capacities and generally are more malleable and amenable to treatment (Steinberg & Cauffman, 1999). Having a separate juvenile system is meant to allow for those developmentally immature to face some consequences for their criminal behavior while also attempting to respond to their developmental needs through treatment and intervention.

A separate system is supported by developmental and criminological theory and research that show some youths' criminal behavior is due to adolescent-specific behaviors, such as impulsivity and immature decision-making. For these youths, their criminal behavior will desist when they mature—they represent adolescent-limited (AL) offenders. Other young offenders show a life-course persistent (LCP) pattern of problems that begins before adolescence and continues after maturity (see Moffitt, 1993; Moffitt & Caspi, 2001; Moffitt, et al., 2002).

Some scholars suggest that youth criminal justice systems attempt to differentiate responses to youth crime by providing harsher, justice-based responses to those whose pattern indicates LCP offending (e.g., violent and repeated violent offences) and diversion or relatively light sentences for those youths whose offending reflects an AL pattern (Feld, 2000; Jeglum-Bartusch, Lynam, Moffitt, & Silva, 1997). However, the research that developed these separate offending trajectories is based on boys' data (Moffitt, 1993; Moffitt & Caspi, 2001; Moffitt et al., 2002; Patterson, Debaryshe, & Ramsey, 1989; Patterson, Forgatch, Yoerger, & Stoolmiller, 1998; see Silverthorn & Frick, 1999; Silverthorn, Frick, & Reynolds, 2001, for a discussion). If youth justice policies are attempting to differentiate the response to LCP and AL offending, is this response appropriate for girls' offending trajectories?

While there is much less research available for girls' offending trajectories compared to boys', there has been a recent increase of interest in the area. Silverthorn and Frick (1999) hypothesized that since Moffitt's (1993, Moffitt et al., 1996, 2002) trajectories were based entirely on boys' data, they may not reflect girls' offending patterns. The authors used past research on girls' offending to argue that women's adult criminality cannot be predicted by childhood problem behavior, but by adolescent problems only. That is, girls and women's serious problems (mental health and criminality) begin to appear only after puberty. After puberty, the number of problems for girls increases substantially (more so than for boys). They argue that girls with this delayed-onset delinquency share the same negative childhood correlates as the LCP boys (e.g., neurocognitive dysfunction, poor parenting practices, family criminality). They argue further that girls with delayed onset offending have poor adult outcomes, including legal and mental health problems. In an effort to provide empirical support for their hypothesis, the authors tested adjudicated girls and boys who met the criteria for conduct disorder (Silverthorn, et al., 2001). They found that boys tend to display either childhood onset or adolescent-onset delinquency, whereas girls were much more likely to show adolescent-onset delinquency. The delayed-onset girls were similar to childhood-onset boys in personality variables such as callousness and impulse control.

Critical response to Silverthorn and colleagues has come from Moffitt and Caspi (2001), who tested their theory on the girls in their birth cohort. Whether they analyzed the data by gender or together, the LCP youths had negative family backgrounds, whereas AL youths did not. The vast majority of delinquent girls had adolescent-onset problems, and did not have adverse family backgrounds. Risk factors for male and female were found to be similar in a study by Fergusson and Horwood (2002), who examined boys and girls' trajectories in a 21-year longitudinal study. These authors found that there was variability in terms of early or late onset of problems *within* the AL group; that is, girls seem to show adolescent-onset delinquency before boys show adolescent-onset delinquency. The risk factors for trajectory membership (whether LCP or AL) were the same for both boys and girls. These findings supported an earlier effort by the same authors (Fergusson, Horwood & Nagin, 2000), in which they concluded a single, 2-trajectory model could describe both boys and girls. To the extent that the YCJA (or any legislation dealing with youth crime) can discriminate between LCP and AL youths, there is little evidence that this discrimination will be more or less effective with female than male offenders.

CONCLUSIONS

For most of the 1900s, youth justice was a welfare-based system that viewed youthful offending as a symptom of delinquency caused by social ills and/or inadequate parenting. By the mid-1960s, there was a clear change in policy towards young offenders; as in the adult criminal justice system, crime control and public protection became important principles of the youth criminal justice policy. In North America, the result of this change in policy is the adultification of the youth criminal justice system. The YCJA is the most recent manifestation of this principle.

Because of the distinctive offending patterns, the effect of adultification of the juvenile justice system on male and female young offenders may be different. Using the YCJA as a recent manifestation of adultification, we attempted to predict the affect of this policy shift on female young offenders by first profiling their offending behavior and then anticipating the effects of the legal changes given that pattern. It became quite clear that predicting the effect of this policy shift is profoundly complicated by the serious paucity of research on young female offenders (e.g., Odgers & Moretti, 2002). This research deficit is particularly striking given the rapid movement towards "just desserts," "crime control," and "public protection" in youth criminal justice policy. Some of the research questions that must be addressed before we can confidently predict the effect of this policy shift on young female offenders include: How will the policy and consequent laws affect the growing number of girls involved in moderately serious personal injury offences? Will the mental health outcomes for girls be affected by the movement to crime-control and adultification of youth justice? Based on potentially different offending trajectories, does the law accurately distinguish between girls who should and girls who should not remain in the juvenile justice system?

Section 3(1)(c), as part of the Declaration of Principle in the *Youth Criminal Justice Act*, stipulates that accountability for crime should be balanced with the special needs of the young person. Section 3(1)(c)(iii) declares that measures taken against young people should respect their gender, as well as other special needs. Given this declared sensitivity to the offenders' gender, we urge researchers in the field to investigate the postulated questions so that we may guide policy makers to respond appropriately to girls' special needs.

REFERENCES

Anand, S. S. (1999a). Preventing youth crime: What works, what doesn't, and what it all means for Canadian juvenile justice policy. *Queens Law Journal, 25*, 177–249.

Anand, S.S. (1999b). Catalyst for change: The history of Canadian juvenile justice reform. *Queens Law Journal, 24*, 515–559.

Anand, S. S. (1999c). The good, the bad, and the unaltered: An analysis of bill C-68, the Youth Criminal Justice Act. *Canadian Criminal Law Review, 4*, 249–270.

Bill C-7, *Youth Criminal Justice Act*, 1st Session, 37th Parliament, 2002.

Bolton, J., Caskey, J., Costom, S., Fowler, R., Fox, S., Hillman, K., Taylor, R., & Yarin, R. (1993). The young offenders act: Principles and policy—the first decade in review. *McGill Law Journal, 38*, 939–1052.

Butts, J. A., & Harrell, A. V. (1998). Delinquents or criminals: Policy options for young offenders. The Urban Institute Crime Policy Report

Campbell, K., Dufresne, M., & Maclure, R. (2001). Amending youth justice policy in Canada: Discourse, mediation, and ambiguity. *The Howard Journal, 40*, 272–284.

Canadian Centre for Justice Statistics. (1999, November). *Canadian crime statistics 1998* (Catalogue No. 85-205-XIE). Ottawa, ON: Author.

Canadian Centre for Justice Statistics. (2000, December). *Canadian crime statistics 1999* (Catalogue No. 85-205-XIE). Ottawa, ON: Author.

Canadian Centre for Justice Statistics. (2001, December). *Canadian crime statistics 2000* (Catalogue No. 85-205-XIE). Ottawa, ON: Author.

Carrington, P., & Moyer, S. (1998). *A statistical profile of female young offenders.* Department of Justice, Canada.

Cauffman, E., & Steinberg, L. (2000). (Im)maturity of judgment in adolescence: Why adolescents may be less culpable than adults. *Behavioral Sciences and the Law, 18,* 741–760.

Conway, H. (July 30, 2001). Ontario's recommendations for the YCJA: Towards abolishing the youth system.

Feld, B. (1993). Juvenile (in)justice and the criminal court alternative. *Crime and Delinquency, 39,* 403–424.

Feld, B. (1998). Juvenile and criminal justice systems' responses to youth violence. *Crime and Justice: An Annual Review, 24,* 189–261.

Feld, B. (1999a). A funny thing happened on the way to the centenary. *Punishment and Society, 1,* 187–214.

Feld, B. (1999b). Transformation of juvenile courts—Part II: Race and the "crack down" on youth crime. *Minnesota Law Review, 84,* 327–395.

Feld, B.C. (2000). Legislative exclusion of offences from juvenile court jurisdiction: A history and critique. In J. Fagan & F. E. Zimring (Eds.), *The changing borders of juvenile justice: Transfer of adolescents to the criminal court* (pp. 83–144). Chicago: University of Chicago Press.

Fergusson, D. M., & Horwood, L. J. (2002). Male and female offending trajectories. *Development and Psychopathology, 14,* 159–177.

Fergusson, D. M., Horwood, L. J., & Nagin, D. S. (2000). Offending trajectories in a New Zealand birth cohort. *Criminology, 38,* 525–551.

Goldson, B. (1999). Youth (in)justice: Contemporary developments in Policy and Practice. In B. Goldson (Ed.), *Youth Justice: Contemporary Policy and Practices* (pp. 1–27). Vermont: Ashgate.

Grisso, T. (1998). *Forensic evaluation of juveniles: A manual for practice.* Sarasota, FL: Professional Resource Press.

Grisso, T. (1996). Society's retributive response to juvenile violence: A developmental perspective. *Law and Human Behavior, 20,* 229–247.

Hylton, J. H. (1994). Get tough or get smart? Options for Canada's youth justice system in the twenty-first century. *Canadian Journal of Criminology, 36,* 229–246.

Jeglum-Bartusch, D., Lynam, D., Moffitt, T. E., & Silva, P. A. (1997). Age is important: Testing general versus developmental theories of antisocial behavior. *Criminology, 35,* 13–47.

Juristat. (2000, May). *Youth court statistics, 1998/99 highlights* (Catalogue No. 85-002-XIE, Vol. 20, No. 2). Ottawa, ON: Author.

Juristat. (2001, May). *Youth court statistics, 1999/00* (Catalogue No. 85-002-XPE, Vol. 21, No. 3). Ottawa, ON: Author.

Juristat. (2002, March). *Youth court statistics, 2000/01* (Catalogue No. 85-002-XIE, Vol. 22, No. 3). Ottawa, ON: Author.

Juvenile Delinquents Act, R.S.C. 1970, c. J-3.

Kent v. United States (1966), 383 U.S. 5411966.

Loveday, B. (1999). Tough on crime or tough on the causes of crime? An evaluation of Labour's Crime and Disorder legislation. *Crime Prevention and Community Safety: An International Journal, 1,* 7–24.

Maxim, P. S., & Whitehead, P. C. (2000). *Youth in conflict with the law.* Scarborough, ON: Nelson Thomson Learning.

Micucci, L. (1998). Responsibility and the young person. *Canadian Journal of Law and Jurisprudence, 11,* 277–309.

Moffitt, T. (1993). Life-course persistent versus adolescent-limited antisocial behavior: A developmental taxonomy. *Psychological Review, 100,* 674–701.

Moffitt, T., & Caspi, A. (2001). Childhood predictors differentiate life-course persistent and adolescence-limited antisocial pathways among males and females. *Development and Psychopathology, 13,* 355–375.

Moffitt, T. E., Caspi, A., Dickson, N., Silva, P., & Stanton, W. (1996). Childhood onset versus adolescent onset antisocial conduct problems in males: Natural history from ages 3 to 18. *Development and Psychopathology, 8,* 399–424.

Moffitt, T. E., Caspi, A., Harrington, H., & Milne, B. (2002). Males on the life-course-persistent and adolescent-limited antisocial pathways: Follow-up at age 26. *Development and Psychopathology, 14,* 179–207.

Odgers, C. L., & Moretti, M.M. (2002). Aggressive and antisocial girls: Research update and challenges. *International Journal of Forensic Mental Health, 1,* 103–109.

Patterson, G. R., Debaryshe, B. D., & Ramsey, E. (1989). A developmental perspective on antisocial behavior. *American Psychologist, 44,* 329–335.

Patterson, G. R., Forgatch, M. S., Yoerger, K. L., & Stoolmiller, M. (1998). Variables that initiate and maintain an early-onset trajectory for juvenile offending. *Development and Psychopathology, 10,* 531–547.

R.v. W.(D.), [2002] B.C.J. No. 627. (Youth Court) (Q.L.)

Salekin, R. T., Rogers, R., & Ustad, K. L. (2001). Juvenile waiver to adult criminal courts: Prototypes for dangerousness, sophistication-maturity, and amenability to treatment. *Psychology, Public Policy, and Law, 7,* 381–408.

Scott, E. (2000). Criminal responsibility in adolescence: Lessons from developmental psychology. In T. Grisso & R.G. Schwartz (Eds.), *Youth on trial: A developmental perspective on juvenile justice* (pp. 291–323). Chicago: University of Chicago Press.

Silverthorn, P., & Frick, P. J. (1999). Developmental pathways to antisocial behavior: The delayed-onset pathway in girls. *Development and psychopathology, 11,* 101–126.

Silverthorn, P., Frick, P. J., & Reynolds, R. (2001). Timing of onset and correlates of severe conduct problems in adjudicated girls and boys. *Journal of Psychopathology and Behavioral Assessment, 23,* 171–181.

Steinberg, L., & Cauffman, E. (1996). Maturity of judgment in adolescence: Psychosocial factors in adolescent decision-making. *Law and Human Behavior, 20,* 249–272.

Steinberg, L., & Cauffman, E. (1999). A developmental perspective on serious juvenile crime: When should juveniles be treated as adults? *Federal Probation, 63,* 52–57.

Steinberg, L., & Schwartz, R. G. (2000). Developmental psychology goes to court. In T. Grisso & R.G. Schwartz (Eds.), *Youth on trial: A developmental perspective on juvenile justice* (pp. 9–31). Chicago: University of Chicago Press.

Uniform Crime Reports. (2000). *Crime in the United States 2000.* Washington, DC: US Government Printing Office.

Von Hofer, H. (2000). Criminal violence and youth in Sweden: A long-term perspective. *Journal of Scandinavian Studies in Criminology and Crime Prevention, 1,* 56–72.

Young Offenders Act, 1980–81-82–83, c. 110.

─────16─────

Girls, Aggression, and Delinquency
Research and Policy Considerations

JENNIFER L. WOOLARD

Historically, research and policy on juvenile offenders in the United States has been primarily the study of males despite the fact that over one in four delinquency arrests involve female offenders (Federal Bureau of Investigation, 2002). When attention has been directed to females they have been typecast in the policy realm as status offenders and in research as demonstrating primarily internalizing disorders. Both characterizations of the female offender are incomplete, ignoring those girls engaging in aggressive and delinquent acts and the system-level influences on their identification and treatment. In this chapter I review some issues that delinquent girls raise for both research and policy. First, I describe how policy makers and researchers might approach the phenomenon of girls' delinquency from different vantage points but with common interests. Then, I briefly highlight three areas that might benefit from policy-relevant empirical research: the nature and extent of offending, system processing, and treatment and intervention.

FRAMING THE ISSUES

Although the system was intended to act as a benevolent but firm parent, in practice the system did not operate that way. In the late 1960s

JENNIFER L. WOOLARD • Department of Psychology, Georgetown University, Washington, DC, United States, 20057.

and early 1970s a significant set of procedural reforms followed several U.S. Supreme Court decisions describing the juvenile justice system as "the worst of both worlds"—failing to provide the promised rehabilitation while simultaneously failing to provide many of the due process protections found in the adversarial adult system (e.g., *Breed v. Jones*, 1975; *In re Gault*, 1967; *In re Winship*, 1970; *Kent v. U.S.*, 1966). If *Gault* (1967) heralded the "due process" era of reform that extended many of adult defendants' rights to juveniles, reform in the post-*Gault* era moved the juvenile court further away from its original rehabilitative model toward a punishment framework in which public safety equaled or surpassed the traditional goal of best interests of the child. A variety of legislative initiatives created changes in jurisdiction and sentencing practices that try more youths as adults and confine them for longer periods (Reppucci, 1999). These legislative changes were based in part on concerns for public safety, but they also represent changing views on how "adult-like" certain juvenile offenders are. Practically speaking, a segment of the adolescent population has been legally redefined as adults and prosecuted in adult criminal court. Contrary to the rehabilitative approach to the immature or developing adolescent, these changes suggest that certain youth are by definition *not* immature; or if they are, it is now irrelevant.

However, much of this rhetoric has occurred with a particular delinquent in mind—the violent male offender. Female delinquents rarely enter the picture, although recent stories in the news media have begun directing attention toward the "bad girls"—perhaps the latest version of the super predator that dominated policy discussions in the early 1990s (Chesney-Lind, 1997). It is unclear whether the wave of fear of crime that apparently followed male super predators and provided rhetorical support for policy change will return, perhaps in lesser form, as anecdotes about violent girls emerge. Likewise, the history of delinquency theory and data is that of boys but a growing number of scholars over the past several decades have drawn attention to girls. To some degree, girls have been operating under the radar screen in policy and research, but that may be changing. This paper reviews the current controversies in research on female delinquents and speculates on some the policy and practice-related questions that could usefully be informed by empirical research.

The premise that empirical research can play an important role in policy formation and evaluation necessitates mutual influence between the two realms. Encouraging psychology's involvement in public policy, Darley (2002) recognizes that "to have an impact on public policy, we need a theory of how public policy is made, one that we can scan for entry points for what we know (p. 15)." I believe it is difficult to identify a coherent juvenile justice policy toward female delinquents that we can scan, much less enter. Even so, the following three questions that policymakers might pose to researchers could serve as entry points.

1. *How do I protect public safety?* Are violent girls like violent boys? How do I ensure that I am protecting the public from delinquent girls now and in the future?
2. *How should I manage female offenders?* Should our processing response (e.g., arrest, adjudication, and sentencing) to boys and girls be similar or different? What, if any, special management issues arise for female offenders? Should our treatment and programming responses to males and females be similar or different?
3. *How should I allocate resources?* I have limited funding dollars for juvenile justice in general and female delinquents in particular. Should there be any special money allocated for female delinquents? Why?

These three questions represent fundamental issues at multiple levels within the juvenile justice system. The first question references overall goals of the juvenile justice system. The policy shifts described earlier have quite literally changed the goals of the juvenile justice system. States have modified their mission or purpose statements to include protection of public safety and/or juvenile accountability as one of the system's primary goals (Snyder & Sickmund, 1999). Offender rehabilitation may or may not explicitly remain. National debates about the justice system are rare; they more often occur at the state level because each state designs and runs its own juvenile justice system. States vary in the attention they have directed toward female offenders.

The second question refers to the implementation of justice system goals. Broad parameters of procedure are set in state law, but written or unwritten procedures for daily system operations vary by state agency, local office, or courtroom. Juvenile justice procedures encompass multiple discretion points about diversion, pretrial detention, petition filing, adjudication, and sentencing. Management issues range from secure confinement in pretrial or post-adjudication facilities to non-secure settings, community-based alternatives, and treatment programs. Again, female offenders present common and unique features compared to boys. The existence and availability of treatment programs and sentencing options vary by jurisdiction and funding levels. Some locales have initiated female-specific interventions (e.g., Office of Juvenile Justice and Delinquency Prevention, 1998b), but the patterns are inconsistent.

Finally, the allocation of resources is the engine that drives the translation of policy goals into practice. Resource allocation for female offenders can be affected by all three branches of government. Policymakers can specify studies, laws, and procedures that explicitly target female offenders. Executive branch agencies promulgate the regulations and administrative practices that interpret those laws and develop initiatives specific to female offenders. The judicial branch can use its powers to set formal or unwritten rules for processing and treating female offenders within the courtroom, or direct other agencies to engage in certain activities.

Researchers share common interest with our hypothetical policymaker but approach the issues differently. The first question about public safety is recast as causes and correlates of delinquency and risk of recidivism. The second question of offender management encompasses several research directions on the ways in which girls are processed through the system, the impact of justice system involvement on health and recidivism, and the implementation and outcome of interventions. The third question about resource allocation can be informed by efficacy and cost-effectiveness research on prevention and intervention strategies.

Researchers should not be content to answer existing policy questions, but should serve a critical role in shaping the policy debate. One way is to identify the assumptions that underlie policy but remain unarticulated, either through deliberate effort or negligence. For example, two issues regarding female delinquency take on the appearance of fact but pose rather vexing questions for theory and research. Daly (1998) refers to these as the gender ratio and generalizability problems. The gender ratio problem is the "fact" that girls commit disproportionately less crime than boys. The generalizability problem is the "fact" that most delinquency theories were generated to explain male delinquency. Both of these problems present significant challenges to researchers and have sparked rather intense debate in the literature. Both also have broad implications for policy-relevant decisions about goals, process, and intervention, but I hypothesize that policy makers see neither problems in the same way that researchers do. They probably accept the first fact as a system reality, tempered by the emerging "bad girl" phenomenon, and consider the second as less than relevant for policy and practice. Researchers can connect academic issues and policy concerns by demonstrating that theories about the cause of delinquency underlie the policy response to delinquency.

Another avenue for research focuses our lens on juvenile justice as a system within a larger historical and organizational context. We can conceptualize the juvenile justice system as a systemic intervention of care and control. A hallmark of the juvenile justice system, discretion provides the opportunity for individualized justice and discrimination, both of which come into play for female offenders. Research on gender bias and the role of status offenses in girls' justice system involvement is one example of the larger systems issues that research is positioned to investigate.

In the next section I attempt to integrate the hypothetical policymaker's questions and the researcher's theoretical and empirical interests. What follows is a brief review of existing research on offending behavior, system processing, and treatment interventions. For each I identify several issues that might benefit from empirical research and policy attention.

THE NATURE AND EXTENT OF OFFENDING

Debate continues on whether girls' crime can be explained by existing theory (referred to as "males plus" or "add and stir" approaches), a female-specific set of theories, or an integrated approach (Daly, 1998; Hoyt & Scherer, 1998). Feminist theorists have made important contributions, and existing theories on males provide a good starting point because both approaches push research to consider multiple levels of influence. For these reasons, the integrated approach shows the most promise of allowing for both similarities and differences among males and females. Rather than searching for gender neutral or gender specific theories, it will be more productive to identify variables and concepts that operate similarly and differently for delinquent girls and boys (Daly, 1998; Hoyt & Scherer, 1998).

An ecological, developmental approach to understanding females in context supports good descriptive research on girls' lives as well as complicated analyses of offending careers and trajectories. Research has begun to examine whether the predictive validity of risk factors for aggression such as exposure to family violence and offending parents and peers vary as a function of gender. Reviewing empirical studies that tested etiological factors or theories of female delinquency, Hoyt and Scherer (1998) identify several focal areas, including abuse, family structure and functioning, peer relationships, and academic correlates. They conclude that the research corpus is contradictory and insufficient to sustain confident generalizations about the causes and correlates of female delinquency.

Questions remain about the stability of predictive factors and their impact on offending rates over time. Analytic tools for testing fit and model equivalence across samples are being used to evaluate how constructs differ in the quality and quantity of their contribution to female offending. Moffitt's (1993) theory differentiates delinquent offending into two developmental trajectories. Life-course persistent offenders begin their antisocial behavior in childhood and persist throughout adulthood, sharing background experiences of inadequate parenting, neurocognitive problems, troubled environments, and poor relationships. Adolescence-limited offending trajectories coincide with pubertal development and represented normative acting out behavior in response to a "maturity gap" between biological development and social rights and responsibilities. Originally tested with males, the authors hypothesized that fewer females would engage in delinquency, but the majority who did would follow the adolescence-limited trajectory with causes similar to those of males. Silverthorn and Frick (1999) argued that all girls' delinquency corresponded to the high-risk backgrounds of life-course persistent males, regardless of onset timing. Moffitt and Caspi (2001) concluded that life course persistent females differed from adolescent-onset females according to theory, findings largely consistent with previous work (e.g., Caspi, Lynam, Moffitt, & Silva, 1993; Mazerolle, Brame, Paternoster, Piquero, & Dean, 2000). Research on early onset offenders is important and expanding (e.g., Hipwell et al., 2002) but they represent a small, albeit attention grabbing, proportion of female offenders (1% in Moffitt & Caspi, 2001). The need for research on adolescent-onset offenders and status offenders is equally pressing.

Statistical advances notwithstanding, methodological limitations constrain the value of existing research on causes and correlates of female delinquency. Females were not often the true target of large scale delinquency studies and therefore limited to secondary analyses. Studies often rely on either self-report or official statistics leading to varying definitions of delinquency, aggression, and violence that reduce cross-study comparability. Regardless of the definition used, most studies fail to sample across the spectrum of offending (e.g., status and delinquency, chronic offenders, violent offenders).

DIFFERENTIAL PROCESSING: A SYSTEM OF CARE AND CONTROL

Gender-based patterns of delinquent behavior and system processing are perhaps the clearest example where policy and research interests coincide but data sources contradict. The gender ratio issue that boys offend at a greater rate than girls is clear on the surface but murky in the details because even basic descriptions of incidence and prevalence are complicated. The first complication accrues from definitional differences. Whereas scientists work more in terms of behavioral and psychological constructs, delinquency is a legally defined status. Within the legal framework of delinquency there are two broad categories of acts: delinquent acts and status offenses. Delinquent acts would be violations of criminal law if adults engaged in them; they include crimes against person (e.g., murder, assault, and robbery), crimes against property (e.g., arson, burglary, larceny) and other minor offenses. Status offenses are specific to juvenile status and are not violations for adults. These include running away from home, being "troublesome" or "incorrigible," skipping school, and drinking alcohol, among others. The second complication arises from data sources. Generated from law enforcement or other justice system agencies, official data track those juveniles and offenses that are officially processed in some capacity. The most common form of official delinquency data is arrest data. Self report data represent behaviors disclosed by the juveniles themselves.[1]

Data from official law enforcement sources clearly demonstrate differential offending rates.[2] Boys have higher incidence and prevalence of offending in almost all delinquent offense categories; this gap increases as offense seriousness increases. Girls comprise the majority of arrests for status offenses, and most girls are arrested for status offenses. Gender differentials in violent and status offending persist but in much diminished form among self-report data which may or may not conform to legal definitions (Chesney-Lind, 1997; Daly, 1998). Because this section of the chapter targets justice system processing specifically, we focus on data from official sources.

In 2001, girls were responsible for 1.7% of all arrests compared to boys at 12.0%. Girls comprised 12.2% of the more than 1.27 million arrests of persons under 18. Gender-based patterns of juvenile arrest become clearer when offense-specific rates are considered. Of all juvenile arrests, girls accounted for 18.2% of violent crime and 31.5% of property crime.[3] The pattern reverses for traditionally "female" offenses such as running away (59.4%) and prostitution (64.1%).

The answer to questions about whether girls are increasingly violent depends on the basis of comparison in official arrest data.[4] Examining the gender distribution of violent crime arrests over time, females do appear to engage in increasing amounts of violent behavior. Between 1992 and 2001, the juvenile male violent crime arrest rate dropped 25.8%. The comparable female rate increased 12.2%. Arrests for other assaults increased

---

[1] A third source of data derives from victimization surveys that ask victims to report on characteristics of their offenders.

[2] These numbers are calculated from Tables 39, 40, and 42 from the FBI's *Crime in the United States, 2001.*

[3] These percentages represent Index crimes of violence (murder, forcible rape, robbery, and aggravated assault) and property (burglary, larceny-theft, motor vehicle theft, and arson).

[4] Numbers in this paragraph come from Tables 32 and 33 of the FBI's *Crime in the United States, 2001.*

17.8% for males and 65.9% for females. Girls' proportion of total violent crime arrests also increased from 12.7% to 18.2%. When examining the distribution of arrest patterns within gender, increases appear much less dramatic. The proportion of serious violent crime arrests among all girls' arrests has remained fairly stable (2.7% versus 2.6%) and increased somewhat for minor assaults (from 8.2% to 11.5%). These data undercut arguments based on available data from the mid 1990s that seemingly dramatic increases in official reports of female violence are comparable to those of male violence and result primarily from increased likelihood of arrest for minor assaults and family conflicts (Chesney-Lind, 2001). Even so, changes in enforcement practices are probably an important factor in the accelerating arrest rate for violent crime but evaluation studies are uncommon.

Some argue that the gender-based differentials in official delinquency statistics as compared to self report data occur because the juvenile justice system has had a different policy goal for females since its inception (Chesney-Lind & Shelden, 1998; Odem & Schlossman, 1991). As a result, girls have come into the juvenile justice system through different types of surveillance or social control, and for different reasons than boys. Historically, the system has demonstrated an ambivalence toward girls cloaked in a parens patriae, paternalistic system. Examining how Los Angeles dealt with female delinquents at the turn of the 20th century, Odem and Schlossman (1991) argue that the court's major goal was the social control of girls' "social hygiene" or sexual behavior through offenses ranging from "staying out late, to flirting with sailors, to engaging in premarital sex" (p. 190). Los Angeles area female delinquents were subject to compulsory gynecological examinations, mandatory venereal disease testing, and forced hospital-based treatment for those who tested positive. Historical data also suggest that girls may have come to the attention of the juvenile justice system in different ways from boys: in the Los Angeles study, a significant proportion of referrals were instigated by parents and the school system, not law enforcement.

Persistent overrepresentation of girls among status offenders and the lower proportion of law enforcement referrals for girls do suggest that the juvenile justice system operates differently according to gender, at least with respect to status offenses. Girls are more likely to be processed for status offenses than boys, but the data are equivocal on gender bias in other aspects of processing such as likelihood of adjudication and sentence severity (Chesney-Lind, 1997; General Accounting Office, 1995; Horowitz & Pottieger, 1991; Hoyt & Scherer, 1998; Snyder & Sickmund, 1999). MacDonald and Chesney-Lind's (2001) longitudinal study of Hawaiian juvenile courts determined that girls were less likely to be handled formally in early stages of the judicial process, but once adjudicated delinquent status they were more likely to be given formal dispositions for less serious crimes. In contrast, a cross sectional GAO study (1995) found little gender disparity in court processing of noncriminal offenders. Conflicting findings across studies may result as much from methodology as the underlying nature of the phenomenon.

Over the past 25 years, the juvenile justice system has moved explicitly from a system of care, at least in theory, to a system of control in theory and practice. This is not to say that boys do not still need the care aspect of the system but that the system has largely abandoned the care ethic and rhetoric for most male delinquents. Whether through paternalism, a desire to regulate behavior that violates gender stereotypes, or inattention, there is some vestige of the care system remaining for female offenders. Feminists argue that "care" has been used differentially as social control, resulting in disparate impact in terms of status offenses and the regulation of sexual behavior. But a system of care also offers the mechanism for providing rehabilitative services that respond to the needs of girls. The promise and peril of caring for girls depend largely on implementation practices.

INTERVENTION AND TREATMENT

Significant program development and evaluation gaps exist for delinquent girls (American Bar Association & National Bar Association, 2001; Chesney-Lind & Shelden, 1998; Horowitz & Pottieger, 1991). To justify the development of programming specifically targeted at girls, practitioners and policy makers say there must be a sufficient number to warrant the attention and expense. The number of cases in which females are detained before trial increased 65% between 1988 and 1997 to 60,000 cases (Scahill, 2000), yet many jurisdictions have only one wing of an institution reserved for females in which all ages and offense types are housed. Girls are not likely to be a homogeneous group with one set of programming needs, even during relatively short pretrial detention stays. Fewer females than males are committed to post-adjudication residential placements but the numbers are growing. Between 1988 and 1997, the number of cases in which females were ordered into residential placements more than doubled to over 22,000 (Scahill, 2000), yet there is little detailed information on the types of programming utilized within these placements (Community Research Associates, 1998). A recent meta-analysis of over 200 interventions was unable to identify gender-specific components of effective programming (Lipsey, 1992).

Ironically, we must hope for the worst, that larger numbers of females enter the system, before we can argue for the best—programming and treatment options that meet their needs regarding sexuality and reproduction, family and relationship violence (Acoca, 1998), sexual abuse (Chesney-Lind, 1997; Widom, 2000), and differential mental health concerns (Cauffman, Feldman, Waterman, & Steiner, 1998). Girls may also be involved in the child welfare/dependency systems for themselves or their children.

As a part of this process, we need to distinguish risk markers from risk factors (Mulvey & Woolard, 1997; Offord, 1997). Risk markers precede the occurrence but cannot be changed (e.g., gender). Risk factors precede, correlate, and are shown to have a causal relationship. Risk markers are useful for identification of potential offender. Risk factors provide potential leverage points for intervention. Renewed attention must focus on protective factors and their potential to moderate or mediate risk potential for initiation and maintenance of girls' delinquent behavior (Schmidt, 2001).

Not all commentators are convinced that gender-specific programming is warranted. Kempf-Leonard and Sample (2000) question whether effective girl programming is distinct from effective youth programming. They identify four themes of recent calls for girl-specific programming that are not specific to gender: safe and reflective therapeutic environments, attention to personal development, skills training for independent living, and comprehensive community-based interventions over time. The criticism is not based on ideology but rather a lack of specific hypotheses and data. The paucity of details on female-specific program characteristics lead the authors to conclude that gender-specific services may be driven by good intentions but undermined by lack of specific details.

Once any treatment options for girls are developed, protocols for risk assessment, classification, and best practices will not lag far behind (e.g., OJJDP, 1998a). The relative dearth of empirical data on girls' offending trajectories is matched by the paucity of information on treatment efficacy. Matching offenders to appropriate treatment types requires research in both areas but we must be cautious about searching for a technology of intervention (Mulvey & Woolard, 1997). We are unlikely to find intervention strategies for girls (or boys) that are completely robust to different service provider and community realities. Decision makers could be more effective if they understood the contextual factors that predict program and treatment success.

CONCLUSION

Delinquency researchers investigate a phenomenon with inherent policy relevance. It is possible to conduct research on female antisocial behavior without considering the influence of policy, but the societal response to female offending is integrally involved in the development, maintenance, and desistance of offending behavior. Likewise, policy does not require empirical verification and may ignore it even when available, but could be strengthened by data and evaluation.

Theory and model testing could maximize its relevance by attending to policy and practice issues in the design phase, rather than consigning them to the implications paragraph of a discussion section. First, research must investigate the common and unique predictors for multiple policy-relevant outcomes, including delinquent behavior, arrest and system involvement, treatment efficacy, and recidivism risk. The models overlap but are unlikely to be structurally or quantitatively equivalent. Second, research must pay attention to the small but apparently growing number of girls who enter the justice system for serious violent behavior, but not at the expense of the majority of girls engaged in minor forms of delinquency. Third, we must investigate intervention pathways or trajectories to understand patterns of system involvement and their impact on treatment efficacy. Fourth, methodological concerns such as varying definitions of delinquency and aggression, sampling issues, and data source differences should be explicitly accounted for, because methodological issues directly affect the strength of our conclusions and our relevance to policy.

These issues combine to make our task as policy-relevant researchers all the more daunting at the outset. Although the research and policy orientations are somewhat disparate, I do believe there is a nexus of interests to be served through rigorous, theoretically-driven research that broadens the parameters of the debate about female delinquency. Empirical research serves a critical function by providing data to inform the policy debates. It is well positioned to begin addressing the hypothetical lawmakers' questions about the nature of female offending and the justice system process. It is less able to provide even rudimentary data on treatment efficacy that could guide funding decisions. Research can also expand the relevant questions our hypothetical lawmakers ask by examining systemic issues such as gender bias and developmental trajectories. Unrealized potential remains for interdisciplinary collaboration among social scientists and policy analysts to conduct research that is mindful of a political context in which some questions are asked, others are answered, and a few ignored.

Girls' offending behavior should not be ignored any longer, but policy and programming are more usefully informed by systematic research than stereotype and anecdote.

REFERENCES

Acoca, L. (1998). Outside/inside: The violation of American girls at home, on the streets, and in the juvenile justice system. *Crime & Delinquency, 44,* 561–589.

American Bar Association & National Bar Association (2001). *Justice by gender: The lack of appropriate prevention, diversion, and treatment alternatives for girls in the justice system.* Washington, DC: Author.

Breed v. Jones, 421 U.S. 519 (1975).

Caspi, A., Lynam, D., Moffitt, T. E., & Silva, P. A. (1993). Unraveling girls' delinquency: Biological, dispositional, and contextual contributions to adolescent misbehavior. *Developmental Psychology, 29,* 19–30.

Cauffman, E., Feldman, S. S., Waterman, J., & Steiner, H. (1998). Posttraumatic stress disorder among female juvenile offenders. *Journal of the American Academy of Child and Adolescent Psychiatry, 31,* 1209–1216.

Chesney-Lind, M. (1997). *The female offender: Girls, women, and crime.* Thousand Oaks: Sage.

Chesney-Lind, M. (2001). Girls, violence, and delinquency: Popular myths and persistent problems. In S. O. White (Ed.), *Handbook of youth and justice* (pp. 135–158). New York: Kluwer Academic/Plenum.

Chesney-Lind, M., & Shelden, R. H. (1998). *Girls, delinquency, and juvenile justice* (2nd ed.). Pacific Grove, CA: Brooks/Cole.

Community Research Associates (1998). *Juvenile female offenders: A status of the states report.* Washington, DC: Office of Juvenile Justice and Delinquency Prevention.

Daly, K. (1998). Gender, crime, and criminology. In M. Tonry (Ed.), *The handbook of crime and punishment* (pp. 85–108). New York: Oxford University Press.

Darley, J. (2002). Gaining traction for psychology in the public arena. *APS Observer, 15.*

Federal Bureau of Investigation (2002). *Crime in the United States, 2001.* Washington, DC: Federal Bureau of Investigation.

Fergusson, D. M., Horwood, L. J., & Nagin, D. S. (2000). Offending trajectories in a New Zealand birth cohort. *Criminology, 38,* 525–552.

General Accounting Office (1995). *Juvenile justice: Minimal gender bias occurred in processing noncriminal juveniles.* Washington, DC: Author.

Hipwell, A. E., Loeber, R., Stouthamer-Loeber, M., Keenan, K., White, H. R., & Kroneman, L. (2002). Characteristics of girls with early onset disruptive and antisocial behaviour. *Criminal Behaviour and Mental Health, 12,* 99–118.

Horowitz, R., & Pottieger, A. E. (1991). Gender bias in juvenile justice handling of seriously crime-involved youths. *Journal of Research in Crime and Delinquency, 28,* 75–100.

Hoyt, S., & Scherer, D. G. (1998). Female juvenile delinquency: Misunderstood by the juvenile justice system, neglected by social science. *Law and Human Behavior, 22,* 81–107.

In re Gault, 387 U.S. 1 (1967).

In re Winship, 397 U.S. 358 (1970).

Kempf-Leonard, K., & Sample, L. L. (2000). Disparity based on sex: Is gender-specific treatment warranted? *Justice Quarterly, 17,* 89–128.

Kent v. United States, 383 U.S. 541 (1966).

Lipsey, M. W. (1992). Juvenile delinquency treatment: A meta-analytic inquiry into the variability of effects. In T. D. Cook , S. Cordray, H. Hartmann, L. V. Hedges, R. J. Light, T. A. Louis, & F. Mosteller (Eds.), *Meta-analysis for explanation* (pp. 83–127). NY: Russell Sage.

MacDonald, J. M., & Chesney-Lind, M. (2001). Gender bias and juvenile justice revisited: A multiyear analysis. *Crime & Delinquency, 47*, 173–195.

Mazerolle, P., Brame, R., Paternoster, R., Piquero, A., & Dean, C. (2000). Onset age, persistence, and offending versatility: Comparisons across gender. *Criminology, 38*, 1143–1172.

Moffitt, T. E. (1993). "Life-course-persistent" and "adolescence-limited" antisocial behavior: A developmental taxonomy. *Psychological Review, 100*, 674–701.

Moffitt, T. E., & Caspi, A. (2001). Childhood predictors differentiate life-course persistent and adolescence-limited antisocial pathways among males and females. *Development and Psychopathology, 13*, 355–375.

Mulvey, E. P., & Woolard, J. L. (1997). Themes for consideration in future research on prevention and intervention with antisocial behaviors. In D.M. Stoff, J. Breiling, & J.D. Maser (Eds.), *Handbook of antisocial behavior* (pp. 454–460). NY: Wiley.

Odem, M., & Schlossman, S. (1991). Guardians of virtue: The juvenile court and female delinquency in early 20th-century Los Angeles. *Crime and Delinquency, 37*, 186–203.

Office of Juvenile Justice and Delinquency Prevention (1998a). *Guiding principles for promising female programming: An inventory of best practices.* Washington, DC: Author.

Office of Juvenile Justice and Delinquency Prevention (1998b). *Juvenile female offenders: A status of the states report.* Washington, DC: Author.

Offord, D. R. (1997). Bridging development, prevention, and policy. In D. M. Stoff, J. Breiling, & J. D. Maser (Eds.), *Handbook of antisocial behavior* (pp. 357–364). NY: Wiley.

Poe-Yamagata, E., & Butts, J. A. (1996). Female offenders in the juvenile justice system: Statistics summary. Pittsburgh, PA: National Center for Juvenile Justice.

Scahill, M. C. (2000). *Female delinquency cases, 1997.* Washington, DC: U.S. Department of Justice, Office of Juvenile Justice and Delinquency Prevention.

Schmidt, M. G. (March, 2002). Protective factors: The potential for female youth. Paper presented at the American Psychology-Law Society conference. Austin, TX.

Reppucci, N. D. (1999). Adolescent development and juvenile justice. *American Journal of Community Psychology, 27*, 307–326.

Silverthorn, P., & Frick, P. J. (1999). Developmental pathways to antisocial behavior: The delayed-onset pathway in girls. *Development and Psychopathology, 9*, 43–58.

Snyder, H., & Sickmund, M. (1999). *Juvenile offenders and victims 1999 national report.* Washington, DC: U.S. Department of Justice, Office of Juvenile Justice and Delinquency Prevention.

Widom, C. S. (2000). Childhood victimization and the derailment of girls and women into the criminal justice system. In *Research on women and girls in the justice system: Plenary papers of the 1999 Conference on Criminal Justice Research and Evaluation—Enhancing Policy and Practice Through Research* (Vol. 3, pp. 27–36). Washington, DC: U.S. Department of Justice, National Institute of Justice.

Girls and Violence
The Never Ending Story

MARION K. UNDERWOOD

For it is important that awake people be awake,
or a breaking line might discourage them back to sleep;
The signals we give—yes or no, or maybe—
should be clear: the darkness around us is deep.

William Stafford (1998)

Females carry children for nine months then care for them ... Females also care for the elderly and the sick. Consequently, the overall damage to the society due to the criminality and/or antisocial behavior of females may be greater than the prevalence rates of offending or antisocial behavior among females would lead us to believe.

Kratzer & Hodgins (1999), p. 69

Evil runs rampant in this world when women are asleep at the wheel.

Adriana Trigiani (2003)

After decades of girls' violence taking place in private places and being shrouded in darkness, girls who fight have become the subject of widespread public concern, of academic research, and of policy debates. As the chapters in this volume make abundantly clear, scholars have shone much light into the dark place that is girls' violence, and the result has been tremendous progress in our understanding of girls and aggression. As much as we have learned, though, any account of girls and aggression will be a never ending story, for several important reasons. First, scholarship

---

MARION K. UNDERWOOD • School of Behavioral and Brain Sciences, University of Texas at Dallas, Richardson, Texas, United States, 75083.

on this topic has moved rapidly from a paucity of data to an overwhelming amount of new information, sometimes in the absence of theoretical frameworks for integrating and understanding results. The story of girls' violence will quickly become even more rich and complex. Second, because girls are violent often in the context of relationships and because women are primarily responsible for rearing children, violent girls may become inept or even violent mothers, and transmit violence and aggression to their children. Third, because so few girls and women engage in serious violence as compared to boys, gender specific interventions are in the very early stages of development. Experts are unsure as to how to help the minority of women who behave violently, thus their behavior and its heart-wrenching consequences will likely continue.

This closing chapter will highlight three themes that emerge across these contributions in an attempt to knit together the story of girls and violence, with the hope of identifying still unanswered questions and future directions for research. First, I will consider how the manner in which girls are socialized might account for the forms their violence takes. Next, I will consider the fact that girls' violence often takes place in the context of close relationships. Last, I will identify the most important implications for intervention raised by these contributions.

GENDERED SOCIALIZATION AND GIRLS' VIOLENCE

Compelling evidence suggests that at least in North American cultures, girls are socialized to be nice, non-aggressive, empathic, and concerned about others (see Zahn-Waxler, 2000, for a discussion). These socialization processes may account at least in part for why the base rate of violence is so much lower for girls than for boys. Gendered socialization may also explain the particular forms that girls' aggression takes and account for special characteristics of the fewer girls who do behave violently.

Because girls are socialized to take care of others and to define themselves in terms of others' evaluations, they may be more vulnerable to preoccupied attachment and to forms of aggression that serve to "coerce and maintain engagement" (Moretti, Da Silva, & Holland, this volume). Clinical experience and preliminary data suggest that disruptions in the mother-daughter relationship may be particularly problematic for girls and might contribute to their subsequent aggression and violence (Levene, Walsh, & Augimeri, this volume). Because girls may be staking their souls on how others perceive them, they may become hypersensitive to signs of rejection in relationships (Downey, Irwin, Ramsay, & Ayduk, this volume). This hypersensitivity coupled with a poor capacity for emotion regulation may lead women to engage in relational and even physical aggression against those they care for the most (Downey et al., this volume). As girls mature and continue to be socialized according to a hidden curriculum that dictates being nice, avoiding conflict, and withdrawing from competition, they may be inclined to view status and power in terms of appearance and others' estimations of them (the "pretty power hierarchy," see Artz, this volume) and be poorly prepared to cope with competition with peers (Artz, but see also Benenson, Roy, Waite, Goldbaum, Linders, & Simpson, 2002). When girls feel furious and wish to express their anger or pursue their social goals, they may resort to relational rather than physical aggression, because relational aggression inflicts harm in the arena they most value (Geiger, Zimmer-Gimbeck, & Crick, this volume). The extent to which relational aggression contributes to physical violence remains unknown. Gendered socialization and the hidden curriculum may take different forms in different cultures, and racism may compound ethnic minority girls' difficulties with understanding social nuances and dealing with frustration (Jackson, this volume). Even when girls do engage in moderate levels of violence in their mid-teens, many desist almost entirely in acts of violence that can be detected by the justice system by young adulthood (Lanctôt, Emond, & LeBlanc, this volume). Perhaps girls' violence decreases in response to the continued influence of the hidden curriculum of gendered socialization or other forces we do not yet understand, or perhaps girls' violence evolves into aggression against intimate others that is harder for the justice system to detect.

How can theories of gendered socialization help us understand why some few girls move beyond relational aggression to engage in physical violence? If there is a hidden curriculum that leads most girls away from violence, what are the forces that compel some girls to become violent? That these forces may be particularly strong is suggested by the fact that when girls do behave violently, they have many more associated problems than boys do. This may be an example of a phenomenon called "the gender paradox," that members of the gender group least often affected by the disorder are often the most severely disturbed (Loeber & Keenan, 1994). The logic of the gender paradox is that to develop a highly gender-atypical disorder, in this case to overcome the gendered socialization processes that work against a girl becoming violent, individuals must have strong risk factors that contribute to a whole host of problems. The theory of the gender paradox is confirmed by the fact that risks may be greater for children who engage in the form of aggression that violates gender norms (Crick, 1997) and who experience gender atypical forms of victimization (Leadbeater, Dahmi, Hogland, & Dickinson, this volume). Also, justice involved girls have more mental health problems than justice involved boys do (Antonioshak, Fried, & Reppucci, this volume), and female offenders have often been victimized themselves and may engage in violence as a way of coping with abuse environments (Odgers, Schmidt, & Reppucci, this volume).

Girls who overcome gendered socialization may be compelled to violence by truly extraordinary forces. For many girls in the justice system, these forces include being the victim of abuse or violence themselves. Sadly, violent girls may be undermined by the same stereotypes that drive gendered socialization. Gender stereotypes pressure young women to become responsible as homemakers, laborers, and volunteers, but gendered, malign, antisocial policies leave them few opportunities and offer few resources when they struggle to meet these obligations (Reitsma-Street, this volume). For all of these reasons, girls' violence reflects difficulties not only within individuals, but serious problems at the societal and cultural levels (Artz; Jackson; Reitsma-Street, this volume). Existing systems and policies may be poorly prepared to help violent girls because they do not take into account the special features of girls' violence, one of which is that it often takes place in the context of close relationships.

THE RELATIONAL CONTEXT OF GIRLS' VIOLENCE

When girls and women engage in violence, they often do so in very specific circumstances, often in the context of close relationships. Many of the contributors to this volume concur that it is critically important that we understand the specific triggers in relationships that lead girls and women to aggression (see especially Vaillancourt & Hymel, this volume). Girls and women are vulnerable to behaving aggressively toward relationship partners when they perceive relationships to be threatened and have poor skills in regulating negative emotions (Downey et al., this volume). When threatened, high rejection-sensitive early adolescents have been shown to get into more fights and have more interpersonal problems, engage in indirect aggression as retaliation, and report that they would engage in risky behaviors they firmly believe to be wrong for the sake of maintaining a dating relationship. High rejection-sensitive women report more conflicts with romantic partners, such that their partners consider ending the relationship, show more hostility toward partners, and report that they would engage in behaviors they believe to be immoral for the sake of keeping a romantic relationship. They also engage in self silencing, and for women who are incarcerated, experience depression, use illegal substances, and engage in a wide variety of antisocial behaviors (see Downey et al., for a review).

Perhaps in part due to this rejection sensitivity, when they behave violently, girls and women hurt those close to them. Girls' aggression is likely to be expressed in small, same-gender peer groups (Pepler et al., this volume). Competition for access to relationships may be particularly uncomfortable for girls and women (Artz, this volume). Immigrant or ethnic minority girls may feel especially desperate to fit in, to not seem FOB ("fresh off the boat"), and violence may be their way of demanding respect or of assuring that they are not targeted by violence themselves (Jackson, this volume). Girls involved in the justice system have often been violent toward known peers or romantic partners, and their aggression may also arise as a result of dysfunctions within relationships (Antonioshak et al., this volume). Girls, when violent, are more likely than boys are to assault a partner or a family member, which suggests that the risk of girls' violence is more to their close associates and perhaps themselves than to society as a whole (Odgers, this volume). These special features of girls' aggression suggest that intervention programs may need to be designed to meet girls' specific needs.

IMPLICATIONS FOR INTERVENTION

Because so few girls are violent as compared to boys and because juvenile justice systems have been designed with the young male offender in mind (Woolard, this volume), most contributors to this volume agree that gender specific interventions are in the very early stages of development. Several of these investigators cite at least preliminary evidence that girls may not improve, and in fact, might get worse in response to gender neutral interventions (Antonioshak et al., Pepler et al., both this volume), although young girls and boys seemed to benefit equally from one gender neutral intervention delivered in school classrooms (the WITS program, see Leadbeater et al., this volume). In contrast, experts in criminology disagree as to whether the current evidence suggests that effective programming for adjudicated girls is really any different from effective programming for all youths (see Woolard, this volume). One recent review pointed out that four components proposed for girl-specific programming are likely helpful for both genders: supportive therapeutic environments, consideration of developmental issues, training in skills for independent living, and broad, community based interventions that continue over time (Kempf-Leonard & Sample, 2000).

What do the papers in this volume add to the debate about gender specific interventions? First, it is important to develop assessment instruments that can determine which girls are most at risk so that these girls can be targeted for prevention and intervention efforts (Odgers et al., this volume). These instruments may need to be different from those that have been developed for boys, because girls' risk factors may differ; for example, early relationship disruptions may be important risk factors (Levene et al., this volume; Moretti et al., this volume). Violence risk assessments for girls may also need to be sensitive predictors for different kinds of outcomes. Though many violent girls desist as they move into adulthood (Lanctôt et al., this volume), lack of recidivism does not necessarily equal positive adjustment, particularly for girls and women who may suffer mental health problems and be prone to hurting those closest to them (Odgers et al., this volume).

What do these contributions suggest for the content of intervention programs to reduce girls' violence? Given that some girls' and women's violence may relate to rejection-sensitivity and difficulty with regulating emotions, girls might benefit from learning strategies for self- and attentional-control (Downey et al., this volume). If girls are indeed more prone to preoccupied attachment and to forms of aggression that force others to maintain engagement, girls might benefit from learning strategies for recognizing when they need reassurance and meeting their needs for closeness without behaving aggressively (Moretti et al., this volume). Although intervening to reduce relational aggression is described as in its very early stages (Geiger et al., this volume), existing research provides clues for effective programs. For example, children can be effective in terminating bouts of malicious gossip by challenging others' negative evaluative statements immediately and firmly (Eder & Enke, 1991). Parents can be taught how to be sensitive to their daughters' involvement in social aggression, to recognize what the triggers might be (for example, being called fat or ugly, see Levene et al., this volume), and to refrain from modeling social aggression for their daughters. Because girls seem reluctant to see some of their aggressive behavior as a response to racism, girls might benefit from being helped to understand that some of their frustration and peer problems may result from racial discrimination. Intervention programs should address systemic racism and bullying (Jackson, this volume).

At the level of juvenile justice systems and social policies, modifications are needed to change policies that confine the opportunities of disadvantaged girls (Reitsma-Street, this volume), to offer safe havens for victimized girls, and to support girls' efforts to obtain education and pursue constructive future goals. On the basis of research on normative female development, the Office for Juvenile Justice and Delinquency Prevention (1998) recommended that programs for girls include special components to enhance self-esteem, foster positive body image, teach empowerment, and enhance interpersonal relationships. These programs may need to be augmented further to meet the needs of adjudicated girls by offering them a way out of abusive environments, by being careful that programs do not promote deviant peer associations, and by considering girls' individual problems while addressing a broader range of concerns that many girls share (Antonioshak et al., this volume).

Unfortunately, many of these recommendations conflict with recent trends toward the adultification of the juvenile justice systems in Canada and in the U.S. (Connolly, Wayte, & Lee, this volume). Recent changes in juvenile justice laws will likely result in violent girls being more likely to be sentenced as adults, and violent girls with associated mental health problems being less likely to be treated (Connolly et al., this volume). Because these changes are fairly recent, it will be important for investigators to document the effects of these changes in juvenile justice laws on the treatment and outcomes for violent girls in the juvenile justice system.

THE RESEARCH AGENDA FOR THE FUTURE

The contributions to this volume make clear that scholars and policy makers have been awakened to the need to understand girls' violence, and have made vast progress in a short time in understanding possible developmental origins and outcomes of girls' and women's aggression. Some authors have provided compelling research evidence for risk factors (for example, Downey et al., on rejection sensitivity and Moretti et al., on preoccupied attachment). Others have reviewed limited data available and make suggestions for research programs (Geiger et al.). Some offered important sociological analyses based on interview data (Artz; Jackson; Reitsma-Street). Others presented data suggesting that interventions with children can be effective in reducing girls' violence (Pepler et al.; Leadbeater et al.). Some described what gender specific assessment devices might look like (Levene et al.; Odgers et al.) and what the content of gender specific interventions might be (Levene et al.; Antonioshak et al.). Others offered analyses of how legal systems currently treat violent girls (Connolly et al.; Woolard).

The interdisciplinary approach taken in this book is an important strength, but also represents a significant challenge. How can scholars working from different perspectives proceed in doing research that will help violent girls and shape the policies that affect their lives? Skeptics might survey the state of the research literature on violent girls, compare it to the wealth of large, well-designed longitudinal studies of aggressive boys, and the treatment programs designed and evaluated to treat violent boys, and say we simply do not know enough to intervene with aggressive girls and that we should concentrate instead on designing the highest quality, basic, developmental research to understand the origins and outcomes of girls' violence. Although basic developmental work certainly should proceed, we cannot afford to wait to begin intervening and altering policies and systems to meet girls' needs, because the stakes are just too great. Clinical and sociological perspectives are not only refreshing in their consideration of contextual factors, they lead to practically helpful ideas and testable hypotheses that might guide more empirical inquiries. Still, what seems to some like stating the obvious or speaking truth to power might make the hard-core methodologists from different disciplines squirm.

All scientists will need to be careful to design studies that speak to challenges that clinicians and policy makers face daily (Woolard, this volume). Policy makers want to know how to protect public safety; researchers can oblige with well-designed studies of offending among girls, which might help identify protective as well as factors. Juvenile justice professionals need to know how they should manage female offenders; scientists can help by conducting program evaluations to test which components are most helpful for girls. Policy makers at all levels seek guidance on how to allocate resources; researchers can help by carefully documenting the costs of gender-specific programs and balancing these against the cost of girls not desisting from violence.

Thanks in large part to the efforts of these and other investigators, we have all become more alive and awake to the importance of understanding and preventing girls' violence. Fewer girls may be violent as compared to boys, but those girls who do fight are equally at risk. It is vitally important that scholars continue to depart from comparing girls to boys, and instead, study girls' aggression and violence in its own right and for its own sake, by carefully examining developmental trajectories and intervention strategies for young women. Violent girls challenge us, disgust some, and force us to examine our assumptions about gender. Aggressive girls may engage in "relational hypocrisies" (Zanarini & Gunderson, 1997) that make them respond poorly to gender neutral interventions, make them get worse before they get better (see Leve & Chamberlain, in press), and drive even the most patient of seasoned treatment professionals crazy. Violent girls are provocative and they compel us to make provocative claims, only some of which can be currently supported by data, but their frightening behaviors force us to move ahead to intervene to stop their behavior. Piecing together the rest of their story will not be easy, but it will be worthwhile, in honor of girls' tremendous capabilities, not only as relationship partners and caregivers, but also as creators and inventors and stewards of our collective future. In the words of Andrienne Rich (1991) from her poem "Final Notations", which some understand as a meditation on mothering,

You are coming into us who cannot withstand you
You are coming into us who never wanted to withstand you
You are taking parts of us into places never planned
You are going far away with pieces of our lives

It will be short, it will take all your breath
It will not be simple, it will become your will.

REFERENCES

Benenson, J. F., Roy, R., Waite, A., Goldbaum, S., Linders, L., & Simpson, A. (2002). Greater discomfort as a proximate cause of sex differences in competition. *Merrill-Palmer Quarterly, 48*, 225–247.

Crick, N. R. (1997). Engagement in gender normative versus gender nonnormative forms of aggression: Links to social-psychological adjustment. *Developmental Psychology, 33*, 610–617.

Eder, D., & Enke, J. L. (1991). The structure of gossip: Opportunities and constraints on collective expression among adolescents. *American Sociological Review, 56*, 494–508.

Kempf-Leonard, K., & Sample, L. L. (2000). Disparity based on sex: Is gender-specific treatment warranted? *Justice Quarterly, 17*, 89–128.

Kratzer, L, & Hodgins, S. (1999). A typology of offenders: A test of Moffitt's theory among males and females from childhood to age 30. *Criminal Behavior and Mental Health, 9*, 57–73.

Leve, L. D., & Chamberlain, P. (in press). Girls in the juvenile justice system: Risk factors and clinical implications. To appear in D. J. Pepler, K. Madsen, C. Webster, & K. Levene (Eds.). *The development and treatment of girlhood aggression.* Mahwah, NJ: Erlbaum.

Loeber, R. & Keenan, K. (1994). Interaction between conduct disorder and its comorbid conditions: Effects of age and gender. *Clinical Psychology Review, 14*, 497–523.

Office of Juvenile Justice and Delinquency Prevention (OJJDP). (1998). *Guiding principles for promising female programming: An inventory of best practices.* Washington, DC: Author.

Rich, A. (1991). Final notations. *An atlas of the difficult world: Poems 1988–1991.* NY: Norton.

Stafford, W. (1998). A ritual to read to each other. *The way it is: New and selected poems.* St. Paul, MN: Graywolf Press.

Trigiani, A. (2003, May). *Guts, blind faith, and sun block.* Commencement address delivered at St. Mary's College, Notre Dame, IN.

Zahn-Waxler, C. (2000). The development of empathy, guilt, and internalization of distress. In R. Davidson (Ed.), *Anxiety, depression, and emotion: Wisconsin Symposium on Emotion, Volume II* (pp. 222–265). NY: Oxford University Press.

Zanarini, M. C., & Gunderson, J. G. (1997). Differential diagnosis of antisocial and borderline personality disorders. In D. M. Stoff, J. Breiling, & J. D. Maser (Eds.), *Handbook of antisocial behavior* (pp. 83–91). New York: Wiley.

Index